EXAMINING ALTERNATIVE MEDICINE

An Inside Look at the Benefits & Risks

Paul C. Reisser, M.D.
Dale Mabe, D.O. Robert Velarde

InterVarsity Press
Downers Grove, Illinois

InterVarsity Press
P.O. Box 1400, Downers Grove, IL 60515-1426
World Wide Web: www.ivpress.com
E-mail: mail@ivpress.com

InterVarsity Press® *is the book-publishing division of InterVarsity Christian Fellowship/USA*®*, a student movement active on campus at hundreds of universities, colleges and schools of nursing in the United States of America, and a member movement of the International Fellowship of Evangelical Students. For information about local and regional activities, write Public Relations Dept., InterVarsity Christian Fellowship/USA, 6400 Schroeder Rd., P.O. Box 7895, Madison, WI 53707-7895.*

Cover photograph: William Whitehurst/The Stock Market

ISBN 0-8308-2275-5

Printed in the United States of America ∞

Library of Congress Cataloging-in-Publication Data

Reisser, Paul C.
  Examining alternative medicine : an inside look at the benefits & risks / Paul C.
Reisser, Dale Mabe, Robert Velarde.
    p. cm.
  Includes bibliographical references.
  ISBN 0-8308-2275-5 (paper : alk. paper)
    1. Alternative medicine. I. Mabe, Dale. II. Velarde, Robert, 1969- III. Title.
R733 . R437 2001
615.5—dc21

                                                                    2001024032

20   19   18   17   16   15   14   13   12   11   10   9   8   7   6   5   4   3   2   1

17   16   15   14   13   12   11   10   09   08   07   06   05   04   03   02   01

CONTENTS

1

A NATION
TAKES NOTICE

On a fall afternoon in 1977 a nurse tending to children on a pediatric ward struck up a conversation with a young physician who was midway through his family practice residency. She had just returned from a medical conference entitled "The Physician of the Future," a gathering attended by more than two thousand health care professionals, and it had clearly affected her. Indeed it almost seemed that she had "gotten religion" at this meeting, as she spoke with enthusiasm about a new paradigm that would soon revolutionize our understanding of health and disease.

The future of health care, she explained, lay in the concept of "holism," an understanding that the whole person—body, mind and spirit—was much more than the sum of several organ systems. Indeed it would soon become much more important to understand the patient who had the illness rather than the illness that had the patient. Prevention, lifestyle, stress reduction and self-awareness would gradually displace drugs and surgery. Eventually we would begin to define *health* in more optimistic terms—not merely as the absence of disease but as a state of increasing energy, productivity, insight and personal transformation.

This sounded intriguing. After all, didn't the scope of family practice extend not only to the whole patient but also to his or her family, work, relationships and even community? The nurse handed the resident a copy of a document called the *Journal of Holistic Health,* which was in fact a transcription of the previous year's conference. At first he merely glanced through it, but then he began to read it more carefully with increasing concern. This movement appeared to have a lot more on its mind than just changing dietary habits, encouraging exercise and helping people cope with stress.

The conference director, in his opening remarks, had declared that this gathering "is part of a process that is bringing about a new way of thinking, a new science merged with religion." The director of the Institute of Noetic Sciences at Stanford University, James Fadiman, Ph.D., proposed that "we are not primarily physical forms. We are primarily energy around which matter adheres." Richard Svihus, M.D., president of the California Academy of Preventive Medicine, announced that the holistic health movement "is desired by higher forces and consciousness within the universe." Harold Bloomfield, a psychiatrist who wrote the bestselling *TM: Discovering Inner Energy and Overcoming Stress,* extolled the benefits of Transcendental Meditation. Dr. Elisabeth Kübler-Ross, widely recognized as the world's leading authority on the dying process, stated unequivocally that "death does not exist" and that after transitioning from this life you will have the opportunity "not to be judged by a judgmental God, but to judge yourself." Many others with multiple initials after their names, impressive titles and engaging anecdotes described healing through aligning the body's invisible energies, developing psychic abilities and, above all, altering, expanding and transforming consciousness.[1]

The pediatric nurse really had gotten religion—but not a gospel that would have set well with Luke, the doctor who authored the New Testament books of Luke and Acts. It was instead a gospel better suited for Luke Skywalker, master of the Force, the impersonal energy pivotal to the plots of the *Star Wars* films. The holistic health movement appeared to be yet another banner under which the we-are-all-energy, all-is-one, I-am-God-and-you-are-God spirituality of the New Age movement was approaching the gates of Western culture and expecting to be welcomed with open arms.

The resident decided to examine the holistic phenomenon in more depth, subsequently attending two large gatherings sponsored by the organizers of the Physician of the Future conference. For the most part, the speakers were interesting, energetic and sincere in their desire to promote health. But these experiences also left no doubt that in the "new medicine" the spiritual agenda—at least as it was presented by its most visible and active proponents—was of utmost importance. Furthermore, a few questions posed to some of the speakers made it abundantly clear that this spirituality, which presented itself as generously inclusive of all religious traditions, did not in fact embrace the core teachings of the Old and New

Testaments. It did not embrace the omnipotent, one true God who is distinct from and Lord of his creation, the rebellion and inherent sinfulness of humankind, the atoning death of Christ on the cross or our need for individual repentance.

If you asked a speaker about Jesus, you might hear that he was a master teacher, enlightened healer or bearer of the Christ consciousness. If you mentioned atonement, you would be gently informed that Jesus demonstrated "at-one-ment," a unity with God that exists within all of us. If you brought up repentance, you would be told in no uncertain terms that what we really need is enlightenment, a direct experience of our own divinity. If you bore down on that distasteful event at Golgotha, the air would suddenly become chilly.

The resident completed his training and joined a busy family practice. Over the next several years he wrote and spoke about the holistic health movement, voicing concern over its spiritual agenda as well as its more questionable therapies. During that time he noted that many people, including committed Christians who would contend fervently over the interpretation of a grammatical detail in a passage of Scripture, were willing to lay critical thinking aside when dealing with unorthodox healing methods. *Does it work?* and more specifically, *Does it make me feel better?* were often far more important considerations than *Does it make any sense?* or *Is there any reasonable proof?* or *What worldview is this healing system based upon?* or *Does this practice conflict with my faith?*

It also seemed that the holistic health movement was making little impact on the practices of rank-and-file physicians. (It had made somewhat deeper inroads among nurses, however, especially with a healing technique known as Therapeutic Touch.) Furthermore, the "new medicine" appeared to be making little, if any, headway within institutions such as medical schools, government bodies and insurance companies. Holistic health proponents repeatedly expressed an ardent desire to enter the cultural mainstream via research, public policy and finance, but for many years this goal proved elusive. Indeed, despite the expansive optimism of holistic health conferences during the late 1970s, the movement seemed to sputter through the 1980s, keeping itself alive primarily through the allegiance of clients who were willing to spend their own money in the offices of unconventional practitioners. As the 1980s came to an end, it looked as though there would always be holistic voices crying in the wilderness but that the general drift of our culture would probably keep them there.

Alternative Medicine Enters the Mainstream
The resident and family practitioner who concluded that the holistic health movement would remain marginalized in American society (and as a result turned his

attention elsewhere for several years) was Paul Reisser, M.D., one of the coauthors of this book—a book that has been written because that conclusion proved to be completely wrong.

Over the past few years a dramatic turnabout has in fact brought the gamut of holistic therapies, including those with New Age and Eastern mystical flags fully unfurled, squarely into the mainstream of American culture under a new banner: *alternative medicine.* The therapies now gathered behind that banner are no longer wandering in the frontier, no longer a "Ripley's Believe It or Not" novelty, no longer excluded from the health care emporium. Alternative therapies have not only moved squarely into the mainstream of everyday American life and commerce but are actually shaping the mainstream's direction.[2] We need not look far to view the breadth of its influence.

The Media

In the 1970s, books extolling the holistic health movement and its therapies were often produced by obscure companies (or were self-published) and sold primarily at conferences, health food stores and New Age bookshops. A few found their way into the major chains, but they were usually scattered unpredictably amid the self-help, fitness, psychology, New Age or even occult titles. Twenty-plus years later, a serious expanse of rack space at bookstores great and small is abundantly supplied with alternative medicine titles. These are either comfortably intermingled with more conventional books on health and fitness or are provided with their own shelves in a prominently labeled aisle. Furthermore, major publishing houses now produce an ongoing stream of such books, many of them beautifully designed and lavishly illustrated. Perhaps the most significant trend has been the emergence of health advisory books that encompass both conventional and alternative viewpoints, usually placing them on equal footing. A prime example is *The Medical Advisor: The Complete Book of Alternative and Conventional Treatment,* published by Time-Life Books. This handsome volume is encyclopedic in scope, and every topic includes the conventional medical approach to a problem, followed by several alternative options: ancient Chinese, homeopathic, herbal and so forth.[3]

Magazines such as *Alternative Medicine* and *Natural Health* reach thousands of subscribers and newsstand browsers every month with the latest developments in alternative medicine. Columns featuring high-profile spokespeople reach even larger audiences through mass-market periodicals.

Video presentations, whether broadcast or packaged for home viewing, have effectively showcased alternative practitioners. The Public Broadcasting

System (PBS) has been particularly active in this area, breaking ground in the early 1990s with Bill Moyers's series *Healing and the Mind* and its companion book of the same title. PBS specials featuring Andrew Weil, M.D., a popular author and teacher of "integrative medicine" at the University of Arizona School of Medicine, have offered articulate distillations of the material in his book *Spontaneous Healing*. Even more prominent in the PBS program schedule, including encore presentations during fund drives, has been Deepak Chopra, M.D., whose platinum-selling books have introduced mainstream America to the world of *ayurveda,* India's metaphysically driven healing tradition. Dr. Chopra has held court with millions of viewers in specials such as "Body, Mind and Soul: The Mystery and the Magic" and "The Way of the Wizard."

Perhaps the greatest boon to alternative medicine has been the Internet, which fosters not only instant access to information on any subject but also ongoing interaction and the option to buy and sell products of every description. The growth of alternative medicine websites has been explosive over the past few years. In late 1997, entering the words "alternative medicine" into the Yahoo! search engine yielded some two hundred listings. Less than two years later, the same search led to more than five hundred listings, and the number continues to grow. The Excite search engine indicates that over a million listings match at least partially with the words "alternative medicine."[4] Platforms such as America Online and Lycos send inquirers to broad-based launching pads devoted to this subject, from which they can begin looking in dozens of different directions. The overwhelming majority of these stopping points on the World Wide Web actively promote alternative therapies or products. Only a handful offer caution, criticism or evenhanded analysis.

The Federal Government

The National Center for Complementary and Alternative Medicine (NCCAM) was created in 1992 by congressional mandate as the Office of Alternative Medicine (OAM), one of several coordinating centers within the Office of the Director of the National Institutes of Health (NIH). Its stated mission was to "encourage and support the investigation of alternative medical practices, with the ultimate goal of integrating validated alternative medical practices into health and medical care."[5] It has not served as a referral agency for any alternative treatment, organization or practitioner.

In 1993 the OAM began awarding research grants to fund exploratory pilot projects and also established ten specialty research centers at universities and medical centers to study alternative approaches to specific disease problems. (Nine of these are based at mainstream, high-profile facilities, such as Stanford University and Harvard Medical School. One, Bastyr University, is a school of naturopathy, whose curriculum is focused primarily on teaching alternative modalities.)[6] The OAM also established a research database program, which has assembled an electronic collection of some one hundred thousand research citations on complementary and alternative medicine topics. The OAM's clearinghouse began disseminating information to the public, media and health professionals, including fact sheets, information packages and a toll-free information line (888-644-6226).

During its first year of existence the OAM operated on a $2 million budget—a paltry 0.02 percent of the NIH's $10.7 billion budget during the same year. By fiscal year 1997, however, that amount had grown to $12 million. In 1998 the OAM's budget was $20 million, and in true exponential style Congress appropriated $68.4 million for fiscal year 2000, with $72.4 million under consideration for 2001. It also changed the OAM's name to the National Center for Complementary and Alternative Medicine (NCCAM), and in so doing upgraded its status. As a center within the NIH, the NCCAM has more horsepower—not only a more impressive budget but also greater status and autonomy in initiating and funding research projects.

A perusal of the NCCAM's current mission statement, fact sheets, website (<nccam.nih.gov>) and, most importantly, past and present staff and advisers should leave little doubt that this agency, like the OAM that preceded it, is neither commissioned nor planning to serve as a consumer watchdog. The NCCAM has no regulatory powers. It will not recommend standards of practice for alternative practitioners, investigate fraud or issue warnings regarding practices found to be worthless or harmful. Much of its output thus far has emphasized the importance of subjecting alternative therapies to appropriate scientific assessment. This is certainly a laudable goal, and hopefully NCCAM funding will underwrite studies that will clarify the safety and efficacy of treatments that thus far have been validated primarily by tradition and anecdote.

But it is worth noting that many who have shown great interest in the NCCAM's activities and who helped chart its early course are themselves enthusiastic proponents of alternative therapies. One of the early congressional supporters of this project, Representative John E. Porter (R-Ill), who has chaired the subcommittee that oversees funding for the NIH, wrote that he saw the OAM as fulfilling a definite mission: "As I see it, the most important contribution the OAM can make to the practice of medicine is to provide that link between alternative and conventional medicine. . . . Therefore, it is important to continue making contacts on Capitol Hill and to deliver the message: *alternative medicine is integral to biomedical research, provides effective results, and is a priority for spending decisions.*[7] James Gordon, M.D., director of the Mind-Body Center in Washington, D.C., and passionate advocate of alternative therapies in the book *Manifesto for a New Medicine,* has served as chairman of the Program Advisory Council for the OAM. Wayne Jonas, M.D., coauthor of a recent book extolling classical homeopathy's capacity to "promote healing and restore health,"[8] served as the first director of the OAM. Such close ties with those who are proponents of alternative therapies leaves a definite suspicion that the NCCAM may tend to approach its subject not just with an open mind but with open arms as well.

Another clear indication of positive regard for alternative medicine in the federal government was Congress's passage and continued support of the Dietary Supplement Health and Education Act (DSHEA) of 1994. Heavily promoted by the manufacturers of nutritional supplements and those who market them, the DSHEA revised the definition of these compounds to include not just the familiar alphabet soup of vitamins and minerals but virtually any substance that could be swallowed: "an herb or other botanical, an amino acid, a dietary substance for use by man to supplement the diet by increasing the total daily intake, or a concentrate, metabolite, constituent, extract, or combination of these ingredients." More importantly, the DSHEA has allowed product labels to claim effects on the "structure or function" of the body, or general well-being, as a result of taking the supplement. Such "nutritional support" statements cannot claim to treat any specific disease, but—very importantly—they also need not be approved by the Food and Drug Administration (FDA).

As a result the label on a bottle containing the herb St. John's wort, for example, can announce that it helps "maintain normal healthy mental function" but cannot state that it "treats depression." The latter claim would cost the manufacturer hundreds of millions of dollars in research and other expenses in order to satisfy the substantial burden of proof demanded by the FDA before a new drug enters the marketplace. Instead, a simple disclaimer, now familiar to anyone who has strolled down the supplement aisle at the grocery store, converts a potentially huge expense into a tidy profit: "This statement has not been evaluated by the Food and Drug Administration. This product is not intended to diagnose, treat, cure or prevent any disease." Largely as a result of this new freedom of manufacturers and distributors to make sweeping but purposely vague claims, the average American is now exposed to a steady diet of advertising for all manner of supplements (especially herbal preparations), which in turn has led to a dramatic increase in their consumption.

Nurses, Physicians and Journals

In the bygone days of the holistic health movement in the 1970s unconventional therapies were promoted primarily by healers of all persuasions, homeopaths, acupuncturists, naturopaths and a wide assortment of others who nearly always practiced somewhere outside the mainstream of the medical establishment. Many nurses, however, carried alternative practices directly into high-profile medical centers. Tens of thousands of them learned Therapeutic Touch, a technique introduced in 1975 by New York University professor Dolores Krieger, R.N., Ph.D. Now taught at more than eighty universities and hospitals, Therapeutic Touch claims to detect and adjust invisible energies flowing within, and emanating from, the human body.

The few Western-trained physicians who embraced the holistic health movement were likely to be viewed by their professional colleagues as having broken ranks or chosen to march to a different drummer. But in the 1990s the drumbeats of complementary and alternative medicine became so loud and pervasive that large numbers of physicians could not help hearing them.

Physicians receive an avalanche of mail every week, including both mainstream journals and advertiser-supported professional magazines and newspapers. (The latter are sometimes called "throwaways" because they are unsolicited. However, they are widely read because they tend to be more practical and user-friendly than their more academic counterparts.) Over the past few years, an unprecedented number of articles about alternative therapies has appeared in all of these publications.

One might have expected a tone of caution, or at least healthy skepticism, among them, but instead they have uniformly cast this phenomenon in a positive light. Phrases such as "unproven claims" and "more studies are needed" have been abundant, but physicians have routinely been encouraged to investigate and utilize alternative therapies or at least to adopt an uncritical stance toward them when the subject comes up with patients. Cautions about possible risks have been rare, and critical evaluation of the underlying assumptions of alternative therapies have been virtually nonexistent.

A striking example of this new acceptance appeared in the November 1996 *American Family Physician,* the official journal of the American Academy of Family Physicians (normally a reliable source of medical information). Its cover article, "Alternative Medicine and the Family Physician," offered a positive overview of the length and breadth of alternative care, admonished family physicians to "convey a sensitive acceptance and an openness to . . . their patients' interest in alternative therapies," and encouraged practitioners to explore this realm themselves. An accompanying editorial strongly endorsed physician involvement in alternative therapies, while cautions or concerns about the scientific validity of any of the approaches mentioned were nowhere to be found.[9]

Primary care physicians have also received complimentary copies of the monthly journals *Alternative and Complementary Therapies* and *Alternative Therapies in Health and Medicine,* and many no doubt have subscribed to them. These periodicals contain review articles and scientific studies of variable quality, and in some cases they wade comfortably into metaphysical and promotional material. Similarly, a newsletter for health care providers, *The Integrative Medicine Consult,* offers findings from the medical literature, reviews of particular therapies, synopses of various alternative approaches to specific medical problems and patient handouts—nearly always with a positive perspective. Only the *Scientific Review of Alternative Medicine,* launched in 1998 by Wallace Sampson, M.D., a long-time critic of unconventional therapies, has established as its specific goal the critical analysis of specific alternative practices and the movement in general.

By far the most significant articles to be published about alternative medicine in the medical literature have appeared not in the throwaways but in two highly prestigious American medical journals. On November 11, 1998, the *Journal of the American Medical Association* (or *JAMA,* as it is widely known among physicians)—a publication definitely not known as a splashy source of news—made front-page headlines across the United States. This week's edition was not announcing the spectacular success of a new cancer-vanquishing drug or a groundbreaking advance in the treatment of coronary artery disease. Instead it had devoted an entire issue, including letters to the editor, book reviews and editorials, to alternative medicine.

Lead articles included studies of herbal remedies for irritable bowel syndrome and obesity, chiropractic manipulation for the relief of tension-type headaches, acupuncture treatment for an HIV-related nerve disorder, and the effects of a classical Chinese practice called moxibustion (the stimulation of specific points on the skin with heat generated by burning certain herbs) for correction of the breech (feet-first) position of a baby prior to delivery. There was also a report on a yoga-based intervention for carpal tunnel syndrome, a review of the current scientific literature regarding saw palmetto extract as a treatment for prostate enlargement, a discussion of medical malpractice issues related to alternative medicine, and editorials examining in measured language the impact and implications of this phenomenon on public health and the practice of medicine in the United States.

One year previously the editors of *JAMA* had selected alternative medicine as the topic for its annual "coordinated theme issue." Each year the editorial board and senior staff of *JAMA,* and the editors of its sister publications known as the *Archive* journals *(Archives of Internal Medicine, Archives of Family Practice* and several others) rank the most important topics to be addressed during the coming twelve months. Only one is chosen for the theme issue, and previous editions had dealt with such far-reaching topics as managed care and quality of care. In 1996 alternative medicine had placed a distant sixty-eighth out of seventy-three subjects under consideration. By 1997 it was among the top three of eighty-six topics. As a result, one year later *JAMA* and nine *Archive* journals simultaneously published more than eighty articles about alternative therapies.

Undoubtedly this dramatic foray of alternative practices into the American Medical Association's family of publications must have delighted those who have carried the torch for holistic health since the 1970s. But it was one particular article, the centerpiece of the November 11 *JAMA* issue, that caused *USA Today* on the same date to post the banner headline "Nation Embraces Alternative Medicine" on page 1. That study, written by David Eisenberg, M.D., with a team of researchers from Harvard Medical School and calmly titled "Trends in Alternative Medicine Use in the United States, 1990–1997," was a highly anticipated follow-up to another article published half a decade earlier, also with Dr. Eisenberg serving as lead author. In January 1993 his study entitled "Unconventional Medicine in the United States: Prevalence, Costs, and Patterns of Care" had appeared in the *New England Journal of Medicine,* a publication widely regarded as the premier medical journal in North America, if not the world.[10] It can be stated without exaggeration that the 1993 study was arguably the most influential article on alternative medicine ever published—at least until its 1998 update arrived.

Both studies used a twenty-five- to thirty-minute telephone survey to estimate an individual's use of unconventional or alternative therapies during the previous year.[11] The first study (1993), which polled 1,539 adults, found that one in three individuals (34 percent) used at least one unconventional therapy over the previous twelve months. Of these, 36 percent actually sought help from a practitioner of these therapies. Those who went to a provider made an average of nineteen visits during the previous year, with an average charge per visit of $27.60. Alternative therapies were used most often for chronic as opposed to acute or life-threatening conditions, and when the problem was considered by the individual to be serious, more than 80 percent also sought conventional treatment. Overall, however, 72 percent of those who used unconventional treatments did *not* inform their own medical doctor that they had done so.

Eisenberg and his coauthors extrapolated these survey results into a seismic wake-up call for the health care industry. When generalized to the population at large, they suggested that Americans made an estimated 425 million visits to providers of alternative care, exceeding the number of visits—an estimated 388 million—to all conventional primary care physicians in the United States. The expenditures associated with these vast numbers of contacts with alternative practitioners were estimated to total $13.7 billion, of which $10.3 billion were paid out of pocket (that is, they were not covered by medical insurance). This intimidating number was even more impressive when it was noted to be in the same league with the $12.8 billion spent out of pocket by Americans for all hospitalizations during the same year.

When Eisenberg repeated the survey with 2,055 adults in 1997, the results were even more striking. As reported in the now-famous November 11, 1998, issue of *JAMA,* the number of those who used at least one alternative therapy increased from 34 percent to 42 percent, and the percentage of users who sought care from an alternative practitioner increased from 36 percent to 46 percent, with a similar number of visits during the previous year. The extrapolation of these figures to the entire U.S. population generated headlines across the country. The statistics suggested the following:

☐ Between 1990 and 1997 there was a 47 percent increase in visits to alternative practitioners, from 427 million to 629 million. The latter number exceeded the estimated total number of visits made to all conventional primary care physicians in 1997.

☐ The estimated expenditures to alternative therapists increased 45 percent to $21.2 billion, of which at least $12.2 billion was paid out of pocket. The latter figure exceeded all out-of-pocket hospital expenses during the same year.

☐ The total amount spent out of pocket for alternative therapies (whether or not a practitioner was involved) in 1997 was estimated to be $27 billion, which is comparable to the estimated total out-of-pocket expense for all physician services in the United States.

The role that these studies have played (and continue to play) in the recent surge of alternative medicine into the mainstream of American culture cannot be understated. Beginning in 1993, the statistics in Dr. Eisenberg's *New England Journal of Medicine* article were quoted and requoted in dozens of articles, books, presentations and speeches before health care organizations, educational institutions, governmental agencies and business entities from one end of the country to the other. With each restatement of the impressive numbers emanating from the most esteemed medical journal in the land, alternative medicine gathered more attention, acceptance and adherents. One could reasonably argue that in 1998 Dr. Eisenberg and his colleagues did not merely describe a substantial rise in the use of alternative therapies in the United States; they had actually helped generate a good deal of it themselves.

Medical Conferences and Medical Schools

Also arriving in physicians' collective in basket have been brochures—lots of them—announcing educational conferences on complementary and alternative medicine. These meetings are nearly always mounted by prestigious universities and medical centers.[12] The involvement of high-profile medical schools in these conferences and many others like them reflects one other important component of the mainstreaming of alternative medicine: the establishment of complementary and alternative programs and centers within their corridors, and the inclusion of related curricula during the training of the next generation of physicians. Like most cultural shifts over the past fifty years, what is taught in the classroom today is likely to become standard operating procedure within two decades.

As of 1998, 75 out of 117 medical schools in the United States included some form of training relating to alternative medicine, either as part of the core curriculum or as an elective.[13] In some schools alternative practices are taught as extracurricular activities. For the physician in training thirty years ago, this would have been another trendy distraction to be endured on the way to learning some "real medicine." Today that attitude would be considered Neanderthal. Whether the focus is that of seeking to better understand their patients' beliefs and needs or actually providing hands-on training in an assortment of alternative therapies, this new dimension to medical training is not a passing fad.[14] However, alternative medicine critic Wallace Sampson has argued that the prevailing orientation in these programs has been one of "indoctrination rather than education." In his own survey of American medical schools, he found that more than fifty included courses that approached alternative practices uncritically, while only five actually taught students how to analyze their claims. "At a time when physicians desperately need to know how to scientifically evaluate all the dubious claims that patients are confronted with," Sampson warned, "this training is practically nonexistent."[15]

Perhaps the most telling indication of a dramatic shift in attitude toward alternative practices within the conventional medical community—or at least among those who shape its publications and organizational policies—has been the evolution in the terms used to identify them in the professional literature. Before the 1980s, therapies that wandered outside the fold of conventional thinking and practice were uniformly dismissed as quackery or were even thrown into the more ominous category of health fraud. During the 1980s and early 1990s, the term *unconventional* became more common. This word is definitely less pejorative but still implies some distance from the mainstream and perhaps eccentricity as well. (A little-known but illuminating bit of governmental trivia is that when it was first mandated by Congress, the NIH Office of Alternative Medicine was supposed to be called the Office of Unconventional Medical Practices.[16])

During the mid-1990s, the term *alternative medicine* came into full flower, and today it continues to be the phrase most widely used. Unlike *quackery* or even *unconventional medicine,* it does not imply the superiority of one system over another. The implication of choice gives the word *alternative* a subtle but clearly positive slant. In the late 1990s the term *complementary* became more widely used, often combined with *alternative.* Many medical publications now routinely use the phrase *complementary and alternative medicine,* and its acronym CAM, in their articles on this subject. The implication is that conventional and alternative therapies are not merely "separate if not exactly equal" but that the latter can supply something the former lacks. Finally, in more recent years the term *integrative* has become popular. While the term *complementary medicine* might suggest a less important or subordinate status to its conventional counterpart, *integrative* implies—and in a subtle way, perhaps mandates—the partnership and blending of equally valid methodologies.

This analysis of terms and phrases might seem to be semantic hairsplitting, but there is no question that language plays a key role in molding attitudes, whether among the general public or among professionals, including those in health care.

Insurance Providers

Last but not least we come to an important—but very practical—ingredient in the mainstreaming of alternative medicine. As already noted, Americans (and their counterparts in other Western nations) have been spending billions of dollars out of their own pocketbooks on alternative therapies. Conventional medicine's annual price tag has escalated into the trillion-dollar range in the United States, and not surprisingly, those who pay the lion's share of the bills—the so-called third-party payers, primarily insurance companies and government programs such as Medicare—have been very concerned about containing it. It would therefore seem plausible that they would strive to stem not only the outflow of dollars but also the number of directions in which those dollars might go. This has been borne out by some of the heated, and often highly publicized, conflicts between critically ill patients and insurance companies over coverage of new treatments (for example, bone marrow transplants) that have been deemed experimental, despite sophisticated protocols from respected universities and researchers. The likelihood that third-party payers would be willing to cover unconventional and unproven therapies, many of which tend to involve a multitude of visits, would appear to be extremely low.

But in fact, for alternative therapies the opposite has been true. For example, Landmark Healthcare, Inc., a company that promotes alternative medicine programs nationally, has surveyed more than one hundred health maintenance organizations (HMOs) in the United States and found that two-thirds offer at least one form of alternative care. Among these, almost half of the subscribers took advantage of this coverage.[17] In 1997 Oxford Health Plans, which services more than 1.5 million members in eastern states, launched the first alternative health care program in the U.S. It now offers access to a network of alternative providers, including acupuncturists, naturopaths, massage therapists and yoga instructors. Other major companies have followed suit. In 1998 six major health insurance companies in California alone decided to cover acupuncture and traditional Chinese medicine.[18] Blue Cross of California provides a referral list of massage therapists and yoga instructors, who in turn offer discounts to Blue Cross members (though without actual coverage).

Why would health insurance plans now appear willing—and in some cases eager—to open their wallets to cover therapies that would have been summarily excluded barely a decade ago? Three reasons have been most commonly cited for the inclusion of alternative practices in insurance plans:

The customers want it. Interest in alternative therapies is keen not only among those who are going to be covered by insurance but also among many employers who choose a menu of plans they will make available to their employees. In the Landmark Healthcare survey of HMOs, nearly 40 percent of those who offered alternative therapies reported that these benefits were added primarily because of the interest (or demand) of members and employers. An internal survey conducted by Oxford Health Plans found that 75 percent of its members were interested in adding alternative medicine services to their current plan.[19]

An increasing number of regulations are requiring it. Landmark's survey of HMOs found that among those offering alternative therapies, nearly 40 percent were responding to government mandates or other legal requirements. At least eight states require that health insurers cover acupuncture treatment, and one (Oregon) mandates it for drug-dependent offenders.[20] A 1996 Washington State law required insurers to cover, at no extra charge, services from any type of health care provider for which the state issues licenses. This included chiropractors, naturopaths, acupuncturists and massage therapists. Even though the law was eventually overturned by a federal judge, Washington insurers appeared willing to continue the alternative medicine coverage anyway (though at an extra charge). Given the dramatic increase in public interest in alternative medicine over the past decade, and given the well-established tendency for legislators to listen to their constituents, an ongoing stream of state and federal legislation favorable to alternative therapies is a near certainty.[21]

It may save money in the long run. Because most alternative therapies are essentially low tech (they rarely require expensive equipment and sophisticated technologies), and because many practices promote lifestyle changes (such as regular exercise and stress management), they might prove to be more cost effective than their conventional counterparts, at least for some conditions. Certainly those promoting alternative therapies make abundant claims for their preventive and health-promoting benefits. But the jury is out as to whether they can in fact deliver on this promise and reduce health care costs in the process. In the Landmark Healthcare HMO study cited previously there was no consensus about the net effect of alternative therapies on the overall price of delivering care. About 20 percent of those surveyed believed that alternative medicine benefits ultimately save money, 30 percent felt that they don't change the financial bottom line either way, and 50 percent were convinced that they increase the total cost of delivering care.[22]

Now That Notice Has Been Taken

The enthusiastic embrace of alternative medicine by a sizable number of Americans, along with its apparent welcome among many important governmental, medical, educational and financial institutions, raises a number of provocative questions.

Is alternative medicine an enhancement to health care or a giant step backward? Do alternative therapies mine the riches of ancient civilizations and diverse cultures and deliver them to our doorstep? Can Western practitioners gain from them an appreciation for caring for the whole person—body, mind and spirit? Or are we tossing aside the hard-won medical advances of the past century in favor of medical relics grounded in superstition and ignorance?

Is it possible to make scientific sense out of therapies as diverse, exotic and seemingly incompatible as ayurveda, *traditional Chinese medicine and homeopathy?* Can these and a host of other alternative therapies be subjected to the Western gold standard of proof: the randomized, double-blind, placebo-controlled trial? Or do they, by their nature, defy such analysis and demand instead a new gold standard, framed by the question "Is it safe and does it work?"

Does the apparent efficacy of a particular treatment validate its underlying assumptions about health and illness? In other words, if acupuncture relieves a toothache, are we compelled to accept the notion that an invisible energy called *chi* has been "balanced" by the needling technique? If a homeopathic remedy containing an infinitesimally small amount of ipecac (which in normal doses provokes vomiting) relieves nausea, does the restored appetite validate an eighteenth-century theory that "like cures like"?

Can the practice of ayurveda, *traditional Chinese medicine, yoga and Therapeutic Touch (among others) be separated from their spiritual underpinnings?* As we will discuss later, these practices, and many others in the alternative stable, are deeply rooted in Eastern mysticism, New Age philosophy and, in some cases, spiritism and the occult. Is it appropriate for those who take the Old and New Testaments seriously (or for anyone else) to participate in these therapies, either as providers or recipients of care? Spiritually speaking, is there a kernel of wheat that can be removed from the chaff, or are they inseparable? Is there a potential spiritual risk associated with any of these therapies?

In the next several chapters we will attempt to address these questions and a number of others. Before embarking on this expedition, however, we need to offer a few disclaimers about our general direction and our ports of call.

First, this book will not be an encyclopedia of alternative health practices. We will be examining broad themes in this movement more often than specific variations, although we will take a more detailed look at certain high-profile therapies.

Second, while two of us practice conventional medicine, we are well aware of its weaknesses as well as its strengths. Indeed, as we will discuss in a subsequent chapter, the rise of alternative medicine has to some degree been driven by limitations in Western medicine's capabilities as well as deficiencies in its delivery to the average citizen. The success of many alternative therapies can suggest, at least in certain areas, where conventional medicine has room for improvement.

Third, we are convinced that the basic methods of scientific inquiry and experimentation on which Western medicine is based have been overwhelmingly validated over the past century. Indeed even a cursory review of the history of the world's medicine suggests that we have emerged from a medical wilderness of misinformation and mythology only during the past few generations. Abandoning the unequivocal success of this methodology in order to embrace wildly diverse healing systems raises, in our minds, some very serious concerns.

Fourth, we are equally convinced that the worldview of the Old and New Testaments—and the clear teachings therein regarding God and humanity, rebellion and restoration, disease and health, and most of all the life, death and resurrection of Jesus Christ—are in fact true. And so, while we unequivocally believe in the power of God to heal anyone anytime and anywhere, we do not believe that God would heal in a manner that would be inconsistent with his nature as revealed in the Bible or that would lead people into spiritual error rather than to spiritual truth. If an apparent supernatural healing episode leads an individual to embrace a philosophy or spiritual practice that flatly contradicts the teachings of Scripture, we would seriously question whether that healing in fact came from God.

Some of our greatest concerns about many alternative therapies, therefore, arise from their spiritual ancestry and their enthusiastic promotion of spiritual perspectives that are incompatible with—or even overtly hostile toward—the teachings of Scripture. The experiences of illness and healing can be extremely powerful, if not life changing. Healing was an important component of Jesus' brief earthly ministry, serving not only to demonstrate his compassion for the human race but also to validate his teaching in a most graphic and convincing manner. Unfortunately, the apparent benefits of some alternative therapies tend to validate notions about human beings, the universe and God that are clearly at odds with those taught by Jesus of Nazareth. Therefore, throughout this book we will examine carefully the spiritual implications of a number of alternative therapies.

2

WHAT ARE ALTERNATIVE THERAPIES?

(And What Therapies Are Alternative?)

We have described the explosive growth of alternative medicine in the United States over the past decade and raised some preliminary questions about the impact of this movement as a new millennium begins. But amid the broad strokes we did not broach a more basic question, one that continues to challenge any and all who wade into this topic: What exactly are alternative therapies?

There are plenty of answers in circulation, and many of them reflect the inherent difficulty of separating definitions from one's general opinion of this phenomenon. Speak with an enthusiastic practitioner and you will hear about "ancient and global healing modalities that are expanding and enriching our perspectives on disease, health and wellness." Listen to a die-hard critic and you will be warned about "a lot of superstitious nonsense, pseudoscience, hype and horse manure that is separating millions of willing victims from their hard-earned money." Talk to an avid user of alternative modalities and you can anticipate terms of endearment: "Natural and safe approaches that help my body heal itself, allow me to take control of my own health and avoid drugs and surgery, cleanse me of toxins, balance and boost my energy and treat me as a *whole* person—body, mind and spirit." Ask a time-pressured primary care physician for input, and your feedback will vary from "My way or the highway!" to "Whatever works for you, as long as you stay on your medication" (perhaps with a silent sigh of relief that a number of schedule-busting complaints may now have somewhere else to go). Ask someone who is not acquainted with (or interested in) this subject, and you may hear that alternative medicine is "anything that doesn't involve drugs or surgery," or perhaps you will hear the legendary statement that lawmakers have made about pornography: "I'm not sure I can define it, but I know it when I see it!"

One simple definition, which has served relatively well for a number of years, goes something like this: Alternative practices are those that, in the United States, are not generally taught in medical schools, are not generally practiced in hospitals and doctors' offices and are not generally covered by insurance. David Eisenberg, M.D., for example, used this type of definition in his landmark articles described in chapter one, describing alternative therapies as "interventions neither taught widely in U.S. medical schools nor generally available in U.S. hospitals."[1] The same points answer the question "What is complementary and alternative medicine?" in the "Frequently Asked Questions" fact sheet published by the National Center for Complementary and Alternative Medicine.[2] But as cultural and medical tides have shifted over the past few years, and as alternative therapies have gained wider access to medical schools, hospitals, doctors' offices and insurance companies, this definition has become less meaningful.

Culture, Context and Credentials

Defining what is alternative and what is not alternative has also been complicated by the observation that we must consider culture, context and point of view. For much of the world, conventional Western medicine is the "alternative" to whatever is the local prevailing system of understanding health and illness. Also, in prior centuries, many of Western medicine's best-established precepts would have been considered "alternative" or dismissed outright as nonsense or quackery. An acute awareness of the role that power, politics, prejudice and economics can play in determining what is considered mainstream medicine has led some authors to describe alternative therapies in cultural and sociologic, rather than medical, terms. For example, Dr. Daniel Eskinasi of Columbia University has suggested a definition based upon the degree to which a practice falls outside of various comfort zones in our society:

> I propose that *alternative medicine* be defined as a broad set of health care practices (i.e., already available to the public) that are not readily integrated into the dominant health care model, because they pose challenges to diverse societal beliefs and practices (cultural, economic, scientific, medical and educational). This definition brings into focus factors that may play a major role in the a priori acceptance and rejection of various alternative health care practices by any society.[3]

For example, a health care system that developed outside of mainstream American culture, such as *ayurveda* from India, may not be widely accepted because it does not fit within commonly held assumptions and values. However, a polished advocate, such as Deepak Chopra, M.D., who smoothly translates an unfamiliar system into more comfortable Western terminology, can help move a "foreign" alternative squarely into the mainstream.

James E. Dalen, M.D., editor of the mainstream journal *Archives of Internal Medicine,* has suggested another definition of alternative medicine based upon the sources from which these practices are brought to our culture: "Conventional therapies are introduced by mainstream Western physicians and scientists, whereas most unconventional modalities are introduced by 'outsiders.' . . . American academic medicine has a bias against outsiders who make therapeutic suggestions, especially when they take their message directly to the public."[4]

To some degree this is true. In mainstream medicine, presenting a "medical breakthrough" to the general public before it is reviewed by one's professional peers is viewed with suspicion, usually with good reason. Often the therapy in question is found to be less impressive than advertised when subjected to closer scientific scrutiny.

Conventional physicians *are* more likely to listen to new ideas from a colleague with impressive credentials (as opposed to an "outsider")—at least for a while. But if his or her medical propositions strain credibility, and especially if they represent a one-person crusade, ears will quickly turn deaf, regardless of who is speaking. A prime example is the promotion by Dr. Linus Pauling of high doses of vitamin C to prevent and treat the common cold, cancer and other ailments. Though the winner of two Nobel Prizes, including one in biochemistry, Pauling could not convince the medical community at large to adopt his point of view. Personal accomplishments notwithstanding, he was seen as having gone too far out on a limb, especially when controlled studies did not appear to support his claims. Generally speaking, Western physicians are more likely to accept new ideas when they are supported by well-designed, peer-reviewed research (especially from multiple sources) and are less likely to follow a voice crying in the wilderness, no matter how brilliant he or she might otherwise be.

Categories and Lists

One of the most common, though indirect, approaches to defining alternative medicine is that of grouping various approaches together under broad categories. For example, in 1994 the Office of Alternative Medicine (OAM) of the National Institutes of Health (NIH) generated a series of lists of therapies grouped under seven broad categories in order to facilitate the process of reviewing requests for research grants. The categories were

- [ ] alternative systems of medical practice
- [ ] bioelectromagnetic applications
- [ ] diet, nutrition and lifestyle changes
- [ ] herbal medicine
- [ ] manual healing
- [ ] mind/body control
- [ ] pharmacological and biological treatments

Each category contained numerous therapies, often highly diverse in theory and practice. For example, grouped under "alternative systems of medical practice" were the following:

- [ ] acupuncture
- [ ] anthroposophically extended medicine
- [ ] *ayurveda*
- [ ] community-based health care practices
- [ ] environmental medicine
- [ ] homeopathic medicine
- [ ] Latin American rural practices
- [ ] Native American practices
- [ ] natural products
- [ ] naturopathic medicine
- [ ] past life therapy
- [ ] shamanism
- [ ] Tibetan medicine
- [ ] traditional Oriental medicine

For the average citizen and the health care professional alike, such lists are both intimidating and bewildering: *There are so many of these therapies; could they all be valid? How in the world would I decide which one(s) I might utilize?* The National Center for Complementary and Alternative Medicine (NCCAM), the body that replaced the OAM, has thus far offered little guidance for those with questions such as these. Among its general information publications, there are no descriptions or explanations of these approaches, and certainly no evaluations of their potential benefits and risks. Indeed these materials are infused with a bland open-mindedness that implies that there is little basis to judge one approach to be any better than another. The NCCAM's basic message to the public, at least thus far, appears to be "Figure it out for yourself."

In its short publication "Considering Complementary and Alternative Therapies?" the NCCAM recommends that before selecting an alternative therapy or practitioner, one should consider "the safety and effectiveness of the therapy or treatment, the expertise and qualifications of the health care practitioner, and the quality of the service delivery."[5] How might this be done? Suggestions from the NCCAM and other consumer-oriented materials run a broad gamut: talk to your doctor, talk to the alternative practitioner, consult the *Reader's Guide to Periodical Literature,* check into the *Index Medicus,* search MEDLINE, contact state regulatory agencies, find out about costs, talk to those who have been to a particular practitioner, call the NIH, go to the library, go to the bookstore. In other words, "Good luck, and may the Force be with you."

Such apparent acceptance of alternative therapies by mainstream organizations and publications has not been limited to the NCCAM, as we noted in the previous chapter. Indeed some have observed what appears to be a general reluctance among physicians to scrutinize the rising tide of alternative medicine, perhaps to avoid appearing judgmental and narrow-minded—a phenomenon that some observers have dubbed "medical correctness." In response a few disgruntled but articulate voices have suggested a more rigorous approach to defining alternative therapies. In a September 1998 *New England Journal of Medicine* editorial frequently quoted by critics of alternative medicine, Marcia Angell, M.D., and Jerome Kassirer, M.D., offered some less flattering distinctions between conventional medicine and its alternative counterpart.

With respect to scientific validation, they observed:

> What most sets alternative medicine apart, in our view, is that it has not been scientifically tested and its advocates largely deny the need for such testing. By testing, we mean the marshaling of rigorous evidence of safety and efficacy, as required by the Food and Drug Administration (FDA) for the approval of drugs and by the best peer-reviewed medical journals for the publication of research reports. . . . Many advocates of alternative medicine . . . believe the scientific method is simply not applicable to their remedies.

With respect to reliance on anecdotes (that is, accounts of the response of individual patients to a particular therapy), Angell and Kassirer noted:

> It might be argued that conventional medicine relies on anecdotes, too, some of which are published as case reports in peer-reviewed journals. But these case reports differ from the anecdotes of alternative medicine. They describe a well-documented new finding in a defined setting. . . . We might publish a case report—not to announce a remedy, but only to suggest a hypothesis that should be tested in a proper clinical trial. In contrast, anecdotes about alternative remedies (usually published in books and magazines for the public) have no such documentation and are considered sufficient in themselves as support for therapeutic claims.

With respect to underlying assumptions, they were particularly critical:

> Alternative medicine also distinguishes itself by an ideology that largely ignores bio-
> logic mechanisms, often disparages modern science, and relies on what are pur-
> ported to be ancient practices and natural remedies (which are seen as somehow
> more potent and less toxic than conventional medicine). . . . Healing methods such
> as homeopathy and therapeutic touch are fervently promoted despite not only the
> lack of good clinical evidence of effectiveness, but the presence of a rationale that
> violates fundamental scientific laws—surely a circumstance that requires more, rather
> than less, evidence.

In a final paragraph that has become the rallying cry not only for skeptics and
critics of alternative medicine but for some of its proponents as well, Drs. Angell
and Kassirer threw down a gauntlet of sorts and suggested a more fundamental
approach to the question of defining conventional versus alternative therapies:

> It is time for the scientific community to stop giving alternative medicine a free ride.
> There cannot be two kinds of medicine—conventional and alternative. There is only
> medicine that has been adequately tested and medicine that has not, medicine that
> works and medicine that may or may not work. Once a treatment has been tested
> rigorously, it no longer matters whether it was considered alternative at the outset. If
> it is found to be reasonably safe and effective, it will be accepted. But assertions,
> speculations, and testimonials do not substitute for evidence. Alternative treatments
> should be subjected to scientific testing no less rigorous than that required for con-
> ventional treatments.[6]

Safety and Effectiveness . . . and Reality Checks

Given the bewildering array of alternative therapies in the current marketplace,
why not simply abandon the entire quandary over what is conventional and what
is alternative and simply focus on safety and effectiveness, on what works and what
doesn't? For some types of therapies—for example, the appropriate use of herbs—
this idea certainly makes a lot of sense. But there is a more fundamental question
that might be ignored if safety and effectiveness are the only issues on the table.
Drs. Angell and Kassirer made reference to therapies whose underlying rationale
"violates fundamental scientific laws." This is such an important consideration that
we would propose adding "scientific reality" to the primary questions of safety and
efficacy when evaluating alternative and conventional therapies: What are the
underlying assumptions of the therapy? Do they make any sense, given what we
have discovered over the past century? If they are true, is it necessary to revise, or
even rewrite, every textbook of biology and physiology?

These are not trivial, or even philosophical, questions. For countless millennia
human beings have attempted to understand the causes and cures of disease. Sadly,

until relatively recently the vast majority of their conclusions have not improved upon the body's wondrous powers of repair and recuperation. An overview of the history of the world's medical interventions is well beyond the scope of this book, but for the most part it reads as a long procession of fanciful theories, gods and demons to be summoned or warded off, potions, nostrums, extravagant concoctions, rituals and, worst of all, frequently harsh treatments: bleeding, purging, poisoning, drilling holes in the skull and any other abuse that someone wearing a mantle of authority might conjure up as a possible remedy for disease—provided, of course, that the poor patient could survive it. One could reasonably argue, in fact, that the primary reason traditional Chinese medicine, homeopathy and certain other therapeutic systems have endured is that they generally do little harm, thus offering the patient a chance to recover without contending with additional damage inflicted by the physician or healer. They have also tapped into an extremely important healing resource: the patient's expectation of improvement. As we will discuss throughout this book, confidence and optimism created by the physician or healer play a definite role in the response of many patients to therapies of all types—not only those that make little sense but also those that have been widely validated by vigorous scientific research.

In view of the catalog of sorrows routinely faced by our ancestors, we dare not dismiss the spectacular progress of Western medicine over the past hundred years as mere good fortune, coinciding with advances in hygiene and public health. This progress has been built upon basic principles of biology and physics, and a methodology of research and development, which continue to be verified and validated all over the world. From the vantage point of a physician at the turn of the previous century, today's mainstream medicine, for all of its shortcomings, would look like heaven on earth. There is no question that we have our own twenty-first-century scourges, the cancers and degenerative diseases and viruses that do not yet respond to treatment. We also have deficiencies in our health care delivery system, complex financial pressures, inequality of access to services, frequent lapses in compassion and plenty of medical misjudgments, many with serious consequences. Nevertheless, few adult Americans, or their counterparts in developed countries, have not been successfully treated for an illness or injury that would have been catastrophic or fatal just a few decades ago.

Furthermore, the thinking and methodology that have given us true medical breakthroughs did *not* do so by locating the meridians of traditional Chinese medicine, identifying the *chakras* of *ayurveda,* uncovering the infinitesimal dosing regimes of homeopathy or stumbling upon the invisible "life energies" of Therapeutic Touch and a dozen other popular therapies. Proponents of these practices are eager for Western medicine's research tools to confirm their usefulness, but those same tools would never have discovered them in the first place.

In view of the importance of applying reality checks to alternative practices, we propose identifying and categorizing them according to their compatibility with well-established and widely validated principles of science, especially biology and physics.

☐ Category 1: reality-based practices. These are therapies whose underlying assumptions and practices do not require a departure from well-established principles of biology, physics and human physiology.

☐ Category 2: leaps of logic. Into this category fall therapies that have at least some connection (if only in terminology) to widely accepted principles of biology but then wade into uncharted—or self-charted—territory.

☐ Category 3: "everything you know is wrong." Here are therapies postulating mechanisms of disease and treatment that are a radical departure from well-established principles of biology. Some of these, such as traditional Chinese medicine, are comprehensive and multidimensional systems of health care.

☐ Category 4: invading the supernatural. These therapies explicitly claim to engage and manipulate supernatural forces and entities.

In the next chapter we will review a number of therapies as they relate to each of these categories.

3

A "REALITY CHECK" TOUR OF ALTERNATIVE MEDICINE

As we begin our exploration of alternative practices from the perspective of their compatibility with well-established principles of biology and physics, three important points should be kept in mind. First, some alternative practices may fall into more than one of these categories. This can depend to some degree on the approach and orientation of the individual practitioner. Second, our examples in each category are not an exhaustive listing of every therapy in the current marketplace.

Finally, our analysis of alternative therapies involves somewhat broader strokes than those used in the pursuit of "evidence-based medicine" (EBM), an important movement that has gained considerable momentum in health care over the past decade. As described in a seminal article published in the *British Medical Journal* in 1996, EBM is the "conscientious, explicit and judicious use of current best evidence in making decisions about the care of individual patients. The practice of evidence-based medicine means integrating individual clinical expertise with the best available external clinical evidence through systematic research."[1] "External clinical evidence" can take a variety of forms, but when dealing with specific therapies EBM is particularly interested in the results of well-designed randomized controlled trials (or RCTs), in which patients given certain treatment for a given condition are compared to those who receive no (or different) treatment—ideally in a manner in which neither the patients nor the investigators know who is getting what. (We will discuss this type of study in more detail in the next chapter.) Even more valuable in EBM are systematic reviews of multiple randomized trials, which are considered a gold standard for judging the potential usefulness of a given treatment.

EBM has been generally well-received in conventional settings, as more physicians seek to base clinical decisions on footing more broad and solid than time-honored (but possibly ineffective) traditions, outdated protocols or "what's always worked in our office." Attempts to apply EBM methodologies to alternative therapies are in their infancy, although two recent books are noteworthy for their efforts to summarize some of the available data.[2] As we will see, however, some alternative approaches are far more amenable to EBM assessments than others. Those that fall into our first and second "reality-check" categories—especially those involving the appropriate use of herbs, vitamins and supplements—have enough of a connection to contemporary science to allow for meaningful RCTs to be conducted and analyzed, and for the results to be useful in patient care. As we venture into more exotic categories that include "energy" therapies, ancient systems such as *ayurveda* and traditional Chinese medicine, and psychic/shamanistic approaches to healing, we will find basic assumptions about the causes and cures of disease that do not at all readily adapt to the approaches of EBM.

Category 1: Reality-Based Practices

This first category comprises those therapies whose underlying assumptions and practices do not require a departure from well-established principles of biology, physics and human physiology.

Vitamin and Mineral Supplements
and Herbal Remedies

Does vitamin E help prevent coronary artery disease? Does St. John's wort relieve depression? Can ginkgo biloba improve memory and general mental functioning? Claims abound for these and many other nutritional supplements, which have enjoyed a spectacular rise in sales and use over the past decade. Of all areas of alternative medicine, the potential benefits of taking supplemental vitamins and minerals, or the treatment of specific conditions with herbal preparations, requires the shortest leap of faith. There are no invisible energies with mysterious mechanisms to deal with, only the straightforward (if laborious) task of sorting out what works from what doesn't, determining the physiological mechanisms at work, applying reasonable guidelines for safe usage and clarifying which preparations are properly manufactured. A great deal of information has been gathered already in Europe, where herbal preparations are more widely used by physicians. In the United States the nutritional supplement horse is already well out of the barn, spurred primarily by marketing and broad public appeal. To what degree scientific research will eventually guide or rein in its gallop remains to be seen. This and other issues related to what many refer to as "natural medicine" will be discussed in more detail in chapter seven.

Biofeedback

This technique involves the use of special electronic equipment to gain some degree of control over a body function that we normally do not consciously regulate. In theory, by observing how skin temperature, pulse rate or even brain waves respond to various mental exercises, one can learn how to manage certain health problems. For example, some individuals can learn to abort migraine headaches by controlling the skin temperature of the hand, although the usefulness of this technique may be limited by the expense and discipline required to master it (not to mention the ability to carry out the appropriate mental process in the thick of a busy schedule or a tense confrontation).

For applications such as this, biofeedback really is not an "alternative" therapy at all but rather a mainstream tool with limited applications. However, over the years a small cadre of biofeedback researchers have promoted this technology as a sort of "electronic yoga," a high-tech means of altering consciousness and inducing psychic experiences. In the late 1970s, for example, British psychologist C. Maxwell Cade wrote the following in the preface to his book *The Awakened Mind: Biofeedback and the Development of Higher States of Awareness:* "My work, . . . while fully incorporating the basic biofeedback principles and techniques in all their aspects, has branched off into a singular direction and emphasis—that of combining biofeedback training and monitoring with the ancient art of meditation, so as to try to achieve a maximal mind-body awareness, this in turn leading to the gradual development of higher states of consciousness."[3]

This vision of biofeedback was expressed far more commonly in the bygone days of the holistic health movement, and one rarely hears about mystical applications of this technique in today's alternative medicine marketplace.

Massage

Massage techniques may fall not only into this category but also into the next two as well because under the general term "massage therapy" are gathered an impressive number of techniques with a broad list of claims and assumptions. Blue Cross of California, for example, lists some twenty-four varieties of massage, from

"AMMA" to "trigger point/myotherapy," in its HealthyExtensions booklet of alternative resources and providers. The popular compendium *Alternative Medicine for Dummies* suggests that more than one hundred different techniques fall under the general definition of massage as a "systemic manipulation of the soft tissues of the body."[4]

The massage technique with which most Americans are familiar is the straightforward, relaxing, invigorating experience usually called "European" or, more specifically, "Swedish" massage, which combines a variety of stroking, kneading and percussive maneuvers applied to superficial muscles from one end of the body to the other.[5] For decades this has been a staple of American health clubs, spas and resorts, but until recently it has not been widely integrated into the mainstream health care system in America. Given the state of pleasant and profound relaxation that normally accompanies a thorough massage, its potential benefits for conditions such as chronic pain syndromes, muscle spasm, sports injuries, headache, anxiety and depression do not require any stretch of the imagination. Claims have also been made (with variable research backup) for improvements in hypertension (high blood pressure), arthritis, allergies, sinusitis and recovery from surgery.

All of these applications are worthy of further study, both to refine the use of massage as a treatment modality and to offer a wider range of therapeutic options for a variety of health problems. What may complicate this process in the future, however, is the sheer number of massage techniques, along with the expansive claims commonly made for many of them. As already mentioned, it is common for alternative therapies to claim far-reaching "holistic" effects, and promoters of many forms of massage routinely state that their particular technique balances energy, harmonizes body and mind, improves the function of various organs and so forth. Such representations, along with claims that particular techniques might confer "rejuvenating" or antiaging benefits, likewise can push the boundaries of massage therapy onto the shakier ground of category two (or "leaps of logic") practices.

More problematic is the fact that many massage therapists freely dip into precepts of traditional Chinese and other mystical systems, claiming to manipulate invisible energy *(chi)* through techniques such as acupressure, shiatsu or *reiki,* which we will discuss at length in chapter five. Some employ foot or hand reflexology, a dubious but nevertheless enduring practice that purportedly benefits far-flung organs through manipulation of specific points on the soles or palms. A few wade into more fanciful realms such as polarity therapy, which supposedly balances the body's electrical fields through a variety of techniques, including massage. These practices fall into category three ("everything you know is wrong"), where diagnostic and therapeutic techniques have made a radical departure from well-established principles of biology and physics.

Relaxation Techniques

As with massage, a variety of activities are touted as "relaxation techniques," but not all of them fit into the same category. The objective, of course, is to reduce physiological and emotional tension or agitation without resorting to the more common (and potentially hazardous) use of drugs or alcohol. Obviously, for many people the combination of a hot bath, soft lighting and quiet music serves as a time-honored relaxation method if they will give themselves time and permission to pursue it. But many Americans are also interested in specific techniques to achieve relaxation. For the past quarter century, perhaps the most widely known of these has been the "relaxation response," originally described in a book of the same name by Herbert Benson, M.D.[6] In the early 1970s Dr. Benson had been studying the physiological responses of individuals practicing Transcendental Meditation (TM), whose enthusiasts were proclaiming its benefits as a scientific, nonreligious method of reducing stress. Those initiated in TM were (and still are) given a secret mantra, a word said to be specially selected for the individual to say repeatedly during the meditation session. (Investigative organizations subsequently revealed that the "specially chosen" mantra was invariably the name of a Hindu deity, contradicting the assertion that TM was "nonreligious.")[7] Dr. Benson eventually concluded that there was nothing unique about the TM training process or its mantras, and he devised a much simpler approach without any Hindu underpinnings.

It is well established that human beings react to stressful events—major or minor, physical or emotional, real or imagined—with a well-orchestrated response: adrenaline and other hormones are released into the bloodstream, muscles tighten, pupils dilate, the pulse quickens and blood pressure rises. This has long been known as the flight or fight response, in honor of our distant ancestors' limited range of options when confronted with animal or human predators. An important part of this stress response is its resolution, the physiologic "all clear" signal, the return to a physical and emotional calm when the threat has passed. Unfortunately, most of us in developed countries experience ongoing daily stresses without well-defined flight or fight episodes, and as a result many live in a constant state of low-grade (or even high-grade) physical and emotional alarm. This may cause or aggravate a host of symptoms, including headache, chronic pain syndromes, sleep disturbances, chronic fatigue and intestinal complaints, not to mention those directly related to anxiety, such as palpitations (pounding of the heart), shortness of breath or even panic episodes. Some researchers contend that ongoing, unregulated stress responses cause more than symptoms and in fact eventually damage the body.

In *The Relaxation Response* Dr. Benson described a simple technique designed to evoke a physiologic "all clear" response, a relaxed physical and emotional state in which blood pressure and heart rate gradually fall and tight muscles relax. Like TM, this involves two twenty-minute sessions per day in which one sits comfortably in a quiet place and quietly repeats a word or phrase, disregarding other mental traffic. In contrast to the practice of TM, any neutral or positive utterance will do—"peace" or "one" or "the Lord is my shepherd," for example. This daily exercise is intended not only to produce some immediate improvement in well-being but to defend against a host of stress-driven conditions as well. More importantly, it appears to be a straightforward process, one that does not require a stretch of reason to accept nor a shift in worldview to practice. This cannot be assumed for all relaxation techniques, many of which (such as TM) are basically Eastern metaphysical practices that have been repackaged for Western consumption.

Since publishing his first book, Dr. Benson has expanded his scope of research and practice, not only through writing several books that deal more extensively with the interactions of mind and body[8] but also through founding the Mind/Body Medical Institute and Medical Clinic at the Beth Israel Deaconess Medical Center in Boston. In so doing he has become increasingly interested in the "faith factor" in healing—a topic of great importance to understanding individual responses to both alternative and conventional medicine. We will take a closer look at this subject in the next chapter.

Chiropractic as Physical Therapy

Chiropractic is so well established as a mode of health care in the United States and around the world that one could legitimately question whether it belongs on a list of alternative or unconventional therapies. Approximately fifty thousand chiropractors in the United States carry out an estimated 190 million treatments every year (as of 1997), including treatment of one in three individuals with lower back pain.[9] They are licensed in all fifty states and are reimbursed through Medicare and most major medical insurance plans. Wide use notwithstanding, chiropractic continues to be viewed as alternative not only because of its colorful history (which has included heated conflict with mainstream medical organizations) but also because of the claims and activities of some of its practitioners.

A detailed review of the origins and history of chiropractic is beyond the scope of this book, but many of the bumps in its road through the twentieth century arose from the teachings of its founder, D. D. Palmer (1845–1913). For nearly a decade prior to the birth of chiropractic in 1895 Palmer had been involved with "magnetic healing," which purported to normalize the flow of "animal magnetism" within the human body. As with many of today's "energy" therapies, it was assumed in "magnetic healing" that unimpeded flow of this invisible energy resulted in vibrant health, while disease arose from obstruction of its progress. Palmer renamed animal magnetism "Innate Intelligence" and claimed that its most important pathway in the human body was the spinal cord and its branches. If the spinal column was beset with misalignments, or "subluxations," the Innate could not flow properly and disease would result. In the late nineteenth century this notion was bolstered by the widespread use of the term "spinal irritation" among conventional physicians to explain complaints that otherwise defied analysis. Palmer maintained that restoring the flow of the Innate through realignment of spinal subluxations through hands-on manipulation (the word *chiropractic* literally means "hand work") not only would relieve local pain but was in fact the key to treating all illness.

On September 19, 1895, Palmer manipulated the cervical (neck) spine of a deaf janitor, who regained his hearing instantaneously—or so it was reported. This event achieved legendary status in the history of chiropractic, although there was some lack of agreement among witnesses as to what in fact occurred that day.[10] But with this dramatic launch (one that was incomprehensible from the standpoint of the physiology of hearing), Palmer's movement gained both practitioners and satisfied clients. It also generated a healthy amount of controversy, not only from the conventional medical establishment but also from within its own ranks. From the earliest years of the twentieth century there has been ongoing disagreement among chiropractors regarding the existence of the Innate, the capacity for chiropractic manipulation to treat any and all diseases, the precise definition of subluxations, the nature of the spinal disturbances that can be corrected with manipulation and even what constitutes the most effective and most appropriate types of chiropractic adjustment.

D. D. Palmer's son and successor, B. J. Palmer, proclaimed the virtues of "straight" chiropractic—the "specific, pure and unadulterated" tradition of releasing the Innate Intelligence strictly through spinal adjustments. He contrasted "straight" chiropractors with "mixers," who are the clear majority today. Needless to say, it is the mixers who have gradually helped chiropractic gain credibility within the broader realm of health care. By avoiding the one-cause-of-all-disease doctrine, which marginalizes straight practitioners to the realm of flat-earth proponents, they limit the scope of problems to be treated with manipulation and at the same time take advantage of other treatment modalities. Some have adopted techniques used by conventional physical therapists, such as ultrasound, local heat, exercise and postural training, including assessment of workplace ergonomics (the physical arrangements of chair, desk and computer hardware, for example) that may contribute to overuse syndromes and chronic pain. In so doing, these practitioners have positioned themselves as musculoskeletal consultants within their medical communities. A continued focus on treating painful lower backs—an extremely common problem and a perennial source of new patients—has also led to more formal recognition within the mainstream of health care.

In December 1994 the Agency for Health Care Policy and Research reviewed the current scientific literature and concluded that "manipulation can be helpful for patients with acute low back problems when used within the first month of symptoms. A trial of manipulation for patients with symptoms longer than a month is probably safe, but efficacy is unproven."[11] Other potential applications for chiropractic manipulation continue to be evaluated with variable results. For example, some studies of its effectiveness in managing headache have shown benefit, while others have been equivocal. One recent study failed to show effectiveness in treating children with asthma, and evidence for benefits in other medical problems (such as high blood pressure) is scarce, confirming the general impression among conventional physicians that chiropractic's niche will remain the management of musculoskeletal pain.

Acupuncture Based on Neurological Concepts

In chapter five we will discuss at some length traditional Chinese medicine, which has made significant inroads into the mainstream of health care over the past three decades. Without a doubt, its most visible point of entry has been acupuncture, which continues to fascinate Westerners as an exotic approach to treating a wide range of problems. While widely practiced in the United States, acupuncture's proposed mechanism of action has been considered from every conceivable perspective in books and media resources, not to mention by its practitioners. This is not an esoteric academic issue. The classical Chinese understanding of illness and its treatment (of which acupuncture is but one of many components) is both overtly mystical and highly convoluted, involving elaborate formulas for determining where an invisible energy called *chi* is or is not flowing through equally invisible channels called "meridians."

While Western investigators have found acupuncture to be effective in treating certain problems, most have proposed explanations based upon current understandings of neurological function. This was the case, more or less, in the landmark

1998 NIH Consensus Panel Statement on Acupuncture, which concluded that this technique appears to be effective in treating nausea and vomiting after surgery or chemotherapy, pain after dental operations and probably nausea during pregnancy. In a number of other conditions—many of which are pain-related (headache, menstrual cramps, tennis elbow, lower back pain, carpal tunnel syndrome, fibromyalgia, stroke rehabilitation, addiction and asthma)—the panel concluded that acupuncture might be helpful as part of a comprehensive treatment program. The panel also acknowledged that many studies of acupuncture's effects were beset with design problems and that key concepts such as the flow of *chi* and the meridian system are "difficult to reconcile with contemporary biomedical information."[12]

Indeed it would appear that many, if not most, Western-trained physicians who practice acupuncture acknowledge that its effects are primarily attributable to a mixture of biochemical events in the nervous system—involving small peripheral nerves, the spinal cord and the brain—as well as the release of pain-blocking compounds known as endorphins. They are also likely to express skepticism about the existence of meridians and the flow of *chi* and to be conservative about the types of problems they might treat with acupuncture. But on an operational level, they may generally practice "by the book," choosing points and needling techniques as if the ancient maps had been drawn in the latest edition of *Gray's Anatomy*. Needless to say, practitioners who accept the total package of traditional Chinese medicine will hold few reservations about the range of problems they might treat and will fervently endorse an approach to health and illness based on *chi* and meridians.

As a result, it can be somewhat difficult for the person seeking acupuncture treatment for a specific problem (for example, relief of postoperative dental pain, where acupuncture has demonstrated some benefit) to know for certain where the practitioner is coming from. Will the treatment be an attempt at straightforward pain management or an exercise of Taoist metaphysics? Needless to say, if one is considering an alternative therapy that has a spectrum of spiritual implications, it is important to know something about the orientation of the practitioner.

Category 2: Leaps of Logic
The next category contains therapies that have at least some connection (if only in terminology) to widely accepted principles of biology but then wade into uncharted—or self-charted—territory. An assortment of alternative practices of all descriptions—young and old, famous and obscure, enduring and fleeting, intriguing and silly—flow through this category. We mention a "flow" of therapies in this category because, along with some enduring practices, there are new arrivals and

hasty departures on a regular basis. There are, in fact, far too many to catalog the current crop in any given year, and a fair segment of this year's list will have changed by this time next year.

What these therapies share is an effort to appropriate the terminology and at least some of the widely accepted concepts of modern biology and physical science. What they also have in common is a tendency to take that terminology and run with it in some highly questionable directions. In some cases there is at least a degree of theoretical plausibility to the claims being made and perhaps case reports or even research studies to back them up. Others are based on ideas that appear to be far more imaginative than scientifically plausible.

Without exception, these therapies are promoted with optimism, enthusiasm or outright evangelistic fervor. Nearly all are presented to the court of public opinion before they are subjected to professional scrutiny, thus bypassing the all-important process known as peer review that is a cornerstone of mainstream health research. Sometimes, if a theory or product gains enough public attention, professional review may occur anyway, usually in the form of pointed questions that may undermine the credibility of the entire enterprise. But in most cases, no amount of evenhanded analysis or outright skepticism from mainstream scientists will dampen the enthusiasm of those who extol the benefits of their therapies. Nor will it discourage people seeking health who respond to the infomercials, books, lectures and, most of all, testimonials from satisfied customers that so frequently promote these therapies. Unfortunately, many of them are associated with a variety of potential problems (for the most part physical, rather than spiritual, in nature). These can include the dissemination of misinformation about normal body functions and causes of disease; the diverting of resources, especially money, toward treatments of dubious value; the delay of a more accurate diagnosis (a potentially disastrous consequence if serious problems are present); and, rarely, the causing of actual bodily harm. A number of these are illustrated in the examples that follow.

Dietary Regimes with Unusual Claims,
Nutritional Supplementation with Unusual Claims and
Megavitamin Therapies

These are the mainstays of this category, and their adherents usually set forth their case using one or more of the following propositions:

☐ The food available to most of us at our local markets is nutritionally inadequate or actually harmful. The soil in which our fruits, vegetables and grains grow has been depleted or is contaminated with pesticides and other toxins. The animals from which we derive our meats have been treated with hormones, antibiotics and other drugs, and they may have ingested toxins or even harmful microorganisms. Not only are we missing out on the nutrients we need, but our bodies must work overtime to counteract harmful substances present in our food supply.

☐ A variation on this theme is the observation that Americans and their counterparts in developed countries have long been accustomed to foods containing excessive amounts of fat, sugar and calories in general, not to mention alcohol and caffeine. Furthermore, many of our favorite foods have been shorn of valuable nutrients through refining and processing. Another variation is the idea that the pace and stresses of everyday life demand more of our metabolic and immune processes, so that we may be falling short of the nutrients our body needs to meet these challenges. Additionally, commonly prescribed medications—especially antibiotics, which alter the normal balance of bacteria within the intestinal tract—may interfere with the proper absorption of foods.

☐ Not only is our food supply deficient in vitamins and minerals but the conventional guidelines for these substances—the dietary reference intakes (DRIs) and the recommended daily allowances (RDAs)—underestimate our need for many, if not most, of them.

☐ Finally, a number of common complaints are said to be symptoms of the above-noted nutritional deficiencies: fatigue, headache, aches and pains in muscles and joints, digestive disturbances, allergies, sexual disturbances (specifically impotence and loss of libido), recurrent colds and other infections and difficulty losing (or gaining) weight.

Many of these propositions sound reasonable, but are they in fact valid? The answer is "Yes, no and maybe." Yes, there is no doubt that most of us could improve our food choices—most importantly, the quantity we consume. Indeed one could argue that the greatest nutritional problem of developed countries is the sheer quantity of food available to their citizens. Did our ancestors have better food available to them than we do? Probably not, when one considers the challenges involved in providing a variety of unspoiled foods on a daily basis to the average individual. The sheer number of options available in the average American supermarket would have seemed miraculous a century ago, and indeed it is still spectacular when compared to the daily rations of most of the world's populations. Are the recommended daily allowances for vitamins and minerals valid? For preventing full-blown vitamin deficiency syndromes in most people, probably yes. For preventing other diseases in both male and female, young and old, maybe not—several juries are still out. Should we be concerned about chemicals in our foods? That depends on the chemical, the amount, the food and the person consuming it. Sweeping statements about the perils of additives and preservatives, or about the virtues of additive- and preservative-free foods, tend to strain credibility. Do food choices and micronutrient deficiencies cause all of the symptoms listed above? They can, but not on the epidemic scale that many promoters would have us believe.

Assuming for a moment that the average American diet really does need repair, what might be done about it from an alternative perspective? The process of determining diagnosis and remedy will vary with the type of therapy and the inclinations of the specific practitioner. Symptoms, physical findings and a variety of tests—some of which are of questionable validity—may be used. Blood tests (such as vitamin levels) and hair analysis, neither of which is routinely used in conventional medical evaluations, may be performed. Some therapists resort to arm-pulling tests: the client holds a particular substance in one hand or in the mouth, and its effect is assessed by testing the strength of an outstretched arm. (This approach, usually encompassed in a practice called "applied kinesiology," hinges on concepts of invisible energy flows derived from traditional Chinese medicine. It will be addressed in more detail in chapter six.) A few practitioners use exotic electronic devices that are purported to analyze nutritional needs or food sensitivities. Since with rare exception the products and supplements that are claimed to be useful in resolving these nutritional issues are available in stores or by direct mail without a prescription, many (if not most) individuals self-prescribe their nutritional and supplement remedies.

Basically, the therapeutic approaches fall under four categories:

Selection of different foods. This may involve making more sensible choices at the neighborhood supermarket—selecting items with less fat and sugar; expanding the amount of fruits, vegetables, and whole-grain products in the shopping cart; and preparing meals from fresh foods, as opposed to processed or canned foods. No one would argue with this lifestyle change, which is only "alternative" in the sense that it goes against the convenience-driven grain of our culture. Those who are more persistent (or adventurous) in their quest for nutritional health will seek products that are advertised as "natural," "organic" or "whole" foods. Whether these labels are merely a marketing ploy (and a license to carry a more expensive price tag) or are an indication of quality surpassing that of similar items at the corner store is debatable. The answer may ultimately depend upon the integrity of the particular retailer.

Restrictive and "therapeutic" diets. Many who are convinced that the typical Western diet is unhealthy may gravitate toward various forms of vegetarianism. This can be a healthy and satisfying dietary approach—in fact, arguably more healthy than its carnivorous counterpart—when a wide variety of foods and food groups are eaten. But some individuals progress in their food choices from proactive and selective choices to restrictive or even obsessive decisions. For example, macrobiotic diets borrow from Eastern mysticism in their claim to balance yin and yang (or "contractive" and "expansive") foods. Some enthusiasts claim that their diet prevents cancer, and hard-core adherents may even insist that the diet is not compatible with conventional cancer chemotherapy. Aside from potentially leading a cancer patient away from conventional treatment, macrobiotic regimes raise dietary deficiency concerns even among those who are basically friendly to alternative therapies and lifestyles.[13]

Cancer patients who seek help at alternative clinics (usually in Mexico) will also encounter dietary prescriptions—for example, the Gerson diet or the Hoxsey treatment—that are claimed to have specific tumor-fighting capabilities. Needless to say, mainstream research continues to seek and identify dietary patterns that may increase or reduce the risk of developing cancer over many years. But there is scant evidence that a specific selection of foods, especially one that is extremely restrictive, will successfully and consistently fight a cancer that is already established. (See "Alternative Cancer Treatments" below.)

Megavitamins. Nutritional research continues to probe the boundaries of daily vitamin and mineral requirements, which (at least for some individuals) may be more than the basic RDAs. (These are amounts known to prevent overt vitamin deficiencies, such as scurvy, pellagra and beriberi—diseases that have essentially been banished from developed countries.) Some adhere to the notion that proper nutritional balance and the treatment of disease can be brought about through the use of huge, or "mega," doses of vitamins and minerals. Linus Pauling, Ph.D., who advocated massive amounts of vitamin C for the common cold and other ailments, coined the term *orthomolecular* to refer to medicine—and in particular, psychiatry—that uses this approach.

Supplements and concoctions claimed to be good for "whatever ails you." In describing alternative therapies in category one (reality-based practices) we noted that the use of herbs and supplements to treat specific problems—for example, St. John's wort for depression—is an area of alternative medicine in which well-designed research will no doubt yield fruit. But a steady stream of products continue to flow into consumers' hands and mouths via the airwaves and Internet—products that promoters claim are useful for just about everything, especially fatigue. This ubiquitous symptom invariably heads the list of complaints that satisfied customers testify were vanquished by the product, whether it be royal jelly, potentiated bee pollen, growth hormone, colloidal minerals, wheat grass, green tea extract, barley green, oregano or any of the other unique and special preparations containing vitamins, minerals and herbs hand-picked after "years of careful study."

Many of these products are promoted through infomercials (a number of which dominate weekend programming on Christian radio stations), and some are accompanied by invitations to sell the product through multilevel marketing plans. After listening to a few of these programs, it is difficult to ignore a few common threads: the unbounded optimism surrounding these products, the complaints they resolve, the testimonials they receive and, unfortunately, the frequent doses of misinformation about health and disease they dispense. The marathon can be eye-opening but also exasperating. How can all of these products be good for so many of the same problems? Are people supposed to take several of these preparations at once?

All of these dietary and nutritional therapies encompass a gamut of credibility, but few invoke the radical departures from known biological facts that we will see in category three. The primary issues are whether they have the facts straight, whether the cause-and-effect relationships they propose are reasonable and whether there is adequate evidence to support the claims they are making. For many of these, it is unlikely that such research will ever be carried out, either because the diet or supplement is so obscure or because their underlying assumptions are too implausible to warrant serious study. For some that are more widely used (such as glucosamine-chondroitin combinations for the prevention and treatment of arthritis) there has been enough evidence to suggest a potential benefit that larger-scale clinical trials are under way to clarify their usefulness on a long-term basis. A few (for example, the compound laetrile, which for years was promoted as a cancer treatment) *have* been studied in detail and have repeatedly been found ineffective.[14]

Rather than attempt to produce an encyclopedic reference of the current crop of diets and nutritional supplements, later in this book we will propose some principles for evaluating a given therapy. However, it is worth noting that this particular area of alternative medicine is the one in which purveyors of deliberate fraud most often take refuge. The most vocal critics of alternative practices tend to lump *all* of their targets into this category, but we would at least attempt to make a distinction between those who are knowingly and purposefully deceiving their clients and those who are sincerely convinced of the validity of their practice and product. Admittedly, the tendency for so many diet and nutritional enthusiasts to make extravagant claims, especially when such claims are made about products they are offering for sale, can make the task of distinguishing between these two categories extremely difficult.

Environmental Medicine

This is an expanded variation on the previous theme, picking up where alternative dietary and nutritional therapies leave off. We should point out immediately that the alternative practices that call themselves "environmental medicine" bear little relation to the well-established fields of public health, occupational medicine and toxicology. Rather than postulating that problems with food—choices, contaminants, deficiencies and reactions—are solely responsible for many common symptoms and ills, environmental medicine proposes that these disorders may also be caused by an expansive array of substances and forces with which we come into contact every day. These include chemicals in the air and water, material in the clothes we wear, mercury in dental fillings, organisms (such as the common yeast *Candida albicans*) that are not generally thought to cause symptoms in otherwise healthy individuals, and radiation from electronic devices, appliances and power lines. Those who are diagnosed as suffering from allergic responses to a large number of substances are given the diagnosis "multiple chemical sensitivities"—a disorder whose existence has been challenged by a number of mainstream physicians.

The symptoms commonly attributed to these environmental hazards are remarkably similar to those attributed to dietary and nutritional deficiencies, with fatigue heading the list. Tests used by practitioners of environmental medicine to detect their causes are also similar, if not more elaborate. They include not only a history and exam but also detailed analyses of blood (including "live cell" testing), hair and urine, not to mention the assistance of various electronic devices. And the list of possible therapies in this arena extends far beyond the realm of changing foods or taking supplements. Since few patients can abandon their homes and head for parts unknown to seek a safer environment, their treatment may involve a major investment in air and water purifiers, negative ion generators, oxygen supplementation, clothing that is warranted to be free of chemical toxins and so forth.

In addition, environmental medicine patients frequently are diagnosed as having accumulated toxins of various sorts that must be cleansed or purged from the body, as well as having a weakened immune system that must be fortified, usually with large doses of supplements. Some practitioners focus on the colon as the organ in need of cleansing in order for health to be restored, and so the regular use of enemas containing various substances may be recommended. (For those who are squeamish about being regularly subjected to such procedures, a variety of fiber and laxative preparations may be offered instead.) A more aggressive and expensive approach is the replacement of all dental fillings that may contain mercury, despite the continued insistence of mainstream dental organizations that this practice is unnecessary.

Many components of environmental medicine are extremely difficult to subject to standard research protocols because they hinge on circular reasoning. For example, a number of books (such as *The Yeast Connection* by William Crook, M.D.) propose that the common yeast *Candida albicans* causes a long list of common complaints: fatigue, headache, digestive disturbances, depression and so on. Candida *is* in fact known to cause oral, esophageal, skin and vaginal infections, and occasionally (as in AIDS patients with compromised immunity) to become disseminated throughout the body, with dire consequences. But how might one determine whether any of several common symptoms might be attributable to candida? Make some rather nonspecific dietary changes (cut sugar, bread and other foods that are "yeast promoting"), consume a variety of supplements and perhaps take some candida-combating medication (such as nystatin). If you feel better, you must have had a yeast problem.

This line of reasoning at first glance might seem logical. Indeed it would be wonderful if so many symptoms could be alleviated by banishing candida from our bodies. But unfortunately there are no specific physical findings or diagnostic tests that can reliably link candida to a collection of generalized symptoms (especially those that are known to have numerous other causes), nor is there any evidence that diet changes the population of this organism in or on one's body. And while nystatin and other antifungal medications are useful in treating visible and culture-verified candida infections, their use in these settings does not routinely lead to sudden improvements in a host of common symptoms. The yeast connection is a closed system: a series of interlocking assumptions that reinforce one another but cannot be consistently validated by an independent observer.

We could just as reasonably propose that fatigue, headache, irritability and intestinal distress are commonly caused by a reaction to *Staph epidermidis,* a common organism that normally lives quietly on the surface of the body. We could furthermore assemble the "Staph Connection" diet, compile a regime of supplements, suggest an antibiotic that might help, write a book, go on the radio and offer this new approach to promote health and prevent disease. Through our persuasive presentation, a semilogical explanation and the all-important placebo effect (by which we can expect at least 30 percent of our clients to feel better no matter what we do, as long as we are reasonably convincing), we could collect a sizable number of satisfied patients.

This scenario is not intended to insult those who are genuinely interested in helping others, or even in belittling the placebo effect, which plays an important role in all medical therapies. Rather it is offered as a brief illustration of an important weakness in the logic of many alternative practices.

Alternative Cancer Treatments

Without a doubt most people who discover they have cancer are alarmed, and their worry is fueled equally by fear of the disease and apprehension over the treatment. "Can I beat this tumor and live a normal life?" is an emotionally charged question. So is "Can I survive the surgery or chemotherapy or radiation that the doctors may recommend?" For this reason, and because a successful outcome cannot be guaranteed even with the most sophisticated of conventional therapies,[15] many individuals with cancer seek alternative forms of care. For this particular disorder, there is often a more well-defined gap between "complementary" therapies, which are used to help an individual cope or feel better while conventional therapies deal with the tumor itself, as opposed to true "alternatives," which are intended to displace conventional approaches. Often, however, an alternative regime is sought after all else has failed and the tumor is progressing in spite of conventional care. Research published in the American Cancer Society journal *CA* indicates that the percentage of cancer patients who use complementary or alternative therapies ranges from around 6 percent in the South Atlantic region to nearly 15 percent in the Rocky Mountains. Women are more frequent users than men, as are younger and more affluent individuals.[16]

Alternative therapies for cancer vary enormously in their complexity, underlying assumptions and credibility. Their history in the United States and Europe has been notable for the emergence of a "headliner" therapy that has attracted considerable attention during every decade since the Second World War: Koch antitoxins in the 1940s, the Hoxsey treatment in the 1950s, Krebiozen in the 1960s, laetrile in the 1970s and "immuno-augmentive" therapy in the 1980s.[17] In the 1990s, when alternative therapies flowed freely into mainstream culture, the river of therapies widened considerably. It is not at all uncommon for patients and practitioners to combine a variety of different approaches, sometimes under the roof of a "comprehensive" cancer treatment center. (Many of these clinics are located in Mexican border cities, such as Tijuana, near San Diego, California.)

The basic alternative approaches to cancer treatment include the following:

Dietary changes. As mentioned earlier in this chapter, while conventional researchers labor to confirm which (and how) dietary patterns might increase or reduce the risk of developing cancer, alternative approaches are more likely to claim dominion over the wayward cells. The macrobiotic diet (mentioned earlier as an example of a restrictive eating pattern) is claimed by its proponents to prevent cancer and sometimes to "relieve" it. In an effort to clarify this proposition, the National Center for Complementary and Alternative Medicine has funded a pilot study to investigate the cancer-preventing potential of the macrobiotic diet.

(It should be noted, however, that the principal investigator for this study is Lawrence Kushi, Sc.D., whose father, Michio Kushi, is arguably the leading proponent of macrobiotics in the world.) More commonly, dietary alterations are included in comprehensive alternative regimes. The Gerson diet, for example, originally included a daily gallon of juices made from vegetables, fruits and raw calf's liver, not to mention frequent coffee enemas that were claimed to remove toxins from the body. The updated version of the Gerson regime encompasses a number of other ingredients, including liver extract injections, thyroid and royal jelly supplements, and both ozone and castor oil enemas (in addition to the original coffee preparations).[18]

Nutritional supplements and herbs. These additives, sometimes in massive doses, frequently accompany dietary regimes. In the mid 1970s, for example, Linus Pauling, Ph.D., claimed that high doses of vitamin C—some 10,000 milligrams per day, as compared to a typical supplemental dose of 250 or 500 milligrams—could prevent or cure cancer. However, a National Cancer Institute review of Pauling's research and three subsequent controlled studies conducted by the Mayo Clinic failed to validate this claim. More recently, selenium has become a bestselling mineral supplement after University of Arizona epidemiologist Larry Clark reported that a two-hundred-microgram daily dose appeared to cut in half the odds of acquiring breast, colon and prostate cancer. But like many reports that suggest a promising role for a nutrient in preventing cancer (or any other disease), methodology issues and difficulty in replicating the results have raised some questions. (Also, toxic effects may occur at doses beyond eight hundred micrograms per day—not far above the proposed cancer-fighting dose.) More definitive studies are under way, but conclusive results may not be available for a few years.

The popular herbal preparation called Essiac was originally formulated by a Canadian native healer and then promoted for decades by Canadian nurse Rene Caisse (whose surname spelled backward supplied the name of this product). Though its exact formula is disputed, it reportedly contains burdock, Turkey rhubarb, sorrel and slippery elm. It has yet to demonstrate antitumor activity in animals or humans. Iscador, a derivative of mistletoe, is a popular cancer remedy in Europe despite its somewhat checkered background. It was originally promoted in the 1920s by Swiss physician Rudolph Steiner, who founded the Society for Cancer Research (SCR) and espoused an obscure practice with occult underpinnings that he called anthroposophical medicine. According to SCR materials, for example, the plants respond to the sun, moon and planets, which in turn affect the optimum time to pick them. Again, reputable evidence of Iscador's usefulness in treating cancer is lacking.

"Metabolic," biologic and pharmacologic treatments. These remedies are colorful, unusual and occasionally risky. The Hoxsey treatment, antineoplastins (promoted by Stanislaw Burzynski, M.D., Ph.D.), immuno-augmentive therapy (developed by the late Lawrence Burton, Ph.D.), Kelley/Gonzales Metabolic Therapy, the Livingston-Wheeler regimen, shark cartilage, CanCell, hyperoxygenation therapies, Cell Specific Cancer Therapy and many others currently attract clients via the Internet, alternative medicine books and magazines, health food stores and occasional high-profile coverage on network television. Most claim to detoxify the body, stimulate immune function and kill, weaken or normalize cancer cells. Unfortunately, such claims lack consistent validation in controlled studies. While a review of the research bearing on these treatments is beyond the scope of this book, major organizations such as the American Cancer Society and the National Cancer Institute, as well as watchdog groups such as Quackwatch, publish updated reviews of these and many other therapies on the Internet. Interestingly, the American Cancer Society's assessment of alternative therapies has become considerably less critical in tone over the past decade.

Mental imaging and other mind-body therapies. These low-tech approaches to cancer treatment are generally viewed as complementary to other therapies. In the 1970s and 1980s O. Carl Simonton, M.D., and his wife, Stephanie Simonton, were highly visible in the holistic health movement because of their work with relaxation and visualization techniques for cancer patients. In their book *Getting Well Again* they described how patients seem to fare better after using a variety of techniques to upgrade their outlook on their chances of survival and ultimate health. One of the Simontons' best-publicized methods was that of imagining white blood cells as wolves or other aggressive carnivores attacking weak, disorganized cancer cells.

More recently surgeon Bernie Siegel, M.D., has become prominent as the author of bestselling books such as *Love, Medicine and Miracles* and *Peace, Love and Healing,* and as an advocate of psychological and spiritual adjustments to deal with cancer. His themes include building positive self-regard, reducing stress, taking responsibility for health (and illness) and encouraging supportive relationships and spiritual growth from whatever perspective one might hold. On one level, much of Dr. Siegel's material is sensible and at times refreshing, particularly in his assessment of the many counterproductive communications from doctors to their patients. But chaff is scattered indiscriminately among his wheat. His comments about taking responsibility for health drift toward the idea that illness is a message sent by an "inner intelligence" for a specific purpose (potentially leaving the impression that cancer is one's own doing). The patient is to consider, for example, why he or she "needs" the cancer. Siegel's conviction regarding the power of belief strays into "It doesn't matter what you do, medically or spiritually, as long as you believe it" territory. He enjoys the input of an "inner guide"—George by name—who advises him on various important matters, and Siegel encourages readers to seek a similar entity themselves.

Dr. Siegel has been criticized for implying that attitude impacts immune function and, more specifically, cancer survival, especially when one study showed that breast cancer patients who participated in Dr. Siegel's "exceptional cancer patient" (or E-CaP) groups did not survive longer than comparable nonparticipants.[19] However, survival time is not the only issue in the life of persons with cancer; the quality of their lives and relationships is extremely important as well. Of all the complementary and alternative approaches to cancer care, those that support mind, heart and spirit are the most likely to benefit patients and their families—provided, of course, that they do not lead them away from the Great Physician himself. As we will see throughout the course of this book, this is not a trivial concern.

Iridology

This unique approach to medical information gathering is based on the premise that the iris—the colored portion of the eye that controls the amount of light arriving at the retina—displays in considerable detail the status of every organ system in the body. By comparing photographs of the patient's iris with elaborate diagrams, the practitioner of iridology is supposedly able both to detect previous health problems and to identify current problems. A careful assessment of the iris is also reputed to predict where trouble may develop in the future.

According to most iridology resources, this practice was born in the early 1880s when a Hungarian physician, Ignatz von Peczely, first published charts of the iris based upon clinical observations. (These were inspired by a childhood episode in which he accidentally broke the leg of a pet owl and subsequently noted a distinct change in the bird's iris.) Iridology eventually spread throughout Europe and then to North America. For many years the most widely quoted American iridologist was chiropractor Dr. Bernard Jensen, who wrote two voluminous textbooks on this subject and reportedly claimed that iridology offers "much more information about the state of the body than do the examinations of Western medicine."[20]

Needless to say, iridology is neither taught in medical school nor practiced (with very rare exception) by optometrists or ophthalmologists. Its basic assumption—that the iris's connections with the central nervous system allow detailed messages to be sent to it from the rest of the body—contradicts a well-established body of anatomical and physiological knowledge. The elaborate neurologic pathways necessary for this technique to be viable have yet to be demonstrated in spite of decades of neuroanatomical studies of the eye and central nervous system. Iridologists have generally sidestepped the neurological details in favor of a simplistic observation that the iris is in fact connected to the autonomic nervous system. But merely being connected to the system does not mean that the entire body is being monitored.

Even more troublesome for iridology's credibility is its insistence that each iris reveals what is happening on its particular side of the body. That is, the right iris shows problems on the right side of the body, and the left iris shows problems on the left side. This contradicts a fundamental observation that incoming nerve impulses from one side of the body nearly always cross to the opposite side on their way to the brain. Dr. Jensen proposed, in response to this objection, that the optic nerve serves as the final messenger between the nervous system and the iris. This explanation would allow for a second crossing of information back to the eye on the same side of the body. But the explanation falls short on two accounts. First, the optic nerve has been shown without question to be only a one-way messenger, carrying information from the retina to the brain, not in the reverse direction. (Indeed the optic nerve is not known to connect directly to the iris at all.) Second, only half of the fibers of the optic nerve cross to the opposite side of the brain.

Perhaps iridology's greatest vulnerability is that its diagnostic prowess can be put to the test using a relatively simple experimental design. Its performance in the simplest controlled studies has not been impressive. One of the most damaging to its reputation was carried out by researchers at the University of California, San Diego, and published in the *Journal of the American Medical Association* in 1979. Three iridologists (including Dr. Jensen himself) and three ophthalmologists examined iris photographs of 143 subjects, of whom 48 had overt kidney failure. When the number of false positives (normal people who were identified as having disease) and false negatives (diseased people who were identified as being normal) were compared to the number of correct answers, the level of accuracy was found to be worse than could have been achieved through chance.[21] Dr. Jensen later criticized this study, arguing that its use of a specific laboratory test—the serum creatinine level—to demonstrate kidney disease was invalid. Yet serum creatinine is used and accepted worldwide as a meaningful indicator of kidney function.

Equally unimpressive results were obtained in a 1981 Australian study of an experienced iridologist who was unable to diagnose any of thirty-three established health problems in fifteen patients using iris photographs. And in a 1988 study five Dutch iridologists were unable to identify which of seventy-eight patients had gallbladder disease (half were affected and half were normal). Nor did they agree with each other in their diagnoses.

Iridologists and their supporters offer a variety of explanations for these discouraging results. They may refer to their technique as an "empiric" science, based on the experience of its practitioners rather than controlled studies. They may also use disease classifications that are not generally accepted outside of the subculture within which they practice. Terms such as "toxic accumulation" or "lymphatic congestion" are common in iridology literature, but they are at best vaguely defined and at worst meaningless to the health care community at large. Furthermore, iridologists have an explanation for false positive diagnoses in their claim that they can discern subclinical disease that will emerge in the future. If the patient never develops the problem, he or she can claim that the treatment corrected the underlying imbalance and prevented more serious disease from developing. If the predicted disorder materializes, the technique is validated.

Magnetic Therapies

The belief that magnets might have healing powers has a long and colorful history, dating back to physician and alchemist Paracelsus in the sixteenth century and, some two hundred years later, to Franz Anton Mesmer (1734–1815), whose theory of animal magnetism shares much in common with today's alternative therapies that claim to manipulate invisible energy. Contemporary promoters claim that magnetic fields can be therapeutic for an ever-expanding number of conditions, including chronic pain, neurologic disorders and insomnia. The most common explanations for their purported effects include improved circulation, changes in nerve function and increased oxygen content in bodily fluids—all of which so far are unproven. Some invoke a nonspecific mechanism of "balancing the body's energy field." A more grandiose proposition is that many of us suffer from "magnetic field deficiency syndrome," brought about by a gradual decrease in the earth's magnetic field plus the shielding effects of concrete, steel and other building materials used in modern construction. Elaborate regimes have been described for the alignment of the poles of magnets, taking into account the type of ailment, its location on the body and even the hemisphere in which one happens to live.

Judging by sales figures, consumers are not exactly skeptical of these claims. *Time* magazine and PBS's *Health Week* reported on the use of magnets for pain relief among senior golfers and professional athletes, and magnets now routinely appear in golf shops and advertisements in sports magazines. Magnets are also showing up in mattresses, blankets, car seats, arm bands, neck wraps and necklaces, shoes, "prostate comfort devices" and even an array of products for animals. The largest manufacturer of magnets in the world, the Nikken Company of Japan, distributes some $1.5 billion worth of magnetic products annually ($350 million in the United States) through a multilevel marketing organization. Most suppliers of magnetic devices carefully avoid claiming that they cure specific diseases (*comfort* or *stimulation* are words more commonly used), although a few have run afoul of the Federal Trade Commission for promoting magnetic therapies for HIV, cancer and high blood pressure on the Internet.[22]

The magnets used in these devices are permanent and create what is called a static field, not unlike their counterparts that attach school art treasures to the refrigerator. The penetration of these fields through tissue and their potential effect on normal physiological processes thus far has appeared to be infinitesimally small. This, combined with the suspiciously sweeping claims and shaky explanations provided by their promoters, has cast serious doubt on the usefulness of magnets as medical therapy.[23] However, a 1997 study at Baylor College of Medicine published in the *Archives of Physical and Rehabilitation Medicine* indicated that permanent magnets reduced pain in postpolio patients. The study appears to have been well designed, and its results surprised some skeptics. Another study published in the *Journal of Pain Management* in January 1999 suggested an improvement in chronic foot pain, though with a relatively small number of patients. More recently a pilot study in the March 2000 issue of the *Journal of the American Medical Association* failed to show any difference between real and sham bipolar magnets, applied for six hours per day, three days per week, in relieving chronic back pain among twenty patients at a Veterans Affairs hospital. The authors noted, however, that the significance of their findings might be limited by the small number of patients in the study and that as a pilot study it was not intended to prove or disprove the effectiveness of magnetic therapy in general.[24] The National Center for Complementary and Alternative Medicine has funded research to determine whether magnetic sleep pads might reduce the pain of fibromyalgia, a chronic syndrome often resistant to other forms of therapy.

Assuming that well-controlled studies continue to show improvement in various conditions using permanent magnets, possible mechanisms that make physiologic sense will need to be explored. It should be noted that these therapies are quite different from pulsed magnetic fields created by electromagnets. These not only have a demonstrated physiologic effect in generating a weak electrical current but also are approved by the FDA for treatment of fractures that have been slow to heal. (It should be noted, however, that one study in the British journal *Lancet* found that pulsed-field bone-growth generators were equally effective when the device was applied but not turned on. The authors concluded that its apparent success was related to the inactivity required for its regular use and not to the magnetic field or electrical current that it generated.)[25]

Chelation Therapy

This is actually a conventional therapy that has been appropriated for alternative uses. Chelation therapy involves the intravenous infusion of the compound EDTA (short for ethylenediamine tetraacetic acid) to remove toxic levels of heavy metals such as lead. The use of EDTA for this purpose is not controversial, but for years a number of practitioners have contended that this treatment also removes calcium deposits from arteries and thus helps restore blood flow through clogged vessels. And for as many years the consensus of mainstream medical organizations and cardiologists, based upon the available evidence, is that chelation therapy does not work as an arterial pipe cleaner. If well-constructed research in the future were to prove it safe and effective, chelation would no doubt be used by conventional practitioners, since coronary artery disease remains the most common cause of death in the United States. But for now this therapy remains squarely outside the mainstream.

Classical ("Straight") Chiropractic

The distinction between "straight" and "mixer" chiropractic was described in the previous category. The original doctrine to which straights cling—that all disease arises from subluxations of the spine that supposedly impede nerve function—fits squarely into this category of therapies, which take the biology of the nervous system into uncharted territory. Needless to say, those who would entrust the care of medical problems such as high blood pressure, diabetes or asthma to manipulation of the spine do so at their own peril. And those straights who believe not only that subluxations are the cause of all disease but also that they are directing the flow of Innate Intelligence throughout the body are essentially abandoning any pretense of working with the body's normal physiologic process.

Category 3: "Everything You Know Is Wrong"

In this category we make a clean break with widely accepted and validated principles of science in general and of human biology and physiology in particular. Many of these approaches attempt to provide comprehensive explanations for how the body works, how and why disease develops, and what can be done about it.

Some are thousands of years old and extraordinarily complex. In most of these therapies the descriptions and categories of disease are foreign to Western thinking—so much so, in fact, that studying them within the framework of normal research protocols is extremely difficult. Furthermore, integration of these therapies with Western medicine, or for that matter with one another, requires considerable verbal finesse, mental compartmentalization or simple denial. To put it bluntly, it is difficult indeed to imagine how all of these systems can simultaneously be true.

Most of these therapies conceive of health and illness as contingent upon the proper flow of an invisible "life energy," whose unimpeded flow through the body is considered essential to good health. Elaborate but highly subjective (or even quasipsychic) methods of diagnosis are usually part of the package. Furthermore, the majority of these therapies have deep roots in, or strong connections to, Eastern metaphysical or monistic ("all is one") worldviews. Because these important messages are often buried in what appears to be scientific terminology, their presence and significance may be overlooked by the individual seeking health.

For all of these reasons we will take a detailed look at the general concept of invisible life energies in chapter five. In subsequent chapters four important therapeutic systems based upon this concept—traditional Chinese medicine, *ayurveda*, homeopathy, and Therapeutic Touch—will be examined in depth.

Category 4: Invading the Supernatural

In addition to characterizing alternative therapies according to their congruence with modern biology, we feel that a fourth category should be added for practices that purport to deal explicitly with the supernatural realm. Here we are not dealing with prayer from the creature to the Creator—the humble request for healing, accompanied by a submissive attitude that says, "Your will be done," as described countless times throughout the Old and New Testaments. Instead these therapies are the province of the "materialist magician," the individual described by C. S. Lewis in *The Screwtape Letters* who believes he or she has both access to the supernatural realm and the spiritual "technology" to manipulate it, but who does not acknowledge a sovereign God.

Psychic Diagnosis and Healing, and
Psychic Surgery

These seem to play a less prominent role in the current world of alternative medicine than they did in the holistic health movement of the 1970s. At that time a holistic conference wasn't complete without a visit from Olga Worrall, the grandmotherly psychic diagnostician and healer, or a talk about the life and readings of Edgar Cayce, or some colorful tales about psychic surgeons excising pathologic tissue with a rusty knife or their bare hands. Now such material seems passé. As alternative medicine has achieved mainstream status in our culture, its proponents continue to talk a lot about spirituality but a lot less about spirits. Also, the exploits of psychic surgeons in the Philippines and South America have been generally debunked as crude magic tricks using sleight of hand and chicken entrails. Somehow there is less excitement when illusionists such as the Amazing Randi, or comic magicians such as Penn and Teller, can conjure similar effects on national television.

Nevertheless, there remain some important pockets of psychic activity within alternative medicine. Carolyn Myss, Ph.D., for example, has earned a reputation as a "medical sensitive," one who supposedly can make an accurate diagnosis when given little more than a patient's name. However, her medical acumen is validated primarily by C. Norman Shealy, M.D., a one-time neurosurgeon and icon of the holistic health movement who has coauthored with Myss a highly mystical book entitled *The Creation of Health*. In subsequent solo works Myss generally uses the psychic diagnoses to validate her elaborate and detailed descriptions of the chakra system of East Indian medicine and mysticism.

In this book we have chosen to devote only brief attention to psychic healing, shamanism (see below) and related approaches because they have thus far played a relatively minor role in the alternative medicine movement. Nevertheless, a word of caution about such practices from a biblical perspective is definitely in order. Two strong currents in Scripture have a direct bearing on the worldview and practices of psychic healers.

One is the consistent Old Testament condemnation of practices designed to gather knowledge from invisible sources and to exercise spiritual power apart from God. The message to the Hebrews as they prepared to enter the land promised to them was blunt: "Let no one be found among you who sacrifices his son or daughter in the fire, who practices divination or sorcery, interprets omens, engages in witchcraft, or casts spells, or who is a medium or spiritist or who consults the dead. Anyone who does these things is detestable to the LORD, and because of these detestable practices the LORD your God will drive out those nations before you" (Deuteronomy 18:10-12).

Isaiah, writing centuries later, expressed similar disapproval, tinged with sarcasm: "When men tell you to consult mediums and spiritists, who whisper and mutter, should not a people inquire of their God? Why consult the dead on behalf of the living?" (Isaiah 8:19). Scripture describes such behavior as spiritual prostitution, fruitless consorting with God's invisible adversaries.

The New Testament elaborates on this theme by raising the issue of spiritual deception. Jesus spoke bluntly about the activities of demons, and all four of his biographers described his confrontations with them in vivid detail. He predicted of the period prior to his return to earth, "False Christs and false prophets will appear and perform great signs and miracles to deceive even the elect—if that were possible" (Matthew 24:24). The clear implication is that an overtly miraculous event can appear virtuous and be just the opposite.

Other New Testament writers echoed this warning. John cautioned the early church, "Dear friends, do not believe every spirit, but test the spirits to see whether they are from God, because many false prophets have gone out into the world" (1 John 4:1). Paul, who not only established numerous congregations but constantly battled against their infiltration by false teachers, characterized his adversaries as "false apostles, deceitful workmen, masquerading as apostles of Christ. And no wonder, for Satan himself masquerades as an angel of light" (2 Corinthians 11:13-14).

These and other passages describe the invisible enemy of God and humanity as capable of producing impressive and inspiring displays that are deliberately misleading. This casts a shadow on psychic diagnosis and healing. If one accepts the Old and New Testaments as authoritative, then one cannot assume that an insight gained from an unseen intelligence is necessarily true, nor that a supernatural healing must have come from God.

Such a viewpoint does not imply that psychic healers are necessarily deceitful or malicious. Most manifest a sincere care for those seeking their help. Furthermore, it is certainly unpleasant to think that a psychic healing could be an occasion for spiritual subterfuge. But if healing signs and wonders are consistently accompanied by metaphysical messages that contradict the core of biblical teachings—humanity's estrangement from God, God's rescue through the Messiah and the need for individual repentance and submission to God's authority—then whatever physical benefit results from the healing may be offset by a far more profound spiritual consequence.

Shamanism

The practices of healers, medicine men and women, and priests of long-ago times and faraway places generated considerable interest in the holistic health movement two decades ago and still receive a respectful nod from alternative theorists today. Many see them as an interesting illustration of the role of belief in healing, and some suggest that studying their apparent success might benefit contemporary

Western physicians. But for the true believer, shamanism is not merely an interesting topic for anthropologists or museum curators; it is, in fact, a technique for leaving normal consciousness, and perhaps the body itself, in order to communicate with spirit "helpers" and other beings for the purpose of obtaining knowledge, power or healing. In many ways shamanism is not as much a modality of (very) alternative medicine as it is a spiritistic religion. As such it does not concern itself with satisfying scientific scrutiny,[26] and it certainly has little use for the Judeo-Christian worldview.

Prayer as an Extension of Individual Consciousness

As we will discuss later in this book (chapter fourteen), the appropriation and redefinition of prayer by alternative therapists—especially Larry Dossey, M.D., who has written extensively on this subject—has created some confusion both in secular and Christian circles. Prayer defined as an extension of individual consciousness across time and space can fairly be characterized as an attempt to invade the supernatural.

Transcendental Meditation and Similar Practices, and
Yoga as a Spiritual Exercise

Despite the fact that Transcendental Meditation made heroic efforts to present itself as nonreligious during the 1970s, religious it indeed is, as are any number of meditative practices that are intended to propel one into altered states of consciousness. For one, yoga—that perennial offering of spas and health clubs—belongs in this category. What some might find unsettling is that the yogic exercises are not merely a collection of ancient maneuvers that happen to improve muscle tone and provide some relaxation at the end of a long day; they are, in fact, religious exercises that are intended to induce a particular *experience*—not just a belief—that we are one with Brahman, the Absolute. We will look at these practices within the larger context of *ayurvedic* medicine in chapter nine.

4

WHAT DRAWS PEOPLE TO ALTERNATIVE THERAPIES?

*I*f conventional Western medicine has made such impressive strides over the past century, why are so many people beating a path to alternative medicine's door? The reasons are many, as are the experiences driving those reasons. Encounters with doctors—good and bad, conventional and otherwise—as well as conversations with friends or health care providers rank high on the list. Information gathered from the media, especially the Internet, also may be a part of the equation. Needless to say, it is well worth taking a look at some of the streams that feed the growing river of alternative medicine, because they reflect important trends in our culture. They also reveal some strengths and weaknesses in both the conventional and alternative camps.

Three primary needs (perhaps a better term would be *primal needs*) draw people to alternative health practices:

☐ People are sick, hurting, tired or in some other ways not feeling well, and Western medicine does not seem to have all of the answers. Furthermore, its practitioners seem to have a hard time delivering what answers it does have.

☐ People want to prolong life and prevent health problems in the future. Meanwhile, Western medicine's solutions do not seem to go into enough detail or are too focused on the broad strokes of certain high-profile problems, such as coronary artery disease.

☐ People want to expand their horizons beyond the absence of disease to a state of "super health," encompassing physical, emotional and spiritual well-being.

Western medicine appears to be preoccupied with other matters.

It is important to note that the decision to use one or more alternative therapies may not necessarily be driven by disdain for conventional medicine. A common sentiment is that both-and is better than either-or and that it makes sense to use whatever appears to be the best of both worlds. A recent study in the *Journal of the American Medical Association* investigating this question pointed out that most users of unconventional therapies were not driven by dissatisfaction with Western medicine. Instead the study found that alternative approaches fit well with people's "values, world view or beliefs regarding the nature and meaning of health and illness."[1] Indeed the widespread use of the phrase "complementary and alternative medicine" (or CAM, as it is commonly abbreviated) reflects this viewpoint.

Life Spans and Limitations

Western medicine's wondrous advances in handling acute illness and trauma continue to be its strong suit, and for many critics of alternative medicine they are also the trump card in any debate on this subject. Do the paramedics rush the motorcyclist with a compound fracture to the nearest acupuncturist? Is the child with a red-hot appendix sent home with a prescription for homeopathic remedies? Did ayurvedic practitioners discover the cause of malaria? Will aromatherapy save the burn victim whose blood pressure is plummeting?

Responsible alternative practitioners usually acknowledge the superiority of Western medicine in such situations with little hesitation. Indeed it is not unusual for books promoting alternative therapies to include one or more warnings to seek medical (that is, conventional) attention for conditions that are severe or acute. Andrew Weil, M.D., whose commitment to alternative therapies is intense and articulate (as we will discuss in chapter eight), has made this abundantly clear in his book *Spontaneous Healing:*

> If I were in a serious automobile accident, I would want to go directly to an urgent care facility in a modern hospital, not to a shaman, guided imagery therapist, or acupuncturist. (Once out of danger, I might use other resources to speed up the natural healing process.) Conventional medicine is also very good at diagnosing and managing crises of all sorts: hemorrhages, heart attacks, pulmonary edema, acute congestive heart failure, acute bacterial infections, diabetic comas, bowel obstructions, acute appendicitis, and so forth. You must be able to recognize symptoms of potentially serious conditions, so that you will not waste time before getting needed treatment. In general, *symptoms that are unusually severe, persistent, or out of the range of your normal experience warrant immediate investigation.*[2]

But alternative promoters are quick to point out that there's a lot more to health care than helping people in emergencies and other dire straits. Some important—and very common—problems give conventional medicine a serious run for its money.

"Trench war" diseases. These are chronic disorders such as cancer, arthritis and AIDS, whose biology is complex and whose treatment is difficult. Lack of a clear-cut, visibly superior battle plan from conventional medicine has left a wide opening not just for alternative therapies but also for wildly diverse theories of disease causation. Western cancer researchers, for example, tend to focus on intricate biochemical mechanisms, often presumed to have strong genetic roots, that cause cells to multiply and spread like a fire burning out of control. Alternative practitioners are more likely to propose that a cancerous growth is unleashed by toxins that need to be cleansed from the body, or by disturbances in invisible energies, or by psychological or spiritual conflicts.

"Diseases of civilization." Among these are coronary artery disease, hypertension, obesity, adult-onset diabetes and other ailments that have strong links to lifestyle. Conventional medicine has much to say about this, but too often its efforts are directed at containing damage already done. And even when technology-oriented physicians identify changes in lifestyle that may be helpful (or even life saving), they may lack the time or the communication skills to inspire a patient to stay the course, or even embark on the journey, toward healthy living. This is particularly true when the problem is obesity, which all too often stands squarely between an individual and safer levels of blood pressure, cholesterol and glucose (blood sugar), not to mention relief of lower back pain, osteoarthritis and a host of other problems. Neither cursory advisories ("Go lose fifty pounds") nor carefully crafted dietary regimes are readily followed or commonly successful. Those who are desperate for *anything* that will help rid the body of excess pounds are often more than willing to explore exotic therapies that offer hope and help.

"Feeling lousy" syndromes. Ongoing symptoms, especially in combinations that conventional practitioners usually find unrewarding, frustrating and at times exasperating make up the "feeling lousy" syndromes. Chronic fatigue consistently leads the list, followed by problems such as dizziness, headaches, bloating, numbness and tingling, aches and pains in a variety of locations, shortness of breath, vague abdominal discomfort and declining sexual interest and performance. For a number of reasons, these common symptoms are usually not endearing to physicians.[3]

One reason physicians may not expend much effort in looking at such common symptoms is that they are time consuming. An appropriate assessment of any of these complaints requires a detailed history and examination, and usually other tests as well. They may thus easily become schedule busters, especially when more than one is on the agenda for a given appointment. To make matters worse, all too often they are brought up at the end of a visit as a dreaded "By the way . . ." question—"By the way, doctor, why do I feel so tired all the time?" When the schedule is packed, the phone lines lit and the waiting room full, these complaints usually receive a less than enthusiastic response.

A second reason is that these conditions are frequently difficult to diagnose and thus to treat. Occasionally chronic fatigue or other ongoing symptoms are found to be the result of a medical problem (such as iron deficiency anemia or hypothyroidism) that has a straightforward solution. Sometimes they signal a more serious or complex disturbance, such as cancer. Not uncommonly, a treatable depression will lie at the heart of the problem, but the time-pressured physician may not have the time or inclination to explore that possibility. Even if he or she does so, the patient may find this line of inquiry threatening or even insulting. All too often the symptoms just don't add up (even if the cost of the evaluation does), leaving the doctor with the task of delivering an unsatisfying debriefing: "I don't know what's wrong with you, but it looks like whatever it is won't kill you."

A third reason is that such "feeling lousy" syndromes are not always addressed with much depth or enthusiasm during conventional medical training. Who wants to spend hours learning how to manage and finesse the "worried well" when there are far more interesting diseases to seek and stamp out? It will be a rare occasion indeed when the weekly morbidity and mortality conference or departmental grand rounds presentation at a medical teaching facility focuses on a patient with numerous complaints who turned out to be depressed.

If "feeling lousy" symptoms are the bane of the conventional physician's existence, they are the bread and butter of alternative medicine. Not only are they extremely common but often many of them cluster in the same patient. They also tend to be physiological rather than pathological in nature; that is, they involve a symptom-generating disturbance in the function of otherwise normal tissues, organs and organ systems. And they are frequently intertwined with anxiety and depression. This is not to say that they are any less important or "real" than a clearly defined, pathology-driven disease. But they are often more effectively approached with time, a listening ear, encouragement, optimism ("I have some ideas about what might help") and drugless remedies—for example, lifestyle changes, diet, exercise, counseling, massage, relaxation techniques—that are less likely to create new problems and symptoms. Unfortunately, they also can be fertile ground for all manner of therapies of dubious value that may drain the wallet or, worse, encourage an individual to embrace misleading medical and spiritual ideas.

The complexity of the human body and mind. The physical-spiritual unity that is a human being has such a profound intricacy that no one can have all the answers for every complaint. What happens when a particular patient's problems extend beyond the boundaries of his or her doctor's experience? What if a definitive answer is not available, even from seasoned consultants and reliable textbooks? Admitting that "I'm not sure what this is, but it doesn't appear to be a threat to you" or "We're going to have to watch this and see what happens" can be a humbling experience for a conventional physician. All too often the "I don't know" message comes across with a tone of frustration that says, "You're a crock," "You're wasting my time" or even "Get out of my office." But alternative practitioners, who may not necessarily be driven by the need to make a specific diagnosis, can be a lot more comfortable with such situations and very willing to make a number of recommendations. As we will discuss later, the very act of suggesting *any* treatment with some degree of enthusiasm may bring about improvement. Furthermore, since mystery syndromes often fade away on their own, any treatment (alternative or otherwise) that is given prior to a spontaneous resolution of symptoms will usually receive credit for the cure.

The wages of aging. As we get older, we face difficult physical problems that encompass all of the previous four areas. Ever-increasing numbers of baby boomers are now crossing the midcentury mark, and it is customary for them to anticipate enjoying many productive years rather than to prepare for physical and intellectual decline. Defenders of conventional medicine are often quick to point out that this development is the direct result of Western scientific advances, which now prevent early death from infections and other catastrophes that shortened so many lives a century ago. Nevertheless, as the birthday candles accumulate, so too do the effects of the "trench war" diseases, "diseases of civilization," and "feeling lousy" syndromes. Furthermore, all of the difficulties conventional medicine faces with these problems are compounded in the elderly. Symptoms are more numerous, more time consuming to sort out and more difficult to manage. Often sophisticated treatments, including complex drug regimes, generate more problems than they solve. Many conventional physicians become discouraged by their inability to fix the problems brought to them by their senior patients, especially the harrowing process of intellectual decline wrought by Alzheimer's disease and other dementing processes. For these and many other reasons, it is not surprising that the use of alternative therapies is particularly common in the elderly.

Boomer Baggage

Speaking of the post–World War II set, a number of attitudes that are prevalent among this highly visible and vocal population have encouraged the growth of alternative practices.

Higher expectations. This generation has been raised with a broad-based assumption that life and health should not be limited to the bare essentials. Those who have grown up in Western nations during the second half of the twentieth century have been pitched, in a myriad of ways, the idea that they should "have it your way," whether that be in material possessions, lifestyle or freedom from any bodily or emotional discomfort. When it comes to symptoms, boomers have not exactly been indoctrinated with a grin-and-bear-it mentality, even (or especially) when there is not an obvious cause or treatment. *If my regular doctor can't figure out why I'm having fatigue and aches and dizziness, someone out there must have an answer.*

For more than twenty-five years, a clarion call of the holistic health movement—"health is more than the absence of disease"—has struck a responsive chord in our culture, especially among the boomers. Vibrant health and terminal illness are extremes on a spectrum, and alternative practitioners tend to be more active than their conventional counterparts in promoting the idea that no one should be content to exist at a neutral, disease-free midpoint. Health should mean feeling fine, being energetic, integrated, self-actualized and productive. George Leonard, once senior editor of *Look* magazine and author of the book *Education and Ecstasy,* noted the following:

> The conventional physician considers a person well if he has no symptoms and falls within the normal range in a series of diagnostic tests. Yet this "well" person might smoke heavily, take no exercise, eat a bland, sweet, starch diet, and impress all who meet him as glum, anti-social, and emotionally repressed. To a New Medicine practitioner, such a person is quite sick, the carrier of what René Dubos calls "submerged potential illness." In the New Medicine, the absence of overt disease is only the starting point, beyond which a whole world of good health beckons.[4]

Western medicine has been criticized for its preoccupation with disease and crisis intervention and for being content to return a person from the negative end of the spectrum to a neutral, disease-free condition. Conventional practitioners, especially those who grapple daily with the complexities of serious disease, could argue that their emphasis on the negative, on pathology, is entirely appropriate and that "wellness" is more properly the province of the psychologist, fitness coach or theologian. In a videotaped debate on the wisdom of integrating conventional and alternative medicine in medical school training, Arnold Relman, M.D., editor emeritus of the *New England Journal of Medicine,* presented this viewpoint:

If you view health as simply an ideal state of being in which everything is just fine, and you have no worries, and you have no symptoms, and you're in an optimal state of being, then I would say that medicine's role in achieving that [state] is limited— should be limited. What medicine is mainly about is the diagnosis, the prevention and the treatment of disease. . . . There are many other disciplines and many other walks of life that deal with the existential problems of life. And I think that one of the problems that we have in discussing the role of alternative medicine is that we assume that medicine, conventional medicine, really ought to be responsible for happiness in general, for well-being in general. And I think that that's unrealistic.[5]

But like it or not, most physicians (even those practicing in subspecialties) are responsible to some degree for health maintenance, whether through detecting unsuspected disease or encouraging risk reduction in their patients. Furthermore, large numbers of people seek medical advice regarding symptoms that prove to be heavily influenced by emotions and lifestyle. Doctors are thus logical candidates to give advice on a broad range of habits and life issues that impact health. This might include not only a review of current symptoms but also eating and exercise habits, recent (and possibly stress-producing) life changes, relationships, personal goals and spiritual commitments. All of these components of well-being are, in fact, important in health promotion and disease prevention, whether from a conventional or alternative perspective.

Dr. Relman's comments notwithstanding, Western medicine has in fact attempted to address these diverse areas more effectively. Doing so, however, requires a struggle against several obstacles.

☐ Time shortage: Addressing general well-being may take a considerable amount of time, and primary care physicians (who are the ones most likely to carry out such an assessment) are routinely faced with shortages of this precious commodity.

☐ Financial pressure: Few insurance plans (and certainly not Medicare) reimburse physicians for a lengthy "wellness" evaluation, and not many patients are willing to pay for one themselves.

☐ Individual responsibility: To paraphrase the old saying, "You can lead a horse to water, but you can't make him stop smoking, start exercising or lose weight." Furthermore, many aren't interested in hearing about the water in the first place. This doesn't mean that making the effort to promote wellness isn't worthwhile, but the rewards for doing so may not always be apparent, at least in the short run.

Conventional medicine's training and practice patterns still have a long way to go in raising the profile of wellness promotion as a viable and valuable endeavor for the busy practitioner. Its long-standing emphasis on stamping out disease has left a gap that alternative practitioners have been more than willing to fill—or at least to describe themselves as filling. Unfortunately, in many alternative therapies, wellness has a tendency to be equated with dubious accomplishments, such as having one's "invisible energies" in balance or achieving altered states of consciousness in which psychic or supernatural experiences occur. Furthermore, in our pluralistic culture, can we even reach a consensus on what wellness is? For example, an individual who has dozens of sexual partners every month could from some perspectives be described as having a high level of wellness because he reports being happy and "self-actualized"—even though he is probably permanently infected with a number of organisms that threaten his future. This is but one ramification of postmodernism, a pervasive worldview that declares, among other things, "I define my own reality."

Suspicion of technology, big business and bureaucracy. Although many ex–flower children of the late 1960s now freely roam the corridors of power in our society, not all have lost touch with their wariness of things technological, corporate and institutional. Conventional medicine is definitely wedded to all three and thus highly suspect in a number of areas.

Physicians are generally perceived as more trusting of their high-tech lab and imaging tests than their person-to-person assessment of patients or (heaven forbid) their own intuition. They also appear much more comfortable with prescription pads than with other interventions, especially discussing nutrition and lifestyle, and in fact seem bound by a compulsion that a visit is not complete unless something is prescribed. The fact that the pharmaceutical industry spares no expense in courting them through advertising and a host of other enticements certainly supports this perception. Since surgery has long been a lucrative direction in medicine, and an important revenue center in hospitals, caricatures of men and women in green who swagger down hallways and boast that "a chance to cut is a chance to cure" may ring all too true.

For many boomers and their offspring, the technological-pharmaceutical-surgical complex of modern conventional medicine revives some unpleasant memories of the military-industrial complex of old, which propelled America into its controversial war in Vietnam. This is aggravated by recurring revelations from network news programs or investigative reporters that a hot new drug may in fact cause cancer, liver failure, heart disease or some other calamity. Overall, statistics reciting the annual costs (including deaths) resulting from adverse reactions to prescription drugs are startling and sobering.

Not surprisingly, many alternative therapies are promoted as an antidote to the more unsavory byproducts of modern technology, using adjectives and catch phrases such as "natural" (the most common), "gentle," "organic" (now a bit outdated), "helping the body heal itself," "stimulating the immune system," "restoring balance," "cleansing," "detoxifying" and of course "drugless" and "nonsurgical." This vocabulary is especially common in the world of alternative cancer therapies, where "cutting," "poisoning" and "burning" (that is, surgery, chemotherapy and radiation) are routinely contrasted with less uncomfortable options.

Distrust of authority. Boomers popularized the famous phrases "Question authority" and "Don't trust anybody over thirty," and many of them have carried these sentiments well into their own sixth decade of life. Until relatively recently, physicians were universally cast as authority figures who dispensed "doctor's orders" with the presumption that they would be followed without question. Over the past two decades, the forces of consumerism and managed care have drastically changed this landscape—a development that has both positive and negative repercussions. Be that as it may, a significant number of people in all age groups harbor fears of things medical, worried that their visit to an office, emergency room or hospital might take on a life of its own and become a bewildering, uncomfortable and expensive misadventure. Corrective measures, such as greater attention to informed consent and the routine posting of a patient's bill of rights in health care facilities, have only begun to allay concerns about loss of autonomy.

Many alternative practitioners and promoters have played to this concern, describing their approach as "taking charge of your own health." Since those who seek alternatives nearly always do so on their own initiative rather than being pointed in that direction by conventional physicians, this perception of individual responsibility is not entirely unfounded. Today's well-informed health care consumer is not supposed to accept anyone's advice as gospel truth but rather is encouraged to ask a lot of questions and consider all sorts of options before embarking on medical treatment. Even if the patient follows the conventional doctor's advice, there is no reason why he or she could not access some additional remedies as well. Interestingly, many who express disdain for authority are in fact more than happy to follow, with little questioning, detailed alternative advisories that are based on arcane diagnostic techniques or incomprehensible treatment regimes. In such cases, "taking charge of my own health" may not be so much about defying authority as it is about "following the authority that *I* choose."

A Deep and Widespread Spiritual Hunger

A number of alternative therapies encompass much more than treating illness. Many serve as a gateway to spiritual technologies and worldviews that address primal needs for meaning, knowledge and power.

While alternative medicine celebrates the spiritual dimensions of the therapies gathered under its tent and insists that they play a vital role in health and healing, the major institutions of Western medicine have for all practical purposes marginalized spirituality. Some observers have suggested that this was a good thing, claiming that medical progress was hopelessly stalled until early investigators jettisoned archaic notions that God or other supernatural forces were responsible for illness and health. But in fact, the biblical view of an orderly (even if fallen) creation is far more compatible with scientific inquiry and progress than the Eastern and New Age notion that the physical world is actually a colossal illusion, the shared dream of billions of us who, for the most part, do not grasp our own divinity.

Even though committed Christians can and do utilize the accomplishments of Western medicine in active service to others and obedience to their Lord, the vast majority of patient encounters with conventional medicine are purely secular events. Some physicians deliberately bring prayer into the exam room or operating theater or discuss how a wide-awake relationship with God can make a positive impact on health. But in general, spiritual insight or disciplines are rarely the centerpiece of conventional medical therapy. As a result, the spiritually famished patient is unlikely to find nourishment in the typical doctor's office or hospital.

Conventional Medicine's Delivery Problems

Western medicine's greatest strengths—its methodologies, which have solved problems that have plagued humankind for millennia, and the power of its diagnostic and therapeutic tools—are often underrated, or flatly berated, because of its delivery problems. Much of this difficulty is logistical: a huge number of people need a diverse array of expensive products and complex services every day. Matching this need with responses that satisfy all concerned is extremely challenging. Add to this mix an ever-growing number of regulatory requirements from all levels of government, the ever-present worry that a less-than-ideal outcome will trigger a lawsuit, and increasingly convoluted payment systems, and you have a recipe for potential widespread dissatisfaction. These issues are the topic of ongoing discussion and debate within the health care industry and are largely beyond the scope of this book, except for one vital concern: their impact on the relationship between an individual patient and an individual health care provider. For it is precisely in this arena where alternative practitioners have staked out some major turf in the world of health care, and where conventional medicine will continue to lose ground if it does not go back to basics.

Ask someone who is unhappy with a particular physician, a clinic, a hospital or the entire conventional health care system what has bothered him or her, and you will usually hear complaints centering on one or more issues that are primarily relational.

"He didn't spend any time with me." Without a doubt the greatest folly of contemporary medicine is the notion that a person's health care can be routinely assessed in fifteen-, ten- or even five-minute installments. With few exceptions, even the most straightforward problem usually requires at least *some* conversation, not only to determine what is going on but also to explain clearly what treatment options are available. Such communication is impossible when the practitioner blows in and out of the examination room like the White Rabbit who is late for a very important date . . . somewhere else. When the patient has waited for a half hour (or often much longer) for the appointment, this type of "one-minute management" is irritating and insulting. Unfortunately, the demands of managed care and the increasing costs of running a medical practice have created intense pressure on physicians, both in primary care and specialties, to see more people in less time every day. But even in the "good old days" many physicians entertained the fantasy that they could build rapport and confidence in a few minutes. Decades ago this presumption may have been aided and abetted by patients who were more willing to take the doctor's few words as gospel and were more reticent about asking questions.

Time pressures are frequently aggravated by another fantasy (which, by the way, is not limited to conventional medicine): the "psychic doctor" syndrome. Many patients seem to believe that a physician can instantaneously deliver a meaningful response to a question such as "Why am I tired all the time?" or "What's causing these headaches?" When such a query arrives as a "By the way . . ." question at the end of a visit, the practitioner has but three options. He may address the complaint immediately, which will usually throw the schedule into disarray and further increase the level of irritation of those who are waiting. He may address the complaint at a later appointment, which may not be feasible for the patient or may not be safe if the question involves an ominous symptom such as chest pain. Or he may succumb to a risky temptation—pretend that he knows what the answer might be and prescribe something that is not likely to cause any harm.

The reality is that many people have several health problems in progress at the same time, and each of these may require considerable time to evaluate properly. The wall-to-wall scheduling patterns that are so prevalent in conventional medical offices are poorly suited for a careful review of one problem, let alone a list of them.

"She didn't listen to me." Part and parcel of the time crunch is the need to get on with it and complete the business of the visit without undue delay. If the patients'

complaints are numerous, if their descriptions are convoluted (a common problem for the elderly) or, worst of all, if these complaints are not part of the agenda for that particular visit, then they are not likely to be greeted with rapt attention in the examination room. Even less welcome in many offices are questions, especially those that sound like a challenge to the physician's recommendations: "What are the side effects of this drug?" or "Is there something that I could do instead of taking that medication?" Not only are these time consuming but also, for too many practitioners, such inquiries are not viewed as an opportunity to educate but instead a waste of precious minutes or even a sign of disrespect.

"He was so arrogant." For some physicians the rigors of internship and residency generate more pride and prejudice than humility. In the popular film *Patch Adams,* instilling this high and mighty attitude was depicted as a deliberate goal of the medical school curriculum a generation ago. But if such pomposity from the podium was in fact delivered and widely accepted during Dr. Adams's training, it would meet with snickers or howls of protest from today's medical students. Nevertheless, even those who enter medical school with the most idealistic visions of providing compassionate care to all in need are likely to develop more than a little cynicism during the crucible of medical training, especially when confronted with patients whose behavior is uninspiring. Most physicians in fact feel genuinely respectful toward the vast majority of their patients but still may at times come across as arrogant (or at least uncaring) because of time pressure or poor communication skills.

"They made me feel like a cog in the machine." Even if a primary caregiver creates terrific rapport with a patient, navigating the system that surrounds him or her can be a daunting task. If making an appointment or completing some lab tests is like running a gauntlet, the overall effect of the physician's efforts may be significantly dampened. Ditto if the waiting room feels like a bus station, especially when the patient must spend a lot of time there. And because the detailed work involved in caring for a patient in a clinic or hospital is daunting for all concerned, the customer service side of the equation may become lost in the shuffle. Patient complaints about the amount of time between ringing the call button and the arrival of the nurse can usually be matched in intensity by the laments of nurses about the number and complexity of the patients under their care on any given shift.

"I nearly had a heart attack when I saw the bill." The rising costs of medical care in the United States over the past three decades are legendary, and their impact is particularly harsh on the uninsured. Even those with excellent coverage who spend some time in a hospital are routinely astounded not only by the size of the bill but also by how many different entities want to be paid. The hospital's tab is

normally astronomical, but then come the bills from every doctor who saw the patient and a few who didn't—for example, the radiologist who read the x-rays or the pathologist who reviewed the biopsy. Throw into this mix red tape from insurance companies or the government, then spend a few hours on the phone trying to straighten things out (not including time on hold), and it is not hard to understand why many lawmakers are ready to overhaul the entire system.

All of these problems are cited and recited by some promoters of alternative therapies as evidence that conventional medicine is at its core defective. But at issue here is not Western medicine's basic understanding of the human body and what goes wrong with it. Instead the problem is that of applying that knowledge to individuals in a manner that is effective, compassionate, accessible and affordable. Indeed there is no reason why alternative medicine couldn't succumb (or hasn't already, in some cases) to the kinds of deficits just described.

The Powerful (but Abandoned) Placebo

While practitioners of alternative medicine by no means hold the corner on virtue, the majority of their therapies tend to be kinder and gentler than those of their conventional counterparts. They also are generally more likely to focus on the patient's inner resources for healing, rather than the doctor's armamentarium. Indeed, if there is any area in which conventional medicine's soul has in fact been tainted by its knowledge, it would be in this tendency to rely on technologies— complex diagnostic procedures, drugs and surgery—at the expense of the power of human interaction and the patient's ability to get well on his or her own.

To grasp the profound importance of this observation, we need to consider for a moment the impact of physicians in prior centuries, when there were few truly effective treatments available, as well as the role of healers in societies untouched by Western medicine and its technologies. This has been aptly summarized by Herbert Benson, M.D., in his book *Timeless Healing,* which explores in some detail the importance of the placebo effect in healing.[6]

Derived from the Latin word meaning "I will please," the term *placebo* is commonly understood in two ways. Traditionally a placebo was a substance or treatment that was known by a practitioner to have no physiological effect but that was presented to a patient as a treatment for symptoms that were not responding to other treatments. This was the so-called "sugar pill," usually reserved for the person who was felt to be troubled more by imagined than by real ills. While few contemporary practitioners deliberately attempt to placate their challenging patients with inert substances, the placebo today plays a critical role in medical research. Here the intention is to compare a proposed treatment with one that appears identical but is actually inert. Most studies are designed in such a way that neither patients nor practitioners know who is taking the actual medication, so as to isolate the effect of the drug from other variables. This type of protocol is called a "randomized placebo-controlled double-blind study" and is considered the gold standard in medical research.

Dr. Benson, who has researched extensively and written about a physiological process that he calls the "relaxation response" (see chapter three), persuasively argues that the placebo effect deserves much more respect as a powerful agent of healing. He even gives it a new name—"remembered wellness"—which he describes as encompassing three kinds of belief and expectation: that of the patient, that of the caregiver and that arising from the relationship between patient and caregiver.[7] In a thought-provoking chapter entitled "Medicine's Spiritual Crisis," he describes how for centuries physicians and healers had little to offer their patients—except themselves.

> Throughout history, medicine had to rely on the human spirit and other seemingly mysterious sources of miracles. Let's face it, in the beginning, there was the placebo. And for primitive medicine, the placebo was all there was. Early medicine and its cross-cultural cast of characters—priests, healers, sorcerers, medicine men, witch doctors, witches, shamans, midwives, herbalists, physicians and surgeons—relied exclusively on scientifically unproved potions and procedures, the vast majority of which had no physical value in and of themselves, and some of which did more harm than good. The fact that some patients got better had much more to do with the natural course of their diseases or illness and with the power of belief than with the inherent value of the medicine. . . .
>
> Well into the twentieth century, despite the influence science had begun to wield in other realms of the world at that time, medicine still offered more care than it did cures, more attention than technology. Ironically, the reputation physicians have enjoyed throughout history, privileged and esteemed in every culture and time one can name, was built on and cultivated by the success of remembered wellness and on the three modes of belief-inspired healing: the belief of an individual in a treatment, the belief of the caregiver, or their mutual beliefs.[8]

Dr. Benson provides a thumbnail history of conventional medicine's recent downsizing of the importance of the relationship between physician and patient. Physicians, whether internists, surgeons or psychiatrists, are generally unwilling to acknowledge that the placebo effect—the response to expectation and relationship—plays any serious role in *their* specialty. They have been instilled with a vision of taking action and getting results, reflected (among other ways) in conventional medicine's quasi-military vocabulary: "giving orders," "fighting the infection," "waging a war on cancer" and so on. Reimbursement by insurance and government payers alike is tied to the currency of specific diagnoses, and entities such as "loneliness" or "lack of direction in life" don't enter the equation. And as already described in this chapter, treating symptoms that don't point to a specific diagnosis is not a favorite pastime in conventional medicine. Some would even consider this "junk medicine" and would characterize serious efforts to reassure such patients and bolster their confidence as a colossal waste of time. But as Dr. Benson points out, this gradual, widespread shift from building a relationship with patients to exercising technical prowess has not been without cost.

> Throughout history, society has afforded healers a special deference and admiration. We undoubtedly do this because we so ardently need for them to work magic and produce miracles. But in modern times, we've removed the aura we used to associate with healing. We've come to expect only facts and figures from our doctors, not hocus-pocus, and lately we don't even count on their succor and reassurance, as did previous generations. We disapprove of the deference people paid to physicians years ago, and we try to eliminate the intimidation factor many patients feel when they talk to their doctors. But in the process we may have depreciated our expectations of healers—the same expectations Hippocrates, the father of Western medicine, knew were important to our healing when he said, "Some patients, though conscious that their condition is perilous, recover their health simply through their contentment with the goodness of the physician."
>
> Too often today, the sacred trust that should be developed between doctor and patient has been replaced by a set of rushed interactions.[9]

It is in this important realm of relationship building and expectation that alternative practitioners are often able to supply what their conventional counterparts have abandoned. They may listen more attentively to their patients, and they frequently promote themselves as encouraging a more collaborative relationship. They project a great deal of optimism, and at times evangelical fervor, about their particular therapies of choice and about life in general. They use positive buzzwords—"natural," "internal cleansing," "building up the immune system," "helping the body heal itself," "healing the mind and spirit as well as the body" and so on—that may grossly oversimplify or even misrepresent how the body actually works but that nevertheless sound promising. At the same time, many of their therapies, especially those involving the manipulation of invisible "life energies," carry with them an air of exotic, almost mysterious, potency. Diagnoses and treatments may be based on subjective impressions or convoluted theories that are impossible to explain in straightforward terms, but they may be seen as tapping into profound truths and unexplored realms of healing. This can be particularly powerful after one has heard more than one doctor say, "I don't know what is causing your problem or what we can do about it." Someone with a complex illness or a laundry list of difficult symptoms may feel a breath of hope when the alternative practitioner announces, "I can find out why you feel so poorly, and I have a specific treatment plan that will get you on the road to recovery."

To top it off, patients of alternative practitioners have nearly always gone out of their way to initiate this type of care. The sense that they are stepping out (often in the face of resistance) to "take charge of my own health" may be emotionally and physically galvanizing. Furthermore, since alternative services are usually not covered by insurance, the patients have literally bought in to their care, betting with their hard-earned money that these treatments are going to work. The psychological and physiological responses to such positive expectations should not be underestimated and no doubt account for a large number of improvements following treatments that otherwise would appear far-fetched or even completely irrational in both theory and practice.

Not all of conventional medicine's loss of the benefits of the placebo effect is attributable to the seduction of physicians by technology or the pressures of managed care and finances. Ironically, conventional physicians who exhibit virtues such as open communication, candor and informed decision making may also diminish their patients' expectations and thus indirectly contribute to the popularity of alternative therapies. In place of the "M.Deity" posture, which says, "I know what's best for you, and that's all you need to know," many doctors have been honestly and candidly admitting the limits of their capabilities and carefully explaining the pros and cons of treatment options. Maintaining this evenhanded approach requires that words like "might" and "maybe" and "I don't know" frequently enter the conversation. Furthermore, an increasing—and quite appropriate—emphasis on informed consent over the past few decades requires physicians to present both the risks and the benefits, to outline not only the desired outcome but also all that might go wrong in connection with a given medication or surgery.

As a result, in far too many situations a conventional physician may not be able to bring the power of positive expectation to bear on the patient's problem. In fact, just the opposite may occur. The process of describing the most common side effects of a drug, for example, may create alarm and apprehension, which themselves can generate any number of symptoms. TV ads for prescription drugs—a new and blossoming phenomenon over the past few years—juxtapose soothing imagery with voice-overs containing dire warnings about possible adverse reactions. The viewer is left with a weird perception: *I really need this drug, even though it'll probably kill me.* Whatever warnings the doctor or a TV commercial did not mention will usually be supplied by the pharmacy, which often attaches its own daunting information sheet and a few cautionary stickers to the prescription bottle.

To complicate the experience of starting a new medication, many people now buy their own copy of the *Physicians Desk Reference (PDR),* a huge compilation of FDA-mandated information for every prescription drug on the market. Unfortunately, the "adverse effects" segment for any given medication invariably contains an intimidating list of every symptom known to humankind, based on reports of those who took the drug during clinical trials. While it is useful to know which side effects occur most frequently, every itch or tingle experienced by anyone involved in any study of the drug shows up on the list, even when the vast majority were almost certainly coincidental. Reading the *PDR* or accessing similar information on the Internet may provide a crateload of facts but little insight. If the doctor has not taken the time to offer some perspective based on a broader understanding of the medication, not to mention his or her own experience with it (and with the particular patient), the first tablet may be accompanied by a major dose of anxiety and one or more unpleasant sensations.

Negative expectations and fear surrounding a proposed treatment (or the person delivering it) can generate all sorts of symptoms or impact the overall course of a health problem—a phenomenon known as the "nocebo effect." This is the placebo effect's evil twin and a force that conventional medicine regularly generates but often fails to acknowledge. Its impact is not limited to responses to medications. Diagnostic tests ranging from a simple blood draw to lying in the claustrophobic tunnel of the MRI scanner all can provoke the adrenaline flow of the flight or fight response, even when the patient quietly endures the entire process. The anticipation of a surgical procedure is even more likely to do so. But even as simple an event as a routine office visit, devoid of any uncomfortable proddings or even undressing, frequently sets off physiological alarms. Primary care physicians and specialists alike are well acquainted with "white coat hypertension," where a person's blood pressure rises in the doctor's office but not at home or in the workplace. Most doctors see this phenomenon as an annoyance, a complicating factor in what should be a relatively straightforward treatment decision. But it should also provoke a more profound question: why does a doctor's office seem so threatening, even when a person knows that nothing uncomfortable is going to happen?

One could reasonably argue that doctor visits during childhood, especially those in which the dreaded shots are given, can set up primal responses of apprehension for the rest of one's life. To some degree, a dislike of things medical is going to be inevitable. Immunizations may be life saving, for example, but they also don't feel good. A number of routine health screening tests throughout life—mammograms, pap smears, sigmoidoscopies—have an annoying tendency to prod into areas we would just as soon be left alone. Few people on the planet relish the idea of a scalpel invading their bodies, even under a general anesthetic. (After all, it's going to hurt when you wake up.)

But even though creating some discomfort is unavoidable, conventional medicine often seems determined to make the entire experience as miserable as possible. Why not instead strive to make the doctor's office, the clinic, the emergency department and the hospital the most safe and sane places in town? Many decades ago Walt Disney noted that the typical "amusement park" was a dismal, shabby, enter-at-your-own-risk zone run by unpleasant individuals, where few people truly were amused. He vowed that he would one day create an entirely different type of destination for families, and the rest is history. As any of the millions of visitors to Disneyland and Walt Disney World can attest, the treatment of "guests" (not "customers") at these destinations is almost otherworldly, the result of intensive training of their employees that creates a unique—and highly profitable—environment. While medical facilities are obviously not amusement parks, hospitals have begun to take patient satisfaction much more seriously, and quality improvements are often provoked by feedback about what went well (and what didn't) during one's stay. (Interestingly, Disney has been putting on seminars for health care organizations to help them improve patient satisfaction.)

An old adage says that "people won't care what you know until they know that you care." There are times, of course, when one is faced with such a complicated medical problem that the services of a true expert are greatly appreciated, with or without a comforting bedside manner. But for the vast majority of interactions between doctors and their patients, the adage is definitely true. Millions of individuals are seeking help from alternative practitioners who seem better equipped than their conventional counterparts to show that they care, even if what they are offering sounds far-fetched. Indeed, in these situations, the adage could be revised: "People won't care whether what you know makes any sense if they know that you care." Unless they are in dire straits (or even when they are), most people are more impressed by the way they are treated than by icy assurances that they are receiving state-of-the-art medicine based on the results of the best double-blind studies. As long as respect, compassion, communication (especially listening) and optimism are manifested more often by alternative providers, millions will continue to beat a path to their door.

5

GOING WITH THE FLOW

The World of Invisible Life Energies

OFFICER ON THE DEATH STAR: This station is now the ultimate power in the universe. I suggest we use it.
DARTH VADER: Don't be too proud of this technological terror you've constructed. The ability to destroy a planet is insignificant next to the power of the Force.
OFFICER: Don't try to frighten us with your sorcerer's ways, Lord Vader. Your sad devotion to that ancient religion has not helped you conjure up the stolen data tapes or given you clairvoyance enough to find the rebels' hidden fort—*gaak!*
[Vader has pointed a finger at the officer's neck, and the officer is now choking and gasping for breath.]
VADER: I find your lack of faith disturbing.[1]

On May 25, 1977, ticket lines began circling the block at theaters across America as an immensely successful epic adventure exploded into popular culture. The release of *Star Wars,* written and directed by George Lucas, marked a pivotal moment in filmmaking. Its special effects, which seem tame by today's standards, were groundbreaking at the time. The film was nominated for eleven Academy Awards, including Best Picture, and won in eight categories. It introduced a new vocabulary and a cast of characters who are now as familiar as Mickey Mouse and Santa Claus: light saber, X-Wing fighter, Jedi, Death Star, Darth Vader, Luke Skywalker, R2D2 and C3PO. The mythology of this film captivated millions and implanted in the public consciousness a concept that has its roots in the mystical traditions of several cultures. The Force, we were told, is an invisible energy that fills the universe, that flows in and around us, that can be used for good and evil purposes. The aging Jedi knight Obi-wan Kenobi explains, "The Force is what gives a Jedi his power. It's an energy field created by all living things. It surrounds us, it penetrates us, it binds the galaxy together." It also proved to be a pivotal element in the story. Two generations of Westerners who know little about Eastern metaphysics and even less about biblical theology can describe in detail how Luke Skywalker single-handedly destroyed the Death Star: he shut off his targeting computer, trusted his feelings and used the Force to hit the impossibly small target that would turn the Death Star into a fireworks show. "May the Force be with you" appeared on lapel buttons and bumper stickers. Christians who misunderstood both the film and the New Testament countered with a decidedly wrong-headed slogan: "The Force is Jesus."

Three years later, in *The Empire Strikes Back,* eager audiences got a more intense lesson in Force metaphysics from Yoda, a Jedi master more than eight hundred years old who attempts to train the impetuous Luke Skywalker. After a series of grueling exercises, Luke is able to use the Force to levitate small objects, but he can't muster the concentration to raise his downed X-Wing fighter out of a swamp. Yoda corrects his misperception that it is too big and then proves his point by levitating the ship himself.

> Size matters not. Judge me by my size, do you? And well you should not. For my ally is the Force, and a powerful ally it is. Life creates it, makes it grow. Its energy surrounds us and binds us. Luminous beings are we—not this crude matter. You must feel the Force around you, between you, me, the rock, everywhere—yes, even between the land and the ship.[2]

He later informs Luke that "through the Force, things you will see . . . other places, the future, the past, old friends long gone."

While he denies that he had any intention of starting a religious movement, Lucas was deeply influenced by the writings of Joseph Campbell regarding the power of mythology, and he definitely desired to express universal mythological themes through the *Star Wars* films. He succeeded spectacularly, using the power of the motion picture to tap into deep currents in a culture that had been disillusioned by Vietnam, Watergate, the threat of nuclear war and the loss of its Judeo-Christian moorings. In *Star Wars: The Magic of Myth,* a companion volume for an extensive *Star Wars* exhibition at the National Air and Space Museum in Washington, D.C., curator Mary Henderson observed:

> Myth is a sacred story, and the world *sacred* means "to be full of power." The original *Star Wars* trilogy appeared at a time when 95 percent of Americans said that they

believed in God, but only 43 percent attended religious services. It is no wonder that these movies with their stories of rebirth and redemption and conquest of good over evil took on the power of myth. Values that had seemed lost to society were given new life in *Star Wars*: chivalry, heroism, nobility, and valor. Luke's character, in particular, reflects the traditions of heroism from the past; these mythological roots enrich his identity and deepen the story's meaning.[3]

For Lucas, the concept of a supremely powerful impersonal Force that could be harnessed by humans (and other creatures) seemed universal as a spiritual theme and thus more useful for his goal of creating mythology than specific gods, or God Almighty. In an interview with Bill Moyers he offered a glimpse of his view of this subject: "I remember when I was 10 years old, I asked my mother, 'If there is only one God, why are there so many religions?' I've been pondering that question ever since, and the conclusion I've come to is that all the religions are true."[4]

Indeed the idea of the Force did not come out of thin air or Lucas's imagination. Under a variety of aliases, it has appeared and reappeared for thousands of years, tapping into another deep-seated, and quite universal, longing of humanity: to have godlike knowledge and power without accountability to a supreme authority. If *Star Wars* reintroduced this concept to the masses by capturing their attention through compelling entertainment, alternative medicine is now doing likewise through an equally compelling interest: the desire for health.

Historians have given the name vitalism to the notion that an invisible, nonmaterial "life force" or "life energy" flows through all things, or at least all living things. This energy is unmeasurable and undetectable (by scientific methodology), it functions in a realm beyond the laws of chemistry and physics, and yet it is claimed to be the basis of all existence. In both religious and healing traditions, it goes by many names. (See table 5.1.)

Authors John Ankerberg and John Weldon note that "this energy is invariably associated with pagan religion and occultic practitioners and has up to sixty different designations depending upon the time and culture."[5] Contemporary proponents of life energy, whether in religious, New Age or alternative medicine circles, contend that regardless of its name, it pervades everything in the universe, unites each individual to the cosmos and is the doorway to untapped human potential. It is at the root of all healing, all psychic abilities, all so-called miraculous occurrences. It is the link between science and religion. It is, in fact, what religions have called God, and it is awaiting our command.

Tradition	Life Energy
Taoism and ancient Chinese medicine	*chi (qi, ki)*
Hinduism and *ayurveda*	*prana*
Polynesian traditions	mana
F. A. Mesmer and subsequent "magnetic healers"	animal magnetism
D. D. Palmer and "straight" chiropractic	Innate Intelligence
Samuel Hahnemann and homeopathy	vital energy
Wilhelm Reich	orgone energy
Contemporary energy therapists	subtle energy

Table 5.1. Energy according to various traditions

Six Basic Principles of Life Energy

In chapters two and three we noted that a number of alternative practices postulate mechanisms of disease and treatment that represent a radical departure from well-established principles of biology. The notion of a flow of life energy is the corner-stone of these approaches, not only supplying their theory of health and disease but also governing the methods and devices used in diagnosis and treatment. But are these ideas based in reality? Can they be scientifically verified, or do they belong entirely to the realm of faith and mythology? Indeed, do such questions even matter? If therapies that claim to function on this basis seem to be working and healing people, isn't that enough? These are some of the issues we will examine in this chapter, along with taking a closer look at one of the more popular forms of energy-based medicine: acupuncture and its offshoots, as understood in traditional Chinese medicine.

To begin, we will set forth six basic principles that are shared by nearly all of the life energy traditions and therapies. (We will use the generic term "life energy" when referring to this entity in general, "energy medicine" when discussing its purported role in healing, and specific names such as *chi* when dealing with a particular practice.)

1. Life energy is the fabric of the universe. Even though we cannot measure it with any modern scientific instrumentation, life energy is said to be omnipresent, flowing from the universe into living creatures, circulating within them in an orderly manner and ultimately flowing out again. (Some pantheistic variations on this theme describe the energy flowing through inanimate objects, such as trees or rocks, as well.) But many writers have taken this idea even further by borrowing the foundational statement of the atomic age—Albert Einstein's formula $E = mc^2$—and then applying it to biology in creative ways. Einstein's famous equation, in simple terms, says that matter can be converted into energy and vice versa. But this conversion occurs only under very specific conditions. When it takes place with strict controls, the result is nuclear power. An uncontrolled conversion of matter into energy, on the other hand, releases the incredible destructive power of an atomic explosion.

Proponents of energy medicine commonly make the following argument: Einstein essentially proved that matter and energy are the same thing. What we perceive to be material objects (whether biological or inanimate) are actually nothing more than congealed energy. As human beings, we are but one form or manifestation of this energy. Hence, energy does not merely flow through us; it *is* us. Conventional medicine, therefore, is mechanistic, old-fashioned and pre-Einsteinian because it treats the body as a material entity. Energy medicine—the "new medicine" that was actually discovered by ancient civilizations—provides us with more effective and natural ways to heal because it views the body as energy and can manipulate energy to change it. A popular speaker during the heyday of the holistic health movement in the 1970s, Dr. Irving Oyle, offered this explanation:

> The idea of the identity of energy and matter has enormous implications for all the healing professions. It gives us a theoretical basis from which to consider therapeutic methods such as acupuncture which purport to restore normal bodily states by manipulating the flow of cosmic energy. If energy and matter are indeed complementary states of a single entity, perhaps it is not unreasonable to hypothesize that by attention to the energy level, we can affect changes in the matter of the physical body.[6]

In order to bolster the idea that manipulating life energy (through whatever means) brings about changes in matter, some life energy proponents take Einstein's formula a step further and in so doing make a major error that undermines their entire line of thinking. They assume that the conversion of matter into energy, and vice versa, occurs in nature and in the human body on a routine basis. In her book *Energy Medicine,* which attempts to synthesize several life energy practices into a single volume, healer Donna Eden states:

> Energy *really* is all there is. Even matter, as Einstein's elegant formula shows, is congealed energy. When you watch a log burning in a fireplace, you are seeing the con-

gealed energy that is the log transform into the roaring energy that is the flame. The flame could then be transformed into mechanical energy, where it might propel a locomotive or run a generator. That generator might, in turn, produce electrical energy. Perhaps, as Einstein believed, there is only a single energy, a "unified field," but if so, it has countless faces.[7]

This statement would cause any high school chemistry student (not to mention Einstein) to cringe. When a log burns, light and heat are produced and the mass of the log seems to disappear. Fortunately, however, a fireplace is not a nuclear reactor. The log is merely oxidized at a rapid rate, and one form of matter (wood) is converted into others (smoke and ashes). Energy is released as a byproduct of the reaction, but not a single atom has been converted directly into energy. (This principle of the conservation of matter during combustion, whether in a fireplace, a candle or the human body, was proved by the French chemist Antoine Lavoisier more than two hundred years ago.) If it were indeed possible to transform a log into energy as defined by $E = mc^2$, the explosion would make a conventional atomic bomb look like a popgun. Certainly the physical body is changed by contact with energy, as anyone who has touched a finger to a hot stove can attest, but to apply Einstein's formula to these interactions and to claim that energy in the human body *becomes* matter (and vice versa) reveals a profound misunderstanding of basic chemistry and physics.

2. *Disease arises from an imbalance or blockage of the flow of life energy in the body.* Most energy-based systems postulate some form of invisible circulation of energy that must be maintained to manifest health. The ancient Chinese described an elaborate system of channels called "meridians" through which the invisible energy *chi* (pronounced "chee") circulates. As we will describe later in some detail, traditional Chinese medicine is built upon the notion that disease arises from deficiencies and excesses in the flow of *chi*, and all of its therapeutic tools are directed toward resolving those disturbances. In Hindu thinking, energy known as *prana* is said to flow through thousands of invisible channels called *nadi*, which cross at a series of seven energy centers known as *chakras*. The *chakras* are typically drawn as a series of small circles (containing esoteric symbols and surrounded by a sunburst-like corona of lotus petals) arranged in a vertical array near the spine and are said to be activated through meditation and other techniques. The founder of chiropractic, D. D. Palmer, called life energy "Innate Intelligence" and claimed that its flow through the nervous system could be blocked by spinal misalignments called "subluxations." (As we noted in chapter two, most contemporary chiropractors do not align themselves with Palmer's original teachings.) The infinitesimally small doses used in homeopathy are commonly claimed to work through their effect on

disturbances in "vital energy." Needless to say, when an alternative therapist mentions an "energy blockage" that is causing symptoms or illness, it is likely that he or she is practicing one or more life energy–based techniques.

3. Although its existence has never been acknowledged by the scientific establishment, life energy and its disturbances can be detected in a variety of ways. Some individuals who describe themselves as "medical sensitives" or psychic healers claim that they can intuitively visualize a person's *chi, prana, chakras* and other manifestations of invisible energy fields. The vast majority of those who deal with life energy, however, rely on somewhat more prosaic methods of diagnosis. Practitioners of traditional Chinese medicine attempt to determine the status of *chi* by evaluating a patient's symptoms and appearance as well as by conducting an elaborate assessment of the tongue and the pulses. Various exercises and meditative techniques, such as yoga and *qi gong,* are reputed to enable individuals to visualize or "sense" the flow of invisible energies. Practitioners of Therapeutic Touch are taught to move their hands above the skin of a patient so that they can "feel" the characteristics of his or her energy and then act on it accordingly. Needless to say, all of these methods involve highly subjective interpretations of sights, sensations and mental images.

For those with a high-tech bent, a number of so-called "electrodiagnostic" or "bioenergetic" devices have been marketed with claims that they can measure electromagnetic energy along acupuncture meridians. Most are variations on equipment designed by German acupuncturist Reinhold Voll in the late 1950s. Voll combined measurements of electrical skin resistance with traditional Chinese medicine to create was is now called "EAV," short for "Electrodiagnosis According to Voll." The assumption is that changes in skin resistance at acupuncture points reflects the state of one's internal organs and overall condition based on the Chinese meridian system. Voll's original diagnostic system involved some 850 points, though his students subsequently simplified the process to about 60. The hardware they developed was dubbed the Vegatest and was subsequently followed by a host of variations from other clinicians and entrepreneurs: Accupath 1000, Dermatron, Interro, Omega AcuBase and many others. Some of these add computer programs and readouts to speed up the diagnostic process and give feedback regarding the suitability of various supplements or homeopathic remedies for the problem identified. (This is usually a "nutritional deficiency" or food allergy, although some practitioners venture to make more serious diagnoses.)

Those who submit to this type of testing should be aware that the use of "black box" devices—contraptions of various shapes and sizes covered with intimidating switches, meters and lights that miraculously diagnose (and often treat) just about anything—have a long and colorful history, including a fair amount of conflict with the laws of the land. In the United States, which has hosted a steady stream of dubious medical gadgets for some two hundred years, there is usually a day of reckoning for these devices (and their manufacturers, marketers and users) with the FDA, the Federal Trade Commission or both. According to medical fraud specialist Stephen Barrett, M.D., marketing the Vegatest and a number of its spinoffs is illegal in the United States.[8] Nevertheless, free enterprise unrestrained by accountability, combined with the Internet and the mainstreaming of alternative medicine, has fueled widespread use of "electrodiagnostic" devices by a number of acupuncturists, chiropractors, dentists, "holistic" physicians, fringe nutritionists and even veterinarians.

4. Life energy can be adjusted, activated, channeled or otherwise manipulated in order to treat illness or maximize health. If disease results from disturbances in energy flow, then correcting the imbalance, blockage or deficit will lead to healing. A significant number of alternative therapies presume to manipulate life energy by one method or another, either by direct physical contact or by some form of invisible transfer from healer to patient. In ancient Chinese medicine, needles or other forms of stimulation at specific acupuncture points are said to cause the life energy *chi* to flow more smoothly or to be rerouted. Massage, exercises, herbs and meditation also are used to manipulate *chi,* and some practitioners of what is called *qi gong* claim to have the ability to project *chi* outside of their bodies for self-defense or healing. Believers in *prana* and *chakras* describe a multitude of breathing, movement and meditative techniques that are said to enhance energy flow. Classical chiropractic theory holds that the spinal manipulations allow the Innate to flow more easily through the nervous system. Sometimes New Age healers will describe an ability to sense and then adjust energy, basing their approach on the teachings of several healing traditions. Others simply claim to be channels for healing energies without referring to any particular system.

Some present-day proponents of alternative medicine take the practices of their predecessors into new ground by claiming that they deal with disturbances in life energy caused by "electromagnetic pollution." Many citizens have followed with considerable interest the ongoing debate over the potential risks of living near electric power lines, although data suggesting that they increase the odds of developing cancer has recently been discredited. In his book and video series *Eight Weeks to Optimum Health* Andrew Weil warns of the dangers of exposure to devices such as electric blankets, hair dryers and clock radios.

But others have gone even further by claiming that electromagnetic fields and other "negative energies" in the environment affect the flow of subtle energies in the body. Donna Eden's book *Energy Medicine* contains a chapter entitled "Swimming in

Electromagnetic Currents," which includes a lengthy explanation of the use of magnets to protect one's subtle energies from electromagnetic fields.[9] Needless to say, this is yet another credibility stretch for life energy theorists, since the invisible flow of *chi, prana* and the rest have remained stubbornly undetectable by reputable researchers—unlike the electromagnetic fields with which they are supposedly interacting.

A more expansive concept, derived from a Chinese practice called *feng shui,* involves a ceremonial process called "space clearing," which is purported to cleanse and purify the energy atmosphere in one's home and workplace, including an adverse condition called "geopathic stress." In her book *Geopathic Stress: How Earth Energies Affect Our Lives,* Jane Thurnell-Read argues that "negative earth energies" are common causes of physical and psychological distress because of their effects on the flow of *chi,* and that crystals, dowsing and kinesiology can be used to combat these negative forces.[10] One website states:

> In Feng Shui terms we call past energy patterns "predecessor Ch'i." It is essential to clear stagnated Ch'i energy left in a place by previous occupants or unfortunate events, in order to remove its continuing influence upon your well being and prosperity and, most important, to protect you from repeating the same experiences associated with unpleasant predecessor Ch'i. To achieve this Space Clearing, a sacred cleansing ceremony to purify the energy of an area, is performed.[11]

Most promoters of life energy therapies make a major point that individuals can adjust their own energy flows by learning a few basic techniques, since the body and the energy itself are said to carry their own intelligence and intention. Donna Eden writes in *Energy Medicine:*

> I . . . cherish and take confidence in knowing the body is designed to heal itself. Your body is engineered so that if you tap into its healing force, that force will lead you toward health. It is not just the personality or the soul wanting the body to get better. The *body* wants to heal, and every cell carries extraordinary intelligence and fortitude. While we all sometimes need outside help and direction, *healing is an inside job.*[12]

5. Alterations of life energy are the source of events that previously have been called supernatural or miraculous. If invisible energy can change the material world or even become matter, we have a ready explanation for miracles. Healings, clairvoyance, psychokinesis and all other events of the paranormal realm merely represent the activity of universal energy, usually under the influence of an enlightened or psychic individual. One of the most expansive theoreticians of the New Age movement, Dr. William Tiller, now professor emeritus of materials science and engineering at Stanford University, offered this dramatic vision of the implications of a universal life energy during a holistic health conference in 1978:

One is that there are new energies which we have never dealt with before in physics; second, that we have within our organisms sensory capacities for cognition of these energies; third, at some level of the universe, we are all connected; . . . fourth, time, space and matter are all mutable. We can perceive events out of our fixed location in space: that's remote viewing. We can perceive events out of our fixed location in time: that's precognition. Some people can materialize and dematerialize objects. If one can do it, eventually all will do it.[13]

This, for all practical purposes, was Yoda's sermon to Luke Skywalker in *The Empire Strikes Back*. Once we begin to understand and use the energy that is available to all of us, the miraculous will become commonplace and the religion of the past will become the science of the future.

6. Life energy is what religions have called God. Many life energy therapists and theorists take the previous five principles and arrive at a bold conclusion: if this energy is both the stuff of which we are made and the life force that flows through us every day, if it extends from one end of the universe to the other and if it manifests intelligence, then it can be nothing less than God. Rosalyn Bruyere, who has been active in energy medicine for decades, has stated this proposition quite clearly: "For me, the terms *God* and *energy* are interchangeable. God is all there is, and energy is all there is, and I can't separate the two."[14] At one of the first conferences of San Diego's Association for Holistic Health in 1976, speaker Evarts Loomis, M.D., proclaimed that "expanded consciousness depends upon the inflow of primal energies variously referred to by different cultures as THE LOGOS, PRANA, CHI, BUDDHA NATURE, NATURE, THE WORD, THE HOLY SPIRIT, COSMIC ENERGY, etc. Who can say that these words are not synonymous?"[15]

With but one more step (or leap) of logic, we arrive at a final stop in this train of thought: since we are energy, and since energy is God, then *we* must be God. The same conferees who heard Dr. Loomis announce that God and energy were the same also heard psychologist Jack Gibb proclaim that "the absolute assumption that a lot of us are making in the holistic health movement is that all of the things that are necessary to create my life are in me. In more than a whimsical sense, I believe that I am God and I believe that you are, and both of those statements are very important." Shirley MacLaine shouted the same message—"I am God!"—to the ocean in an ecstatic moment of what no doubt seemed to be self-discovery, as related in her New Age manifesto *Out on a Limb*.[16]

Obviously, not every acupuncturist or homeopath is eagerly awaiting opportunities to tell patients that everyone in the room is God. And not everyone who believes in the flow of some form of life energy has arrived at the conviction that it is God under an assumed name. But it does not require much probing into the roots of life energy therapies, nor a lot of extrapolation from their primary assumptions, to arrive at a worldview that is entirely harmonious with a host of Eastern mystical traditions, shamanistic practices, "mind science" philosophies of the nineteenth century, some old-fashioned occultism and the current-day New Age movement. As we will discuss later, these worldviews are at their core incompatible with the teachings of the Old and New Testaments. Nevertheless, some energy healers and alternative medicine proponents attempt to include Christianity, or at least their particular take on the life of Jesus, within the scope of their theory and practice.

Evarts Loomis, in his statement just quoted, claimed "THE WORD" and "THE HOLY SPIRIT" as synonyms for life energy. Carolyn Myss, Ph.D., in her book *Anatomy of the Spirit,* attempts to synthesize the Hindu chakra system with the sacraments of Christianity. Jesus is routinely described as the "Master Teacher," the bearer of the "Christ consciousness" and, most important, the example of what can happen when one becomes completely enlightened as to his or her true identity. But for all of this praise for Jesus and expansive vision of what manipulating life energy might accomplish, no one has duplicated the miraculous events— and in particular the healings—recorded in the New Testament Gospels. These cures were plainly visible and impossible to dismiss as trickery: withered hands restored, blind eyes opened, leprosy banished, years of paralysis brought to an abrupt end and the dead returned to life. Periodically a report will surface that in some distant village a guru can levitate objects or that a psychic surgeon is performing miracles of healing. But when cameras and knowledgeable observers arrive, the miraculous event either does not materialize or is shown to have a more prosaic explanation (including, at times, outright trickery). So far it appears that the only place in which mastering the flow of life energy appears to lead to unquestionable supernatural powers is on the silver screen.

Furthermore, just as energy therapists and New Age theorists have attempted to enlist Jesus into their ranks, so some Christians have unwittingly made a similar mistake by approaching the Holy Spirit as if he, too, were a healing energy force. Say the right prayer, lay on hands, anoint with oil or deliver a good whack on the forehead, and the Holy Spirit will be obliged to do our bidding. However, such a concept is foreign to the teachings of the Bible and historical Christianity.[17] Throughout Scripture the Holy Spirit is presented as possessing all of the attributes of God and yet being distinct from the Father and Son. He is one of the three persons of God, not an impersonal force who is one and the same as each person on the planet. While a detailed review of biblical theology of the Holy Spirit is beyond the scope of this book, we will repeatedly set forth a clear principle taught throughout Scripture: God Almighty, Creator of heaven and earth, is the one and only God—and we are not. He is the potter and we are the clay. Yes, he is the loving Father, and he is the Son who came to seek and save the lost, and he is the Spirit who will lead us into all truth. He loves us, hears our petitions and knows our needs before we can articulate them. We cannot begin to comprehend the breadth and depth of his love and compassion. But he is in charge and he takes no orders from those whom he has made. God can, and at times does, heal in miraculous ways, but such healing cannot be called forth through any technique, formula or methodology—certainly not through any practice that contradicts his nature as revealed in the Bible.

Prana: **Energy from the Air**

We will be looking at a variety of life energy concepts throughout the course of this book, but this particular chapter will focus on two expressions of this idea— *prana* and *chi* (also spelled *qi* or *ki).* Both have considerable visibility throughout the world of alternative medicine.

From ancient Hinduism comes the idea that life energy flows from the air we breathe—hence the word *prana,* from the Sanskrit word for "breath." The various schools of yoga place much emphasis on breathing techniques and exercises, known as *pranayama,* which are said to concentrate *prana* from the air and distribute it throughout the body. While yoga is often thought of as a series of exercises for improving flexibility and muscle tone, yogic practices are intended primarily to produce altered states of consciousness. The word *yoga,* in fact, comes from the Sanskrit term for "yoke" or "union," and yogic exercises are ultimately intended to produce an experience of union with Brahman, the impersonal god of Hinduism. The widespread availability of yoga classes in health clubs, YMCAs, physical education programs and universities has unfortunately given these practices an air of innocence and spiritual neutrality they scarcely deserve. One should not take yoga's mystical ties lightly.

Some might argue that the Hindu mystics simply gave oxygen a name before it was isolated scientifically. But modern mystics allow us no such conclusion. One contributor to *A Visual Encyclopedia of Unconventional Medicine* informs us that "in some areas of the world there is a high concentration of prana, particularly at the sea-side, at high altitudes, and in an abundance of sunshine."[18] (Anyone with chronic lung disease can testify that there is no abundance of oxygen at high altitude.) Another author, Yogi Ramarcharaka, describes how one can hang on to *prana* if it seems to be slipping away: "If you feel that your vital energy is at a low ebb and you need to build up and store a new supply quickly, the best plan is to place the feet close together, side by side, and lock the fingers of both hands. This closes the circuit and prevents any escape of prana through the extremities. Then breathe rhythmically a few times and you will feel the effects of the recharging."[19]

Many teachers claim that *prana* is concentrated at seven energy centers or vortices called chakras. The chakras are said to be positioned in the midline of the body from the base of the spine to the top of the head and are assumed to regulate both physiological and spiritual events. Some correlate them with specific body parts (for example, the heart or the throat) or with the endocrine glands, although the ancient mystics to whom we owe this system had no specific knowledge of endocrine function. Contemporary energy healers such as Donna Eden and Caroline Myss have written elaborate descriptions of the chakras as energetic "memory banks." Eden writes, "Memory is energetically coded in your *chakras* just as it is chemically coded in your neurons. An imprint of every important or emotionally significant event you have experienced is recorded in your chakra energy. If I know your *chakras*, I know your history, the obstacles to your growth, your vulnerabilities to illness, and your soul's longings."[20]

"Medical sensitives" who claim to "see" and otherwise interact with other people's chakras thus are given access to information not only about health problems but about their current and past life issues and their spiritual status as well. In an introduction to her book *Why People Don't Heal, and How They Can,* Carolyn Myss writes:

> As a medical intuitive, I describe for people the nature of their physical diseases as well as the energetic dysfunctions that are present within their bodies. I read the energy field that permeates and surrounds the body, picking up information about dramatic childhood experiences, behavior patterns, even superstitious beliefs, all of which have bearing on the person's physical health. Based on that information I perceive intuitively in their energy fields, including the *chakras*, I can make recommendations for treating their condition on both a physical and spiritual level.
>
> The intention behind using energy medicine is to treat the body and the spirit equally.[21]

In addition, some writers describe what is considered among psychics to be the most potent flow of energy within the body: the *kundalini.* Within the spinal column is said to exist an energy conduit. If *prana* is channeled through this canal, from the base of the spine to the base of the skull, one may experience the rising of the *kundalini.* All who describe the *kundalini* warn of its power to destroy as well as heal. Even under the supervision of an experienced teacher, one who manipulates this energy is considered liable to experience severe physical reactions, psychosis or even death.

Needless to say, like the seven chakras, the notion of the *kundalini* is loaded with mystical and even sexual overtones. One form of yoga known as tantra teaches specific techniques to raise *kundalini* through sexual intercourse. Tantric lovers visualize currents of *prana* flowing through them during their meditative embrace, in which they are "using their bodies and the joined magnitude of their complementary forces as a vehicle through which to achieve consciousness."[22]

Another popular energy therapy that claims to manipulate *prana* is Therapeutic Touch, an overtly mystical practice that has made significant inroads into the nursing profession. Because of its extraordinary subjectivism, we will take a closer look at this phenomenon in chapter twelve.

What is the ultimate goal of manipulating *prana?* Learning to relax? Healing the sick? Coping with the stress of life? These may be the immediate intentions of many life energy therapists, but they are child's play compared to the ultimate goal, which is to become God. Swami Vivekananda declares the overtly religious implications of *prana* as he portrays the powers of the fully enlightened yogi:

> What power on earth would not be his? He would be able to move the sun and stars out of their places, to control everything in the universe from the atoms to the biggest suns. This is the end and aim of pranayama. When the yogi becomes perfect there will be nothing in nature not under his control. If he orders the gods or the souls of the departed to come, they will come at his bidding. All the forces of nature will obey him as slaves. . . . He who has controlled prana has controlled his own mind and all the minds . . . and all the bodies that exist.[23]

Chi and Traditional Chinese Medicine

We will look at these imports from China in some detail because, of all the energy therapies, both ancient and modern, they have arguably made the deepest inroads into Western conventional medicine and popular culture. Within one generation the products of traditional Chinese medicine, especially acupuncture and acupressure, rose from utter obscurity to household familiarity in North America and Europe. Acupuncture has progressed from a "Ripley's Believe It or Not" curiosity to a treatment for chronic pain (and a host of other ailments) at prestigious university centers, and it recently garnered a favorable review in a National Institutes of Health Consensus Report.[24] Acupressure techniques appear in magazines at the supermarket checkout counter and medical self-care books in the mall. Applied kinesiology, a homegrown blend of Chinese medicine and American chiropractic theory, continues to be used, among other things, as a logic-defying test for food and drug sensitivities. *Tai chi* and *qi gong* are becoming as common on the exercise landscape as aerobic workouts.

For all of their diversity, all of these flowers in the colorful Chinese bouquet share a common root that may or may not be obvious to those who are sampling the aromas. As a result, without realizing it, many Westerners are slowly conforming their worldview to an ancient metaphysical system called Taoism. Like so many other practices within the realm of alternative medicine, a transformation in thinking comes on the heels of a simple technique for achieving some other purpose, such as relaxing, relieving a headache or feeling more energetic. People who know nothing of ancient Chinese religion will tacitly accept the idea that some sort of energy is coursing through their body in invisible channels. Christians who would be flabbergasted if someone accused them of practicing Taoism are concerned about whether they might be suffering from an imbalance of yin and yang. Traditional Chinese medicine is providing a way for people (including many who consider the Bible as authoritative) to act like mystics without realizing it—and perhaps eventually to *become* mystics.

Traditional Chinese Medicine: Origins, Theories and Diagnostics

The origins of classical Chinese medicine are obscure, buried in thousands of years of tradition. Nevertheless, its first and most important textbook is widely recognized to be the *Huang Ti Nei Ching Su Wen,* or *The Yellow Emperor's Classic of Internal Medicine* (which we will refer to as the *Nei Ching*). Its author, the "Yellow Lord" Huang Ti, is said to have lived from 2697 to 2597 B.C. and reigned as the third of China's first five rulers, although there is some disagreement as to whether he existed at all. The date and authorship of the *Nei Ching* are open to question as well, since its original contents have been thoroughly sifted by commentators over the centuries. While the best editions of the *Nei Ching* date from some thirty-four hundred years after the reign of the Yellow Lord, both the text and its reputed author are the object of highest regard in traditional Chinese medicine. This is not a textbook as such but rather a series of dialogues between Huang Ti and his minister/physician Chi Po. The emperor poses questions about various illnesses, which prompt long discourses that range into general ethics and metaphysics. Historian Ilza Veith comments in her excellent introduction to the *Nei Ching:* "This combination is, as matter of fact, the only way in which early Chinese medical thinking could be expressed, for medicine was but a part of philosophy and religion, both of which propounded oneness with nature, i.e., the universe."[25]

Like so many healing systems that populate the realm of alternative medicine, traditional Chinese medicine is the child of Chinese religion. At their core both share the same ingredients: the Tao, yin and yang, the invisible life energy *chi* and the five elements.

The ancient Chinese produced many philosophical systems, of which two are most familiar to Westerners. Confucianism stressed social order and practical knowledge, laying the groundwork for formal education and etiquette. Taoism, on the other hand, was far more mystical. Its spiritual father, Lao-tzu (literally, "the old master"), expounded on the concept of the Tao, or "the way," an impersonal concept of ultimate reality. Taoism centers on the importance of process and change, the concept that nature and universe flow in an endless course of phases and cycles. Day becomes night, winter turns to spring, warm things cool, wet becomes dry and so on, all in observable patterns. These are not the handiwork of a Creator who cares about what he has fashioned. German acupuncturist Gabriel Stux comments that "the Tao is the Ultimate that creates and unites all things. It is the unstructured continuum from which everything has emanated and which persists in the structured universe. The essence of the Ultimate cannot be more clearly defined conceptually."[26]

Lao-tzu himself made it clear that we are not capable of grasping a complete understanding of the Tao: "The Tao that can be described is not the real Tao."[27] Nevertheless, Taoism urges human beings, who are seen as utterly dependent upon nature, to live in harmony with these cycles and thus to be one with the Tao. The person who does so is promised success, health and long life, while the one who tries to buck the system, so to speak, will suffer failure, disease and an early grave.

Yin and yang are said to be the two foundational forces that generate all of the transformations in the universe. These forces are bipolar, meaning that they are opposites that are not antagonistic. They do not cancel one another but are part of the same whole, much as the North and South Poles are opposite ends of the same planet. The words *yin* and *yang* literally mean "the shady and sunny sides of a hill," but they have come to encompass a wealth of characteristics.

Yin	Yang	Yin	Yang
dark	light	yielding	firm
moon	sun	west/north	east/south
night	day	metal	wood
cold	heat	white/black	green/red
water	fire	rest	movement
dampness	dryness	spring/summer	autumn/winter
feminine	masculine	interior	exterior
below	above	contraction	expansion

Table 5.2. Characteristics of yin and yang

All events in nature and in human lives are said to be influenced by the ever-changing interplay of these forces. Neither is said to exist in an absolute state, but small amounts of each are contained in the other, as illustrated by the familiar ancient symbol *tai chi T'u,* the "Diagram of the Supreme Ultimate."

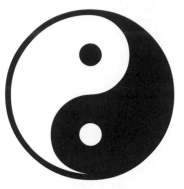

Figure 5.1. The *Tai chi T'u,* the "Diagram of the Supreme Ultimate"

This figure has been impressed into popular consciousness for decades, adorning a large variety of objects from T-shirts to jewelry.

Although yang sometimes is given virtuous characteristics (life, nobility, beauty) and yin negative values (death, commonness, ugliness), they are not considered good and evil principles but only complementary attributes of the same reality. (Similarly, what appears to be good and evil on earth are, in fact, only contrasting aspects of the same unity. The Taoist sage, in theory, sees beyond good and evil.)

The *Nei Ching* applies the interaction of yin and yang to the human body in exacting detail. The inside of the body is yin, the surface yang, the front yin and the back yang. Each major organ of the body is designated as either yin or yang, depending on which force dominates its function. The entire body is divided into lower, middle and upper regions, each of which has yin and yang subdivisions, which in turn contain two specific organs. Health is then defined as the state in which yin and yang are in perfect dynamic balance over a period of time, with disease occurring when there is an excess or deficiency of yin and yang anywhere in the body.

The key to the interplay of yin and yang, and thus to traditional Chinese medicine, is the flow of chi, the Chinese version of invisible life energy—the "life force" that is said to flow through the universe and all living organisms. *Chi* is reputedly inhaled from the air (much like *prana*) and extracted from food and drink. Some "ancestral *chi*" is also inherited from one's parents and purportedly stored in the kidneys. Once inside the body, it finds its way to a network of twelve invisible channels called meridians, ten of which are associated with a particular organ (for example, heart, spleen or liver) and share that organ's yin or yang polarity. Two meridians—Circulation and Triple Warmer—carry the names of nonexistent organs, for which various explanations are given in modern acupuncture literature.

The twelve meridians are duplicated on each side of the body and divided into closely associated pairs. The *Nei Ching* teaches that in health *chi* flows freely through the meridians in a one-way circuit vaguely resembling a road with hairpin turns at the fingertips and toes. Illness occurs when this flow is obstructed or excessive in any area, disrupting the balance of yin and yang. Specific diseases, such as pneumonia and diabetes, were not known to the Yellow Lord, and thus imbalances of yin and yang are given names such as "injuries of the heart" or "injuries of the stomach."

In diagnosing the cause of an illness, the patient's complaints, overall appearance, color and breathing pattern are taken into account, but according to traditional Chinese medicine, the key to correct diagnosis is examination of the tongue and the pulses. The appearance of the tongue is said to reflect a significant number and variety of internal conditions involving the balance of yin and yang and the flow of *chi*. In his book *Encounters with Qi,* David Eisenberg, M.D., notes, "A redder-than-normal tongue with a yellow, greasy coating corresponds to 'excessive internal heat, dampness, and deficiency of bodily vital energy.' A whiter-than-normal tongue with a thin coating reveals 'a deficiency of Yang, vital energy and blood.' There are thousands of permutations and diagnostic combinations. A comprehensive medical education includes the study of hundreds of tongues."[28] Eisenberg notes that Beijing's Institute of Traditional Chinese Medicine has a small room full of display cases containing hundreds of sculpted models of tongues, which are meant to serve as an educational tool for the traditional physician in training.

Even more informative than inspection of the tongue is a careful evaluation of the pulses. At each wrist the radial pulse (the one on the thumb side) is divided into three zones, each of which has a superficial and a deep position. These twelve pulse locations correspond to the twelve meridians and are said to communicate to the examiner information about each of them. All twelve positions are supposed to be felt carefully, and a skilled practitioner supposedly can differentiate some twenty-eight different qualities of the pulse, such as "full," "weak," "floating," "slippery" or "wiry." Pulses are interpreted in light of several factors, including time of day (the hours of 3:00 a.m. to 9:00 a.m. being the ideal hours to examine them), season of the year and sex of the patient (with the woman's right pulse to be examined first, and the man's left).

A detailed survey of the twelve wrist pulses may require thirty minutes or more, but they are said to reward the astute traditional Chinese diagnostician with knowledge of imbalances in any given organ, a precise diagnosis, a prognosis and even warnings of unsuspected disease. There are even seven "fatal" pulses, such as "rolling peas under the finger," suggesting a terminal abdominal infection, and "feather brushing the cheek," indicating a lethal lung infection such as tuberculosis.[29] Needless to say, this miraculous ability of the radial pulses to communicate information about the entire body requires a considerable stretch of the imagination. But it is only one of many points at which the teachings of traditional Chinese medicine are clearly at odds with basic physiology.

Once the practitioner has gathered enough information to determine where *chi* is or is not flowing properly, he or she must use a complex system known as the "Law of the Five Elements" to restore balance. The ancient Chinese, like their tradition-oriented modern-day counterparts, conceived of everything in the world as belonging to one of five categories: wood, fire, earth, metal and water. These were thought to represent tangible components, or "creations," of yin and yang. (They are vaguely similar to the discredited Western notion that all matter consists of earth, air, fire and water.) The Chinese system is far more complex, in that the five elements interact with each other in a specific manner. Each "creates" another (for example, wood creates fire) and is "subjugated" by a third (for example, metal subjugates wood). In addition, each of the five elements is associated with a particular color, season, direction, flavor (the basis of dietary therapies), odor, sound and musical note. And to top it all off, each organ in the human body is related to one of the elements. The overall system is represented in nearly all traditional Chinese medical textbooks by a diagram of interconnected circles and arrows. This is meant to serve as a road map of sorts for routing energies, since surplus *chi* is said to travel only in the directions shown in the drawing. Memorizing the map is felt to be essential for the well-trained traditional therapist.

Traditional Chinese Medicine's Approaches to Treatment

Armed with information about the patient, a thorough assessment of the pulses and a five-elements diagram, what might a practitioner recommend? The *Nei Ching* devotes relatively few pages to therapy compared to those dealing with diagnosis, apparently assuming that the physician would know what to do once the problem was identified. The text identifies five basic approaches, the first of which is treatment of the spirit, guiding the patient toward the Tao in the practice of a modest, tranquil way of life. The second and third are dietary changes and herbal remedies, which would be chosen for their specific effects upon the balance of yin and yang, and the flow of *chi,* in various organs and the body as a whole. Herbal recipes used by traditional therapists in China today are estimated to be hundreds of years old. (The treating physician a millennium ago reportedly had some one thousand herbs at his disposal, and more than two thousand ingredients—not all of them derived from plants—are used by traditional Chinese physicians today.)[30] Herbal broths are complex mixtures of several components, which might include such exotica as boiled scorpion or gecko, concocted and prepared with great care. David Eisenberg, M.D., writes:

> Practitioners of traditional Chinese medicine recognize herbal therapy as the most complex and demanding subspecialty. In order to prescribe herbal remedies effectively, one must first master Chinese medical theory as well as tongue and pulse diagnosis. The dependable recall of thousands of combinations of well-studied herbal preparations is the next prerequisite. Add these skills to twenty or thirty years of experience and you get a respected herbal doctor.[31]

The fourth type of therapy noted by the *Nei Ching* was massage, and the fifth acupuncture, for which Chinese medicine has become most famous—but which is by no means the treatment most frequently used by traditional practitioners in that country. The origin of acupuncture is unknown, but its techniques were refined over many centuries. Needles of all shapes and sizes have been used, some rather terrifying in appearance. At present most therapists use stainless steel needles ranging in length from one-half to four inches. When points of insertion are identified, one or more needles are inserted and advanced until a sensation described as "tingling, distention, heaviness and numbness" is felt by the patient.[32] The needles are then twisted manually or (a modern convenience for the busy therapist) connected to an electrical pulse generator for ten to fifteen minutes. A traditional variant is the practice of moxibustion, in which a smoldering fragment of the plant *Artimisia vulgaris* is placed on or near the chosen acupuncture point. A more popular contemporary variation is acupressure, where simple finger pressure is applied.

What is the puncturing, pressing or smoldering supposed to do? In traditional Chinese medicine, the goal is to correct imbalances in yin and yang by stimulating specific points along the twelve meridians, thereby draining excesses of energy or restoring deficiencies. Various authors recognize anywhere from 365 to 800 points, which are mapped on charts and mannequins and then located on the patient using landmarks of surface anatomy. These are reputed to be the sites of literal holes in the body through which *chi* flows or, alternatively, places where *chi* passes close enough to the surface to be influenced by activity at the surface. Based on training, experience and reference materials at his or her disposal, the practitioner picks the desired points for treatment. Contemporary textbooks are no less detailed or earnest in their presentation of maps and needling suggestions than those of bygone days. One, for example, gives the following example of a diagnosis and its corresponding treatment:

> The pulse diagnosis indicates:
> DEFICIENCY ON XII (Spleen)   Earth organ
> EXCESS ON IX (Lungs)   Metal organ
> First, we draw upon Wood by the control device of supplementing the wood point on the spleen meridian. This starts an energy movement by drawing on the normal towards the deficiency—thus creating a small deficiency on the Wood organ VIII (liver). We now can act upon this artificially created deficiency to draw the surplus from the Metal by supplementing at the metal point on the liver meridian. This treatment involves action at two points.[33]

The manipulations of *chi,* by whatever approach, are supposed to take into account the season of the year, phase of the moon, weather and time of day because these also affect the flow of yin and yang. All things considered, the "prescription" for a given patient is highly individualized—so much so, in fact, that attempts to compare different treatment approaches for effectiveness would appear pointless. Western medicine makes progress, among other means, by setting up carefully planned studies that are designed to ask, "All things being equal, do people with a particular problem fare better with the drug, surgery or therapy being considered, compared with people with the same problem not receiving that treatment (or receiving some other treatment)?" To the traditional Chinese therapist, this would be a meaningless question. Each individual illness is a unique event, with a unique treatment, even when people appear to manifest similar symptoms. Fifty patients with bacterial pneumonia, for example, would receive relatively similar treatment in the West: rest, antibiotics known to be effective against the organism suspected or specifically identified by culture, supplemental oxygen and fluids if needed, and attention to other conditions that might be complicating the problem. None of these cases would be alike in every single detail, but there would be similarities and patterns that any Western-trained physician would recognize, as well as basic parameters for treatment that would be used whether the patient was seen in Los Angeles, London or Lebanon. But fifty patients with pneumonia—even cases involving the same organism—who presented themselves to practitioners of traditional Chinese medicine would receive fifty completely different diagnoses and treatment regimes, all targeting the unique imbalance in *chi* that was supposedly the underlying cause for each person.

Those who are enthused about this one-of-a-kind approach to illness would praise it as "holistic," "attending to the body, mind and spirit in a truly individual way" and "treating the underlying cause, not just the symptoms." Those who are less enamored with traditional Chinese medicine would challenge its treatment strategies as irrational, hopelessly subjective, potentially dangerous for the person who is acutely ill and a serious impediment to any genuine progress or discovery. Yes, every patient with pneumonia, diabetes, warts or malaria has his or her own unique course—but not *completely* unique. Illnesses have identifiable similarities and patterns that lead thoughtful researchers to an understanding both of causes and of meaningful treatments. Yes, it is often not possible to determine why a particular individual developed a particular illness at a particular time. But the study of patterns of illness can lead to the identification of risk factors, which are far more useful in discovering causation and promoting prevention than assuming that one person's medical problem bears little or no relation to another's. It is indeed worth pondering how many millions of lives would have been lost in the past century if the reasoning that led to the discovery of the organisms that cause cholera, malaria, yellow fever and polio, to name a few, had been dismissed in favor of plowing ahead indefinitely with pulse diagnosis, acupuncture and individualized herbal remedies.

6

VARIATIONS ON
A *CHI* THEME

Over the centuries, the idea of manipulating invisible energy in order to restore health, or stimulating one part of the body in order to control another, has been continuously revised and reinvented. Many of these variations are a direct spinoff of traditional Chinese medicine, while others bear a vague resemblance to it but have their own unique take on health.

Ear acupuncture, or *auriculotherapy,* for example, is based on the assumption that meridians begin, end or pass through the outer ear. Apparently because of a vague similarity of the ear to the appearance of a human fetus or newborn turned upside down, some 168 acupuncture points on the ear are said to be associated with specific body parts. (In general, the head and face are represented by points around the earlobe, while the lower parts of the body correspond to the upper segments of the ear.) More than seventy ailments are said to be treatable using ear acupuncture, which has been promoted widely in the United States for managing addictions, especially smoking. Small needles or staples inserted into one or both ears, and then left in place for days or weeks at a time, are supposed to curb one's appetite for tobacco or even food. Less well known are treatments involving points on the face, scalp and tongue, as well as Korean hand acupuncture, in which meridians and body parts are supposedly projected onto the palm.

One alternative energy therapy that is not directly derived from the ancient Chinese is *reflexology,* an offshoot of a practice called "zone therapy," which was introduced by American ear, nose and throat specialist William Fitzgerald in 1915. Reflexologists believe that functions in all areas of the body are reflected in the feet, and conversely that massaging certain areas of the soles will impact specific organs. Reflexology has its own representation of the body on each foot, with facial structures focused in the toes and organs such as colon and bladder nearer the heel. Interestingly, these diagrams are not completely symmetrical. For example, the gall bladder and the right (or ascending) colon is on the right foot, while the heart and the left (or descending) colon is on the left. Like acupuncture, the physiological mechanism for reflexology somehow escaped twentieth-century anatomists and neurologists, but supposedly it involves invisible energy channels (different from the Chinese notion of meridians and *chi*) as well as heretofore undiscovered "reflex" nerve pathways. Since extended foot massage is usually extraordinarily relaxing, it is not difficult to envision how this technique might bring about feelings of improvement for a number of symptoms. Some practitioners believe that similar benefits can be accrued using hand reflexology, and they use similar maps showing representations of the body on the palm.

Many individuals who are squeamish about having their skin punctured (even by tiny needles) have been drawn to *acupressure* techniques, which are in essence acupuncture treatments involving finger pressure rather than the insertion of pointed objects. A number of these acupressure techniques originated in Japan, but all are in one way or another rooted in the mysticism of *chi*. *Shiatsu*, for example, involves not only pressure with fingers on small points of skin but also at times the use of hands, knees or even feet applied to wider areas of the body. By contrast, another Japanese variation, *jin shin jyutsu*, uses very light pressure to maneuver *chi* based upon pulse diagnoses. *Jin shin do*, or the "Way of the Compassionate Spirit," strongly emphasizes an understanding of the metaphysics of Taoism as critical not only to its healing benefits but also to opening an individual's "higher" or psychic centers. This particular technique, in addition to manipulating *chi* through the twelve traditional meridians, teaches the use of eight "psychic channels," or "strange flows," which are affected by meditation, as a means of solving invisible energy traffic problems.

Applied Kinesiology and Touch for Health

A colorful and distinctly American variation was devised by chiropractor George Goodheart, who in 1964 introduced a mixture of Chinese energy flow, acupressure and muscle testing called *applied kinesiology* (AK). (This technique, it should be noted, is unrelated to the mainstream science of kinesiology, which studies body movements and the muscles controlling them. Formal kinesiology has important applications to rehabilitation and physical therapy.) The premise of AK is that the flow of *chi* communicates information about problems within the body to specific muscle groups. For example, subtle changes in the triceps, the muscle that straightens the arm at the elbow, reflect the condition of the pancreas. And the anterior deltoid, which helps flex the shoulder, is said to be related to the gall bladder.

AK practitioners also use muscle testing to determine immediately which foods, vitamins or other substances might help a person get well or which might make a problem worse. The substance is held in the mouth or hand, or simply placed on the body, and then an "indicator" muscle is checked. (Often this involves pulling downward on an outstretched arm.) If the muscle feels stronger, the substance must be beneficial for that person, and vice versa if the muscle becomes weaker. One AK manual states, for example, "If a patient is diagnosed as having a liver disturbance, and the associated pectoralis major tests weak, have the patient chew a substance that may help the liver, such as vitamin A. If . . . the vitamin A is appropriate treatment, the muscle will test strong."[1]

The communication of *chi* to muscle even allows for "surrogate" testing, in which a parent's arm strength can be used to diagnose and treat a child held on the lap. More adventurous proponents of AK suggest that the arm-pulling test can be applied to any and all materials that come in contact with the body (for example, a wristwatch, a pair of sunglasses or even clothing) in order to determine how they might affect one's supply and flow of *chi*.[2]

A popular extrapolation of AK, "Touch for Health," was introduced in 1973 by chiropractor John Thie. Touch for Health adds a simple treatment strategy to AK's muscle-testing techniques: to strengthen a weak muscle (and presumably the unbalanced organ associated with it), simply use a hand to trace the associated meridian from one end to the other, using a gentle, smooth, continuous motion. The technique is reputed to work even if one's hand misses the meridian by an inch or two—or even if it passes above the skin, not touching it at all. The simplicity of this method and the ease with which the general public might use it have kept AK in general, and Touch for Health in particular, alive and well for well over twenty-five years. For example, a report from John Maguire, director of the Kinesiology Institute, describes how Touch for Health techniques have been enthusiastically embraced and taught at the "Mastery University" program of Anthony Robbins, a popular and highly visible motivational speaker, "success coach" and author associated with the human potential movement.[3]

Going Deeper into Mysticism: *Reiki* and *Qi Gong*

Reiki is a Japanese word combining two syllables: *rei,* which is usually translated "universal," and *ki,* a variant spelling for *chi,* the life force we have been discussing. In its introductory material "What is Reiki?" the International Center for Reiki Training adds considerable weight to this word:

> Research into the esoteric meaning of the Japanese kanji character for Rei has given a much deeper understanding of this ideogram. The word Rei as it is used in Reiki is more accurately interpreted to mean supernatural knowledge or spiritual conscious-ness. This is the wisdom that comes from God or the Higher Self. This is the God-Consciousness which is all knowing. It understands each person completely. . . .
> Ki means the same as Chi in Chinese, Prana in Sanskrit and Ti or Ki in Hawaiian. . . .
> Ki is the life force. It is also called the vital life force or the universal life force. This is the nonphysical energy that animates all living things. As long as something is alive, it has life force circulating through it and surrounding it; when it dies, the life force departs. . . .
> Ki is used by martial artists in their physical training and mental development. It is used in meditative breathing exercises called Pranayama, and by the shamans in all cultures for divination, psychic awareness, manifestation and healing. Ki is the non-physical energy used by all healers. Ki is present all around and can be accumulated by the mind.
> It is the God-consciousness called Rei that guides the life force called Ki in the practice we call Reiki. Therefore, Reiki can be defined as spiritually guided life force energy. This is a meaningful interpretation of the word Reiki. It more closely describes the experience most people have of it; Reiki guiding itself with its own wisdom, and being unresponsive to the direction of the practitioner.[4]

Reiki was developed by Dr. Mikao Usui, a nineteenth-century Japanese theolo-gian who for years sought a way to recreate the healing miracles of Jesus. He stud-ied not only Christian but also Buddhist texts in multiple languages, eventually uncovering in a Sanskrit translation what he concluded was a forgotten healing art. During an extended time of prayer and fasting, he reportedly experienced a vision that gave him a deeper understanding of these teachings, which he then synthesized into the system now called *reiki.*

Reiki, from first to last, is all about improving the flow of life energy in the body, though without the complex formulas and interactions of traditional Chi-nese medicine. The practitioner is not considered the source of the energy but merely a "conduit" who holds his or her hands on or over twelve basic locations on the recipient's body during a treatment session lasting about an hour. The patient pays little role in this process other than "formulating an intent" of what he or she would like treated and perhaps feeling a warm or tingling feeling at some point during the session. The process of becoming a practitioner involves an initi-ation of sorts (including ancient secret symbols), during which a *reiki* master "transfers energy" to the student. Apparently other skills or mindsets are less important than this process of opening a "healing channel," also referred to as an "attunement," which is said to allow the individual to use the energy for a lifetime.

One can become a *reiki* master through receiving additional (second- and third-degree) instruction and attunements and then teaching the practice to someone else. According to material published by the International Center for Reiki Training, *reiki* "is not a religion. It has no dogma, and there is nothing you must believe in order to learn and use Reiki. In fact, Reiki is not dependent on belief at all and will work whether you believe it or not."[5] Apparently, however, *reiki* has some intentionality of its own. While most life energy therapies drift toward the idea that we can learn techniques to manipulate this universal force (and thus, in essence, control God), *reiki* apparently intends to be in command of those who interact with it.

> By treating yourself and others, and meditating on the essence of Reiki, you will be guided more and more by Reiki in making important decisions. Sometimes you will find yourself doing things that don't make sense or conform to what you think you should be doing. Sometimes you will be guided to do things that you have vowed you would never do. . . . Over time, you will learn from experience that the guidance of Reiki is worthy of your trust. Once you have surrendered completely, you will have entered the Way of Reiki. . . .
>
> In the end, we must consider that a Reiki Master is not one who has mastered Reiki, but one whom Reiki has mastered. This requires that we surrender completely to the spirit of Reiki, allowing it to guide every area of our lives and become our only focus and source of nurturing and sustenance.[6]

Needless to say, the assertion that this is not a religion is more than a little disingenuous. Proponents of life energy therapies commonly represent them as scientific, empirical and usable by people of all faiths. But the spiritual underpinnings of these practices are ubiquitous, and in *reiki* they are boldly unfurled.

Similarly, *qi gong,* which is not a recent add-on but has been part and parcel of traditional Chinese medicine for thousands of years, literally brings us back to the metaphysical teachings of Yoda in *The Empire Strikes Back.* (It may be no coincidence that the Jedi master portrayed by Liam Neeson in the 1999 *Star Wars* prequel *The Phantom Menace* is named Qui-Gon Jinn.) Literally meaning "energy work," *qi gong* is a mixture of body movements, breathing techniques and meditation that is extremely popular in China. Some estimates suggest that it is practiced daily by more than sixty million Chinese citizens, often in mass groups in public parks.[7] The majority are involved in "internal *qi gong,*" carrying out slow, choreographed movements and careful breathing for twenty to sixty minutes, visualizing *chi* flowing smoothly through their bodies.

In contrast to *reiki,* in which the energy ultimately is supposed to take charge of the individual, *qi gong* participants are convinced that they can direct the flow mentally. "In the philosophy of qigong, a primary aim is to maintain or restore balance and harmony of mind-body," states one introduction to this practice. "Through qigong, one can build up qi and move it to where a disturbance or blockage occurs."[8] Mental focus during *qi gong* also supposedly enables one to store the invisible energy in any of several "reservoirs," from which it can then be properly distributed within the body. Traditional practitioners in China, and their counterparts in the West, believe that the regular practice of internal *qi gong* strengthens immunity and generally decreases the likelihood and severity of illness. While it is not hard to imagine that a daily routine of quiet movement and breathing exercises might have a number of benefits, it would be extremely difficult to prove that *qi gong* confers all of the positive outcomes described by those who practice it.

What has generated some interesting controversy is the claim by some enthusiasts that they can cause *chi* to flow *outside* of their bodies—a process called "external *qi gong*." Some say they can direct their *chi* into others for healing purposes, while others make more flamboyant claims that they can move objects without touching them, cause fluorescent bulbs to flicker or repel attackers without using physical force. According to an extensive report by the Committee for the Scientific Investigation of Claims of the Paranormal (CSICOP), there has been no shortage of *qi gong* masters in China who have accrued wealth and influence through their apparent supernatural healing and psychic powers. But as is typical whenever such claims are put to the test under controlled conditions, and especially when experienced stage magicians are available to scrutinize the proceedings, the miraculous events inevitably turn out to be old-fashioned sleight of hand, suggestibility, fizzles (sometimes attributed to lack of belief among those in the room) or flat-out no-shows. A symposium convened in June 1995 by the China Association for Science and Technology (CAST) and attended by, among others, a contingent from CSICOP repeatedly identified widespread belief in external *qi gong* as China's "major pseudoscience problem." One Chinese scientific journalist and policy expert, Lin Zixin, described rampant superstition in China as a threat to the country's technological development.[9]

Needless to say, traditional Chinese medicine in general, and *qi gong* in particular, is not held in high regard by a major contingent of China's scientific community—a fact that has been given little notice in the West. A prime example of this type of selective attention can be viewed in the PBS series *Healing and the Mind,* featuring Bill Moyers, which originally aired in 1993. Its first segment, "The Mys-

tery of Ch'i," was a wide-eyed look at traditional Chinese medicine featuring
David Eisenberg, M.D., the principal author of the highly influential alternative
medicine studies described in chapter one of this book. Eisenberg has been fascinated with Chinese medicine since his undergraduate years at Harvard University,
and while attending Harvard Medical School, he became the first American medical exchange student to visit China after diplomatic relations were reestablished
with the United States in the late 1970s. He studied traditional medicine in China
intensively for a year beginning in August 1979 and then returned to China in
1983 with a medical delegation to study the concept of *chi*. All of these encounters
made it abundantly clear to him that this mystical notion cannot be teased out of
traditional Chinese medicine.

> MOYERS: When you got here twelve years ago, when you arrived, were you skep-
> tical?
> EISENBERG: Very. I had exactly the same questions.
> MOYERS: What was your attitude toward traditional Chinese medicine?
> EISENBERG: It was really very simplistic—does it work? And if it works, how does
> it work? If it works, how much of it is the placebo effect? Is it just people's belief, or
> do the drugs work, do the needles work, does the meditation work? I asked all the
> same questions that you're asking. And I didn't know a thing about this Ch'i, this
> vital energy. In fact, it wasn't until I was in the traditional medical college here for
> months that my teachers finally drove it home that the whole system is based on this
> odd thing called Ch'i energy. . . .
>   Part of the difficulty in looking at Chinese medicine is that it's like going to med-
> ical school within the confines of a theological seminary. In the West, we separate
> religion and medicine. In Chinese medicine, the medical masters, the people who
> understood material things, were also the spiritual leaders. They never split the two.
> Imagine if Harvard Medical School were placed inside a large theological seminary,
> and classes were taught jointly. That's in large part what Chinese medicine is about.[10]

In the "Mystery of Ch'i" episode Moyers and Eisenberg tour a traditional Chinese hospital, watch exotic concoctions of herbs being prepared, view brain surgery in which the patient is conscious and apparently needs less sedation because
she is also receiving acupuncture, discuss the flow of *chi* in Chinese massage with a
master masseuse and observe a physician who claims to be treating his patients
with doses of his external *qi gong*. In nearly all of these segments they speak in
hushed tones around the traditional healers and later express amazement over all
they have seen. There is an occasional note of skepticism, but it is rather muted,
and the pair make some comments about the importance of controlled studies that
seem more obligatory than heartfelt.

One segment of the program involves an encounter with a *qi gong* teacher,

Master Shi, who holds court in Beijing's Purple Bamboo Park. A small, elderly gentleman, he is supposedly capable of causing his strapping young students to flail or fall away from him purely through the force of his external *chi*. A number of them repeatedly try to push Master Shi over, but they are easily repelled, apparently without much effort on the old man's part. While they claim to be straining and struggling against him, grunting audibly in the process, at one point Eisenberg yells to one, "C'mon, Andrew, it doesn't look real!" Others who have studied this segment in detail have concluded that this was indeed a performance; this would not be difficult to believe, since the participants were students deeply committed to learning Master Shi's secrets. (The old man reportedly instructed them to come to the park every morning at dawn for three years in order to prove they are serious.)[11] Yet the program's presentation of this exhibition, which even Moyers didn't seem to accept as genuine, still left the audience hanging as to whether the aged teacher in the park might actually have some sort of psychokinetic power.

In his book *Encounters with Qi* and in his interactions with Bill Moyers, Eisenberg manifests an ongoing tension between his high regard for Chinese medicine and his rigorous training at Harvard Medical School and UCLA. He repeatedly displays what appears to be a desire—almost a longing—for *chi* and its offshoots (including external *qi gong*) to be validated. But then, like a planet in an elliptical orbit around two suns, he swings back to a Western center of gravity, noting the credibility problems of therapies, the likelihood that prosaic mechanisms such as suggestibility and the placebo effect are at work in Chinese medicine, and the need for more rigorous clinical studies. Nevertheless, as he seems to loop back and forth between Western and Eastern spheres of influence, one can't help suspecting that the latter holds greater sway. Ultimately he clearly desires to bring the two together:

> When I'm asked the question, "What do you think, Doc? Does it [traditional Chinese medicine] do the job?"—I don't know. To know, there has to be a marriage of Chinese medicine and Western medicine. The two sides have to come together, because the Chinese doctors are not trained in science. They don't know about control groups and randomization and statistics. That wasn't part of their theory, any more than Western-style physicians know about Ch'i. . . . You need to apply the sharpest, most insightful science to figure out, "Does it really work, is it helpful, is it safe, does it save money?" That's what needs to happen, and that's never happened before, either in the West or in China. So the offspring of that marriage would be a brand new thing.[12]

A Cautionary Tale: The Debunking of Animal Magnetism

We have spent a considerable amount of time describing the pervasive notion that manipulating invisible life energy, by whatever name it is called, and by any number of methods, will bring about healing. This idea continues to flourish both in primitive and developed cultures, despite widespread agreement that *chi* or *prana* or anything else like it has never been detected, nor in some reasonable way proven to exist, by any reputable scientific body on any continent.

So why does this idea persist, especially in technologically sophisticated societies? One important reason is that the idea of universal life energy taps into deep yearnings for spirituality and meaning, and provides methods to exert spiritual power with few strings attached.

Another important reason is the current reign of no-questions-asked pragmatism in Western cultures, which is manifested by arguments such as the following:

- ☐ "I don't understand it—it just works!"
- ☐ "Millions of Chinese people benefit from this, so there must be something to it."
- ☐ "My sore shoulder got better after the treatment, so I guess it must have gotten my energy flowing like the doctor said."
- ☐ "I felt some warmth where the therapist waved her hand over my body."
- ☐ "Since I started doing the *reiki,* I feel a lot more focused."

Even physicians can fall into this line of thinking when a clinical study appears to show some benefit from a therapy that otherwise does not make a lot of sense. For example, an otherwise reputable family practice journal recently published a study showing some apparent improvement in osteoarthritic knees following treatment using Therapeutic Touch, then pondered the meaning of it all in an accompanying editorial.[13] But in this particular journal, and in countless other articles and books (for both professional and lay audiences) that have given energy therapies an air of respectability, no one appears willing to take a deep breath and ask the obvious question: why should we pay any serious attention, except for anthropological or sociological interest, to theories of health and disease that defy basic laws of chemistry and physics, uproot two centuries of progress in biology and physiology, challenge common sense and frankly appear mythological?

If a world-famous stage illusionist claimed that he had supernatural power and that he could transport a person instantly from one end of the room to the other, should we become true believers when he puts on a convincing demonstration of his alleged power? If he were to persist in his claim, and if we could not quite figure out how he did it, should we walk away convinced that he can defy the laws of physics? Or should we look for a more reasonable explanation: *Yes, he is a master of stagecraft and distraction, and we will figure out what actually happens up there on the stage, perhaps with the help of another illusionist. But he also appears to need psychiatric care.* Most of us would opt for the latter conclusion. But what if at the end of his magic show he said he had developed the capacity to direct healing energy across the room into another person's sore joints or brain tumor? Would he still get the psychiatric consultation, or would he instead be offered a lucrative book contract and an appearance on the Public Broadcasting System?

We would be wise to consider the astute approach of some of our forebears, who faced a similar situation more than two centuries ago when they were called upon to assess the claims and practices of the Austrian physician Franz Anton Mesmer. While better known for the trancelike state he evoked in many of his patients (from which we derive the word *mesmerism*), Mesmer was famous in his own day for proclaiming his theory of "animal magnetism." This life force, like *chi* and *prana,* was supposed to flow throughout the universe and into the human body, where its proper circulation was said to be vital to health. Mesmer proclaimed that magnetic therapy could correct "the unequal distribution of the nervous fluid and its confused movement with its uniform current, and produces that condition which I call the harmony of the nerves."[14]

At first Mesmer used actual magnets as therapeutic tools, but later he decided that his own animal magnetism was potent enough to "magnetize" any other object, such as paper or wood, that he wished to use. Eventually he dispensed with such intermediaries and claimed that he could direct this invisible force to someone several feet away merely by pointing at him or her. The patient on the receiving end would reportedly respond with a "crisis" involving convulsive shaking, groaning, grimacing and eventually passing out. A few such "treatments" led to apparent improvements frequently enough to earn Mesmer considerable notoriety in Paris—so much, in fact, that in 1784 King Louis XVI appointed a royal commission to investigate him and his animal magnetism. The nine-member commission, which included Benjamin Franklin and Antoine Lavoisier (one of the founders of modern chemistry), designed some elegantly simple experiments that showed that the magnetic crises and their subsequent cures were in fact the result solely of the power of suggestion.

For example, one experiment involved a woman who was convinced that she felt warmth in whatever part of her body received magnetic treatment. When blindfolded and then unknowingly exposed to magnetism, she indicated no response to it. When she was told she was being exposed but was in fact not, she reported the customary warmth. Based upon the evidence it gathered, the commission observed that "imagination without magnetism produces convulsions, and . . . magnetism without imagination produces nothing." Their conclusion: "This fluid without existence is consequently without utility."[15] Apparently the findings of the commission were not widely disseminated, however, and thus animal magnetism and "magnetic healing" continued to attract therapists and patients until the early years of the twentieth century.

This episode in medical history is noteworthy because the members of King Louis's royal commission displayed more "street wisdom" than many of their counterparts in the late twentieth and early twenty-first centuries. Mesmer, like most of today's proponents of alternative therapies, had insisted that they focus on the convulsions and cures he had wrought, which he claimed were objective evidence of the effects of animal magnetism. But well aware of the body's capacity for recovery and the mind's role in that process, the commissioners put the horse before the cart and decided that they must first determine whether or not there was reasonable evidence that animal magnetism actually existed. They would consider its potential usefulness in treating illness only after they were convinced that the first question had been answered in the affirmative. Their straightforward experiments demonstrated conclusively that this "vital force" was in fact imaginary. Unfortunately, this approach has rarely been applied to therapies today that make similar claims about life energies in the body.

"There Must Be *Something* to All This"

This chapter has painted a less than flattering picture of the world of life energy therapies because of two primary issues, one scientific and one spiritual. If the flow of invisible, universal life energy (by whatever name) within human beings is the key to understanding health and illness, and if such energy is indeed the fabric of the universe, then the following statements are true:

☐ Whatever we thought we knew about biology and physics is wrong.

☐ Whatever we thought we knew about God from the Old and New Testaments is wrong.

Many alternative medicine enthusiasts would say "Amen!" to both of these conclusions. "Let's get rid of the old mechanistic, reductionistic paradigm and start seeing human beings holistically, as body, mind and spirit. And while we're at it, let's get past this idea of God as separate from ourselves, paternalistic and obsessed with 'sin,' and move ahead to developing our full potential as spiritual beings."

Not everyone would agree with this assessment, of course. As we noted in chapter one, the widely used term "complementary and alternative medicine" implies that we should not think in strict either-or terms and that we can benefit from conventional medicine for some kinds of problems (such as a broken leg) and alternative therapies for others (such as chronic leg pain). Many articles written for lay and professional readers, apparently eager to embrace what seem to be groundbreaking ideas (or at least not to appear narrow-minded), gloss over this issue as they encourage East to meet West in medicine. And there are many firm believers in the Scriptures who regularly participate in energy therapies, either as recipients or as providers. In their view the energy flow is simply another aspect of God's creation, not God himself, and the benefits of manipulating it are wheat that can be separated from the Eastern or New Age metaphysical chaff.

An editorial in *The Journal of Family Practice* seemed to grasp the scientific implications if a particular energy therapy (in this case, Therapeutic Touch, or TT) was actually shown to be effective in some clinical situation:

> Properly executed and blinded TT experiments with positive results are challenges to our overall scientific framework and, most of all, to physics. If the data is convincing, then we have discovered predictive and explanatory failures in our more tested and trusted models of the universe. This would be exciting! A generation of experimental physicists and chemists would turn forests into theses exploring these phenomena. Novel and intense experimentation could forge new rationalistic and reductionistic models of the universe. The upheaval would be titanic. So, is the data convincing?

The authors go on to explain all of the ways in which studies of a therapy such as TT might be tainted.

> The small studies to date are, like all small studies by pioneers in new fields, very susceptible to submission and publication bias. If negative results are not submitted for publication, or if positive results are not published when submitted, then statistical variability will give us the wrong answers. There is also intense political, economic and social pressure. Billions are being spent on alternative remedies, the engines of American capitalism are throttling up, and politicians are receiving the usual financial incentives. Therapeutic touch is widely taught in nursing programs, and many medical schools are adding courses in alternative therapies. . . . Science is never free of politics and commerce; we must weigh those pressures, too.

So what is the answer? According to this editorial, it is to carry out a definitive study of this particular therapy and then let the chips fall where they may, even if the chips are the size of Mount Everest.

> Let us then do a large, well-designed, and well-regulated study of TT. This study should be definitive, and managed by experienced scientists willing to publish both positive and negative results. If the results are negative, then we can return to our existing scientific models, and look for new challenges from other directions. If, however, the answers are positive, then we shall all have a great adventure that will go far beyond mere medicine.[16]

The writers of this piece, in their contemplation of a study that might overturn two hundred years of Western scientific inquiry, have neglected an extremely important axiom: extraordinary claims demand extraordinary proof. This axiom has a very important corollary: talk is cheap.

If one intends to promote an idea—specifically for our discussion, a health care concept—that challenges fundamental and well-established principles of biology, chemistry and physics, the burden is on the challenger to provide evidence that is extremely convincing along several lines:

☐ The effects of the therapy should be observable in more ways than the report of an individual that he or she feels better. Subjective improvement, of course, is important in all areas of health care. But it rarely, if ever, would qualify as extraordinary proof for an extraordinary claim.

☐ The effects should be reproducible by others (*many* others!), especially by researchers who don't have an agenda or something to gain or lose from the outcome. The suggestion in the above-quoted editorial that one large-scale study of Therapeutic Touch would be adequate to launch a "great adventure" into unexplored realms sells the process of scientific exploration short. If researchers all over the world can't duplicate the results, don't rewrite any textbooks.

☐ Any and all other possible explanations for the observed effect must be seriously addressed and ruled out. If the effect can be explained using more conservative mechanisms and theories, the proof that they are not in fact the reason must be very compelling and also reproducible.

A Case in Point: Acupuncture for Pain Relief

To illustrate these principles, let us consider a phenomenon that caught the attention of Western journalists and the general public decades ago and still serves as a focal point for proponents of traditional Chinese medicine: the use of acupuncture to relieve pain during and after surgery.

It is intriguing to consider that one of the pivotal events in the history of alternative medicine was a case of appendicitis. James Reston, an editorial columnist for the *New York Times,* was one of the first American reporters to visit mainland China after relations were reestablished with the United States during the Nixon Administration. In 1971 he viewed a number of surgical operations, including the removal of a brain tumor, in which the patients remained awake and alert—with acupuncture apparently the sole anesthetic. During his visit to Beijing, Reston developed appendicitis, requiring emergency surgery, during which a spinal anesthetic was used. Postoperatively he developed stomach cramps, which were diagnosed as gastritis and treated successfully by an acupuncturist. Reston's report of these incidents in the *New York Times* (August 22, 1971) and in media interviews stirred considerable interest in the United States.

Within the next several months, journalists, scientists and physicians made pilgrimages to China, most reporting their observations in the popular press and a few in scientific journals. The articles reported that thousands of successful operations of all kinds were being carried out in China using acupuncture anesthesia: craniotomies (opening the skull), thyroid surgery, tonsillectomies, caesarean sections, and even lung and open-heart surgeries. Unfortunately, many of these travelers, even those with medical degrees, lacked the experience necessary to evaluate what they were shown. As the scientific community began to take a closer look at the acupuncture phenomenon, questions were raised that had been overlooked by the popular press. Does Chinese medicine work as advertised? How successful is it, especially when compared to other forms of treatment or no treatment at all? Are its effects influenced by such variables as the type of disease, the prevalent beliefs in the culture or the emotional makeup of the patient? Are the specific points used or the type of stimulation really important? If acupuncture works in a significant number of cases, by what mechanism does it do so?

Some particularly insightful commentary was published more than a quarter century ago by John J. Bonica, M.D., a long-time student of the phenomenon of pain who served as chairman of the department of anesthesiology at the University of Washington. Bonica's careful observations of acupuncture anesthesia in China illuminated a number of facts that had been—and still are—misunderstood by other observers. Initial reports, for example, suggested that this form of anesthesia was used in the majority of surgical operations in China. From statistics compiled by the Chinese, however, Bonica calculated that it was being used in less than 10 percent of all cases.[17] Furthermore, while apparently reducing the sensation of pain, acupuncture typically does not totally eliminate pain or other uncomfortable sensations. Some writers have observed that the word *anesthesia,* meaning "absence of sensation," does not truly apply to acupuncture and that the word *hypalgesia,* meaning "decrease in pain," is more appropriate.

Nearly every patient receiving acupuncture during surgery also receives a narcotic or barbiturate injection prior to surgery, or a slow drip of narcotic into a vein during the operation. Local anesthesia is frequently injected into sensitive structures before they are cut or manipulated. Acupuncture does not produce muscle relaxation, making abdominal operations extremely difficult if not impossible (tight abdominal muscles are a formidable barrier), and the unavoidable traction on internal organs may produce nausea and vomiting. To minimize this problem, Chinese surgeons often work with extreme deliberation when acupuncture is the main pain reliever. Emergency surgery is essentially never done using acupuncture. Even with these limitations, however, it cannot be denied that a large variety (if not number) of operations have been carried out with patients awake and alert—a definite advantage in some procedures. Other benefits of acupuncture would include minimal risk, essentially no change in normal physiology and decreased time in recovery. Bonica also reported claims of excellent response in many chronic pain disorders, except for pain caused by advanced cancer or the residual nerve discomfort (neuralgia) following an outbreak of herpes zoster (shingles). Emergency situations in which the patient is apprehensive also did not show impressive responses to acupuncture.

While the November 1997 National Institutes of Health (NIH) Consensus Development Conference on acupuncture did not specifically address the use of acupuncture during surgery in its report, it noted that the medical literature reviewed by the panel suggested that acupuncture was effective in reducing post-operative dental pain and that some reasonable evidence (though sometimes only single studies) showed pain relief in a variety of conditions such as menstrual cramps and tennis elbow.[18] Aside from relief of postoperative and chemotherapy nausea and vomiting (and probably that arising from pregnancy as well), the NIH panel indicated that the quality and quantity of research regarding the use of acupuncture in a wide variety of other conditions was inadequate to provide clear evidence of its effectiveness. This echoed Bonica's assessment of the claims he heard in China for acupuncture's efficacy in a host of conditions, including deafness and paralysis:

> As far as I have been able to ascertain from my observations, discussions, and from reviews of the literature, *the claims for the high degree of efficacy of acupuncture are not based on data derived from well-controlled clinical trials.* In fact, in many health stations and even in some hospitals, no records are kept of either the patient's history or of his response to therapy. In some instances, the practitioner administering the acupuncture could not recount for us the number of treatments and the results obtained with each treatment, simply because he did not have records.[19]

Given the spectrum of research and eyewitness reports indicating that acupuncture can have a definite effect on various types of pain, what explanations might be offered for this effect? The possibilities are numerous, and likely more than one is operating in a given situation. They can be grouped into a few basic categories:

Physiological mechanisms. Pain, like most functions in the human body, is a complex phenomenon. The familiar experience that a specific event (a stubbed toe) results in an immediate reaction ("Ouch!") gives rise to the intuitive notion that there is a simple and direct connection between the offended body part and the brain. But even this seemingly straightforward event involves complicated mechanisms in multiple areas of the nervous system, many of which may be affected by acupuncture. More than thirty years ago Canadian researchers Ronald Melzack and P. D. Wall proposed the "gate theory," the idea that the transmission of pain sensations may be altered by a number of mechanisms in the nervous system before reaching the brain, which itself may alter the perception of the painful input. The NIH Consensus Report notes:

> Many studies in animals and humans have demonstrated that acupuncture can cause multiple biological responses. These responses can occur locally, i.e., at or close to the site of application, or at a distance, mediated mainly by sensory neurons to many structures within the central nervous system. This can lead to activation of pathways affecting various physiological systems in the brain as well as in the periphery.[20]

These biological responses include the following:

☐ Release of substances called endogenous opioids—internal pain relievers with properties similar to familiar painkillers such as codeine. Elaborate studies by Dr. Ji-Sheng Han at Beijing University have identified the activity of compounds called endorphins, enkephalins and dynorphins in both brain and spinal cord.

☐ Release of the neurotransmitters serotonin and norepinephrine—biochemical "messengers" that affect mood and pain perception, among other functions.

☐ Changes in activity of the hypothalamus and pituitary gland as well as the autonomic nervous system. These may have a variety of far-reaching effects on hormone release and blood flow.

☐ The phenomenon of counterstimulation. It has long been observed that the transmission of pain signals from one part of the body can be inhibited by stimulation of another area at some distance from it. (This has been the basis for the use of transcutaneous electrical nerve stimulator units, which send low-voltage electrical pulses through pads applied to the skin. These have been effective for many individuals with chronic pain, especially in the neck and back.)

Neuroanatomist/neurophysiologist George Ulett, M.D., in his book *Beyond Yin and Yang: How Acupuncture Really Works* has summarized these mechanisms as follows:

> In summary, acupuncture stimulates the endogenous pain-modulating systems to release serotonin, opioid substances, and other transmitters at three levels of the central nervous system, the spinal cord, and thalamus, and the cerebral cortex, thus serving to dampen the perception and transmission of nociceptive [pain-generating] signals.[21]

Further research has addressed the question of the acupuncture points themselves. Does it matter where the needles are inserted? Most Western-trained acupuncture practitioners do not believe that points and meridians are real entities. British acupuncturist Felix Mann, commenting on the bewildering number of points at various locations described by contemporary therapists, quipped that if they are to be believed, there is literally "no skin left which is not an acupuncture point."[22] Many of the effects of acupuncture are seen with stimulation of "sham" points, which lie at some distance from the "true" points on traditional maps. Some researchers believe that there are in fact specific locations where acupuncture needling causes a greater physiologic response but that these are limited in number and coincide with known anatomical structures.[23]

Psychosocial mechanisms. As we discussed in the previous chapter, belief, expectation and cultural conditioning play a powerful role in all systems of health care (including conventional Western medicine). Many observers of Chinese medicine have noted that these may be particularly important in the apparent effectiveness of acupuncture and other traditional modalities. This is especially significant when dealing with pain. Important components include the following:

☐ confidence in the practitioner

☐ expectation that the treatment will help

☐ the ritualized components of examination, pulse diagnosis and the needling itself

☐ the patient's level of anxiety or lack thereof

☐ the patient's overall tolerance of discomfort

☐ a desire to please the practitioner by reporting improvement

Experimental design issues. As was noted above, the NIH Consensus Development Conference on acupuncture described significant problems in drawing conclusions from the hundreds of studies in current literature because of poor design. The issues involved in creating a valid study and interpreting it appropriately are numerous. Needless to say, not all studies are created equal, and those that appear to validate extraordinary claims often do not stand up under close scrutiny.

Fraud and trickery. Those who have studied acupuncture's effects on pain, whether proponents or skeptics, have found little to suggest that the entire phenomenon is an elaborate hoax. The same cannot be said, however, about more flamboyant demonstrations of the power of *chi,* such as have been presented to the unwary by *qi gong* "masters." In general, the more extreme the claim or apparently miraculous the occurrence, the more likely that old-fashioned showmanship may be involved.

Life Energies: Articles of Faith

Given these plausible explanations for the apparent effects of acupuncture on pain—or, for that matter, on any number of other conditions—where does that leave *chi* and meridians? Clearly the Western scientific community is not rewriting all of its textbooks based on its experience with Chinese medicine or any other therapy (such as *ayurveda*) rooted in vitalism. The current interest in life energy is not the result of research by scores of neutral investigators in diverse fields. Thus far no one has constructed an airtight proof that such energy exists, nor has anyone demonstrated its effects in reproducible experiments.

Acupuncturists, acupressurists and other energy therapists usually adopt a pragmatic stance: "I don't know how its works—it just does, and that's good enough for me." Some would argue that one need not understand electronics to turn on the television nor master auto mechanics to drive the family car, and that billions of aspirin tablets were consumed before anyone understood how the drug worked. But the workings of automobiles and video equipment can be comprehended by anyone with ordinary intelligence, given enough time and some straightforward instruction. Likewise the mechanism by which aspirin relieves inflamed joints was unraveled using straightforward logic and experimentation. No one swallows a Bayer aspirin assuming that it contains vital life forces or friendly spirits. Classical Chinese medicine, *ayurveda* and other ancient systems stand in sharp contrast to these examples, in that observations from ages past were incorporated into the prevailing religious thinking of that era. Furthermore, human beings are not TVs and cars, and their responses to medical therapies are hardly comparable to the normal effects of pushing the on button on the remote control or turning the key in the ignition. Cause-and-effect relationships in the human body are rarely observed to occur in such a simplistic manner.

A sizable contingent of alternative practitioners is not overly concerned with whether Western science discovers, acknowledges or even pays any attention to *chi*, meridians, *prana* and the other life energy concepts. For them the existence and manipulation of life energy is a matter of faith and practice. As often as they might attempt to tie their ideas (however loosely) to the findings of Western scientific research, the heart and soul of their approach arises from a worldview that is validated by personal experiences, often involving not only healings but also altered states of consciousness. While the specifics may vary, this worldview involves four basic precepts that appear in a variety of ways in Eastern mystical traditions (especially Vedism/Hinduism, Taoism and Buddhism), "mind science" thinking from the nineteenth century, some occult philosophies and, tying them all together, the New Age movement, which attempts to welcome nearly all faiths and philosophies under its very big tent. Needless to say, these four principles stand in sharp contrast to the basic teachings of the Old and New Testaments.

1. All is one. This summary statement of the worldview known as monism is not a theoretical proposition but rather a conclusion that is nearly always drawn from altered states of consciousness (such as those induced through meditation or the use of mind-altering drugs). Under their influence, many individuals experience the disappearance of all distinctions between self and other individuals and objects.

In addition, good and evil are said to be nothing more than different manifestations of the same reality, which various religions and mystics have designated as God or the Goddess or the One or Brahman or cosmic consciousness or any of a number of other entities. Furthermore, what we see around us—the world of people and animals, trees and plants, rocks and rivers, oceans and sky—is not real. Depending upon one's tradition, our everyday perceptions may be described as an illusion (often the Hindu term *maya* is used), a collective hallucination, God having a dream and forgetting to wake up, and so on. Explanations as to *why* this has occurred vary in plausibility, though most involve the notion that we are all little fragments of God who have embarked on an adventure away from the One, to which we will all ultimately return like drops of water finding our way back to a vast ocean. Reincarnation—numerous excursions into human (and animal) forms over thousands or millions of years—is usually an integral part of the story.

This idea of course flatly contradicts a foundational biblical teaching that might be summarized like this: "There is only one God, and you aren't him." David asked:

> Who is God besides the LORD?
>> And who is the Rock except our God? (Psalm 18:31)

Isaiah delivered the message more forcefully:

> This is what the LORD says—
>> Israel's King and Redeemer, the LORD Almighty:
> "I am the first and I am the last;
>> apart from me there is no God.
> Who then is like me?" (Isaiah 44:6-7)

While the Scriptures clearly teach that there is a reality beyond the material realm, beyond the reach of our five senses and our inventions that extend them, they also clearly acknowledge the reality and significance of our lives on this planet. Christians have long been ridiculed for being concerned only about "pie in the sky by and by," without attending to the suffering around them. But in fact it is monism, in all of its various presentations, that deserves this criticism. Why try to improve the lot of the less fortunate when nothing in their (or our) lives is real?

2. *Human beings are, at their core, perfect.* If there is only one reality in the universe and we are one with it, then our true nature must be one of divinity and perfection. Not only is our perception of ourselves as individuals separate from one another an illusion but so is our experience of illness and human frailty. Our innermost self must therefore be a source of infinite wisdom and love, even if our outward behavior suggests otherwise. Many alternative therapies tap into this idea,

whether advocating the contacting of our "higher self" or an "inner guide" or extolling the inherent wisdom of the life energy flowing through our bodies.

Obviously the chasm between this idea and the message of the Scriptures is profound. The entire Bible is the story of humanity's estrangement from its Creator and of the supreme sacrifice of his Son to provide for our reconciliation to him. Along the way the inclination of each one of us to rebel against God and to inflict every form of harm upon ourselves and each other is clearly and painfully spelled out. In his foundational presentation of these ideas to the believers in Rome the apostle Paul drove his argument home with the intensity of a prosecuting attorney:

> As it is written:
> "There is no one righteous, not even one;
>   there is no one who understands,
>   no one who seeks God.
> All have turned away,
>   they have together become worthless;
> there is no one who does good,
>   not even one."
> "Their throats are open graves;
>   their tongues practice deceit."
> "The poison of vipers is on their lips."
>   "Their mouths are full of cursing and bitterness."
> "Their feet are swift to shed blood;
>   ruin and misery mark their ways,
> and the way of peace they do not know."
>   "There is no fear of God before their eyes." (Romans 3:10-18)

Jesus, who is generally highly regarded even in New Age circles as an enlightened healer and master teacher, certainly did not validate the idea of our inner perfection. Following a discussion about whether eating certain foods made a person unclean, he made this provocative statement:

> "Are you so dull?" he asked. "Don't you see that nothing that enters a man from the outside can make him 'unclean'? For it doesn't go into his heart but into his stomach, and then out of his body." (In saying this, Jesus declared all foods "clean.")
>
> He went on: "What comes out of a man is what makes him 'unclean.' For from within, out of men's hearts, come evil thoughts, sexual immorality, theft, murder, adultery, greed, malice, deceit, lewdness, envy, slander, arrogance and folly. All these evils come from inside." (Mark 7:18-23)

3. Our most important purpose in life is to become keenly aware of our true, divine nature. This understanding may go by any of several names: enlightenment, illumination, self-awareness or self-actualization. We will supposedly arrive at such a state over the course of multiple incarnations as we gravitate back toward the One, or we can shorten the process through various meditative techniques and other disciplines. A few writers, especially prominent alternative medicine apologist Andrew Weil, M.D., whom we will discuss in chapter eight, suggest that the judicious use of mind-altering drugs can be an effective means of experiencing the unity of all things and our own true nature. Some who desire to amend their Christian roots revive the early-sixteenth-century origin of the word *atonement* and present it as "at-one-ment." In doing so they shift its emphasis away from reconciliation and the restoration of a broken relationship between ourselves and the God of the Bible, who deeply cares about us, stressing instead the idea that we are already "at one" with the God of Eastern and New Age mysticism, for whom (or for which) this is a nonissue.

In this worldview, enlightenment is the substitute for salvation, the forgiveness of sins by a holy God, without which we remain permanently in darkness, separated from him. Obviously if there is no real need for such reconciliation, then the means by which the Scriptures declare that God provided for it—the death of Jesus Christ on a Roman cross—is likewise a meaningless act of violence or at least has a different meaning from the one Christians have given it for two millennia. The apostle Paul would disagree forcefully:

> You see, at just the right time, when we were still powerless, Christ died for the ungodly. Very rarely will anyone die for a righteous man, though for a good man someone might possibly dare to die. But God demonstrates his own love for us in this: While we were still sinners, Christ died for us.
>
> Since we have now been justified by his blood, how much more shall we be saved from God's wrath through him! For if, when we were God's enemies, we were reconciled to him through the death of his Son, how much more, having been reconciled, shall we be saved through his life! Not only is this so, but we also rejoice in God through our Lord Jesus Christ, through whom we have now received reconciliation. (Romans 5:6-11)

4. Enlightenment leads to healing and other powerful psychospiritual experiences. As an individual progresses in knowledge of the reality that exists beyond the five senses, manipulation of the spiritual and physical worlds can occur by controlling one's consciousness. Knowledge of things unseen, locally or at a distance, both present and future, becomes a possibility. Healings can be brought to pass through any number of hands-on or meditative techniques to redirect "life energy," or through altering our own consciousness about the status of the person who is ill. Some alternative medicine authors have appropriated the word *prayer* to describe a "nonlocal extension of consciousness" to benefit another person. More adventurous (or foolhardy) individuals, especially those who are pursuing careers in shamanism, seek contact with spirit entities who supposedly assist their healing efforts.

The desire for knowledge and power has been universal throughout human history, but even more compelling and enduring has been the lure of transcending the earthbound limits of the five senses and normal waking consciousness. This was, indeed, the basis of the first temptation as described in the book of Genesis. The benefits of disobeying God, purred the serpent, would be twofold: "You will not surely die" and "You will be like God" (Genesis 3:4-5). The tragic consequences of the first humans acting on those false promises have been plainly evident ever since, not only in the Scriptures but in the daily news as well.

A Final Word of Caution

Our look at the underpinnings of life energy therapies has raised a strong concern that those who claim to manipulate *chi, prana* and the others are, knowingly or not, helping to forge a compelling link between our primal desire to recover from illness (or maximize our overall health) and an Eastern or New Age mystical worldview. For this reason we strongly urge that such therapists be avoided, whether they use needles, massage, light touch, hand passes, arm pulling or any other maneuver.[24]

Why such a hard-nosed stand?

First, those who use such techniques have strayed far from the mainstream of objective knowledge about the human body. Their "science" is based on conjecture, subjective impressions, unreliable data, altered states of consciousness and the precepts of ancient religions. It is indeed unlikely that we will ever see a review article on the flow of *prana* in *Scientific American* or recognition by the NIH of the importance of balancing *chi*. Despite frequent efforts to link life energy to quantum physics, no reputable scientific organization endorses any such connection. We challenge anyone who is involved in this type of therapy to take a hard look at its origins, its underlying assumptions and the nature of its supporting evidence.

Second, the literature promoting life energies consistently proclaims, embraces or at the very least acknowledges the validity of Eastern and New Age mysticism. As a result, energy therapists, whether they intend to or not, are carrying out what is for all practical purposes a form of religious practice and are conditioning their patients to accept its underlying assumptions. (Some practitioners actually enter a trancelike state in order to become a channel to direct their life energy of choice into a client.) The idea of the healer manipulating invisible energy in another person may sound innocuous, but the results may be anything but trivial. Brooks Alexander, who founded the Christian research organization Spiritual Counterfeits Project in the 1970s, sounded this warning during the heyday of the holistic health movement:

> It is not difficult to see that . . . psychic manipulation could turn an otherwise benign form of treatment into a spiritual booby-trap. The nature of the doctor-patient relationship implicitly involves a kind of trust in and submission to the healer on many levels. . . . To accept the passive stance of "patient" before a practitioner who exercises spiritual power (either in his own right or as a channel for other influences) could easily result in spiritual derangement or bondage.[25]

All things considered, it is unsettling to see committed Christians practicing life energy therapies. These practitioners typically believe that *chi, prana,* meridians and *chakras* are neutral components of God's creation (similar to electricity and radio waves) and are available for anyone to use. But they either ignore the roots of these ideas or believe—mistakenly, in our opinion—that they can separate the "truth" about energy flow from all of the mystical trappings. The products of natural science—the technologies of electronics, biochemistry and many others—can be validated anywhere in the world by experiments whose results are not tied to the religious beliefs of the researcher. But the "technology" of life energy is defined entirely by the religious belief systems of its originators and promoters.

Christian energy balancers present us with a paradox. They profess a reliance on the Bible as the basis of their faith and yet they carry out the practices of a worldview that contradicts the core teachings of the Scriptures they claim to follow. They are no doubt sincere both in their faith and in their desire to help others, but unfortunately they fail to see the implications of the ideas they promote. To these therapists we offer a heartfelt challenge: take a long look at the world of life energies and your involvement with them. Do you feel comfortable promoting Eastern mysticism, supporting the notion that "all is one" and helping usher in a new age of "miracles" and magic? If not, then it is time to consider limiting your practice to therapies that do not contradict the cornerstone of your faith.

7

GOING NATURAL
The Herb & Supplement Boom

*I*f our world at the dawn of a new millennium looked anything like the visions of the future concocted in the first decades of the last century, most of us would be buzzing around gleaming skyscrapers in our hovercrafts, reveling in our toil-free lifestyle and feasting on artificial nutrients delivered by robotic servants. Or if one subscribed to the bleaker views of more recent years (exemplified by films such as *Blade Runner*), we would be surrounded by unending vistas of urban decay, darkness and eternal rain brought on by overpopulation and pollution-spewing industry. In either case trees, parks, waterfalls, flowers, blue sky and green grass would be nowhere in sight. Obviously neither of these visions bears any resemblance to the world in which we now live. But it is of no small significance that our culture's general outlook on "scientific progress" has, in just a few decades, shifted from naive optimism to caution, suspicion and even outright cynicism.

The same transition could be charted for opinions of "medical miracles," especially medications. In the 1950s new pharmaceutical products were often called wonder drugs. But today's informed patients are frequently more concerned about the risks and side effects, not to mention the cost, of the latest arrivals in their doctors' armamentarium. For this and many other reasons, at least once every week (if not every day) a primary care physician is likely to hear the following question: "Is there anything I can take for this problem that is more *natural?*"

Who would have thought that nature, like a tortoise overtaking a hare, would at the end of the twentieth century take the lead in the race for attention from persons seeking greater health? If you doubt that this has occurred, take a stroll down an aisle or two in the local supermarket (and not just the health food store), roam around the Internet or merely listen to a Christian radio station on any given Saturday morning. *Natural* has become a powerful, if not always entirely legitimate, marketing buzzword for all sorts of products and services. Describing a food, supplement or treatment as "natural"—or better yet, "all natural"—has become shorthand in our culture for "It can't possibly hurt you" and "It's definitely good for you." By implication, any product for our consumption that is artificial, synthetic or otherwise created or modified by human intervention is suspect. This has become evident not only in the realm of foods and supplements but also in health care in general, as many alternative therapies have effectively positioned themselves as more "natural" than their conventional counterparts.

There are elements both of truth and distortion in such impressions. Conventional physicians would readily agree that a major percentage of the problems they see every day would respond dramatically to measures patients could do on their own—losing excess weight, quitting smoking or starting a consistent exercise routine, for example. Such efforts are entirely natural in that they can produce the desired results without a prescription or other medical interventions. Furthermore, most conventional practitioners will readily endorse the value of "tincture of time" in managing many problems they see.

So what might reasonably be considered a natural approach to treating or preventing illness? Opinions will vary, of course, but we would find little disagreement about the following ingredients:

☐ a regular supply of high-quality food from a variety of sources (fruits, vegetables, meats, grains and—for those who can digest it without difficulty—dairy)

☐ uncontaminated food, water and air

☐ regular aerobic exercise—at least a half hour daily

☐ an adequate amount, and satisfactory quality, of sleep

☐ maintenance of weight within reasonable boundaries

☐ basic hygiene: regular bathing and grooming

☐ a clean, safe, temperature-regulated environment

☐ healthy, supportive relationships

☐ meaningful, satisfying work

☐ increased rest during an illness (such as the flu)

☐ increased fluids during certain types of illnesses or medical conditions

☐ vitamin supplementation, at least for some individuals (for example, pregnant women) and conditions (such as pernicious anemia)

☐ avoidance of tobacco and "recreational" drugs

☐ limited use of alcoholic beverages

☐ avoidance of high-risk behavior (including sexual misadventures)

☐ freedom from the presence or threat of violence

☐ a meaningful spiritual life

Pursuing goals such as these is certainly not the exclusive province of the alternative medicine movement. Nevertheless, in everyday conventional practice physicians tend to devote less time and attention to such basic concerns of daily living and instead gravitate toward the diagnosis and treatment of disorders such as diabetes and coronary artery disease that represent more specific targets. Alternative practitioners in general have been more enthusiastic about promoting lifestyle changes that they feel will enhance health and prevent disease. Yet in so doing many have demonstrated a paradoxical orientation toward what should be a natural approach to health.

Promoters of alternative medicine stress that getting back to basics with diet, exercise and health-enhancing behavior is preferable to prescriptions and other medical interventions. Given the proper fuel, environment and basic support, they say, the body's internal wisdom will keep it healthy or the body will heal itself if some sort of imbalance or illness occurs. Or will it? If one believes many of the voices promoting "natural health and healing," it would appear that the body needs a considerable amount of help to function properly, even with the best of surroundings. Some contend that members of different food groups must be combined in specific ways in order to be absorbed properly. Over the past century a host of chiropractors have asserted that the spinal column needs adjustment on a regular basis so that the nervous system (or the Innate Intelligence) can govern the body's functions properly. Traditional healing systems from all parts of the world teach that any number of internal or environmental events can disrupt the flow of invisible "life energy," despite its apparent—or even divine—intelligence. A number of voices in alternative medicine (including that of Andrew Weil, whom we will discuss in the next chapter) proclaim that we need to override our normal patterns of breathing with specific techniques that are purportedly better than doing what comes naturally.

All of these (and many other) proposed addenda to our daily routines have impacted our culture to varying degrees, but none as dramatically as the use of nutritional supplements. Indeed one could argue that the use of vitamins, herbs and other plant-derived substances to prevent and treat illness is what comes to mind most often when one uses the phrase "natural medicine." No other arena of alternative medicine has seen as spectacular a growth, whether measured by number of users or the amount of money they spend. While it rarely carries the spiritual baggage that weighs so heavily in invisible energy therapies, the widespread promotion of nutritional supplements in the public square brings with it a gamut of potential benefits and pitfalls.

Expanding Markets

Instead of regular tortilla chips, why not try St. John's Wort Tortilla Chips to lift your spirits at the end of a long day? Tired of greasy onion rings that may clog the arteries in your brain? How about some Gingko Biloba Rings (actually made from potatoes) to improve your mental function? Feeling a little tense at the party? A bowl of Kava Kava Corn Chips might just mellow you out. In an obvious effort to climb aboard the bandwagon of the exploding herbal medicine business, Robert's American Gourmet Snacks is producing these and other alternative snacks. The company also makes Cats Claw Crunch, containing a Peruvian herb, and Personality Puffs, human-shaped snacks containing rice, corn and some edible flowers with a pinch of St. John's wort and ginkgo biloba thrown in for good measure. Designed by a team of dietitians, herbalists, aromatherapists, a Zen master and a psychologist, the Puffs also feature some suggested steps toward psychological improvement printed right on the package.

Robert's is not the only company producing what have been dubbed "functional foods." Personal Health Development produces Think! Interactive Root Beer, containing ginkgo biloba, ginseng and an assortment of other herbs and vitamins intended to create a sense of calm mixed with stamina and concentration. For those who would like a little succor in their soup bowl, Hain's split pea soup contains about one hundred milligrams of St. John's wort per serving. If the sniffles are at hand, the same company also makes—what else?—chicken broth containing echinacea.

So what's wrong if snacks contain not only herbs that enhance flavor but some that improve emotional outlook as well? Robert Ehrlich, a former Wall Street trader who now heads Robert's American Gourmet Snacks, has stated (perhaps with tongue in or near the cheek), "This innovative approach to incorporating psychological well being through tasty snack foods is part of our company's long-term approach to marketing a complement of social benefits along with our products. If nothing else, the Personality Puffs should create less road rage." However, some nutritionists and clinicians are not amused by this marketing ploy. Psychiatrist Norman Rosenthal, an authority on the use of St. John's wort to treat depression, said of the St. John's wort chips, "They're just ridiculous . . . like having a penicillin pie or an antibiotic apple strudel. If people are really feeling depressed or anxious they should not depend on a potato chip."[1] In fact, based on current therapeutic guidelines and the amount of St. John's wort contained in a bag of the chips (a one-ounce bag contains an average of 150 milligrams of the herb), one would have to consume six bags per day—a whopping 840 calories' worth—for the better part of a month in order to notice any benefit.

This effort to promote snack foods as a form of natural medicine epitomizes the potential and the problems associated with the spectacular boom in the herb and supplement industry over the past decade. At face value it would appear that Americans have become enamored with the prospect of treating common problems—chronic fatigue, digestive disorders, depression, the effects of aging, sexual malfunctions and many others—using nondrug remedies they can buy and try on their own. (In this regard they have lagged behind their counterparts in Western Europe, for whom herbs have long been a common part of the medical landscape.) But if a trip down the supplement aisle at a local supermarket or the proliferation of advertisements, infomercials, articles and books on this subject is not convincing, consider the cash flow.

According to the landmark study on alternative therapies published in the November 11, 1998, *Journal of the American Medical Association (JAMA)*, between 1990 and 1997 there was a 380 percent rise in the use of herbal remedies and a 130 percent increase in high-dose vitamin use in the United States.[2] The study also estimated that $5.1 billion (all out of pocket) was spent on herbal remedies in 1997. Two weeks later *Time* magazine ran a cover article called "The Herbal Medicine Boom." The November 23, 1998, cover read, "It's great business, but is it good for what ails us?" *Time* indicated that American consumers had spent more than $12 billion on supplements of all types in 1997 (more than double that sold in 1994), and current estimates place the number of Americans using herbal supplements at 60 to 72 million.[3]

It should come as no surprise that this dramatic increase in the use of supplements, and of herbal preparations in particular, has caught the attention of the conventional medical establishment. Physicians who have traditionally received little or no formal training in herbal remedies are now reading up on this subject, either because their patients have been asking them questions they can't answer or because their patients have not mentioned their use of herbs and supplements but have had an adverse reaction or interaction with another drug. Mainstream medical journals are now including more articles dealing with herbs, although the general tone of these has been far more cautionary (focusing especially on drug-herb interactions) than promotional.[4] Needless to say, most physicians now routinely ask patients about their use of supplements, especially herbal preparations, as part of a routine history.

In addition, the pharmaceutical industry has decided to wake up and smell the kava kava. Traditionally it has been assumed that there would be little incentive for mainstream drug companies to evaluate the clinical benefits of herbal preparations. After all, the cost of researching and developing a drug and passing FDA muster to bring a new prescription drug to market can run upwards of $200 to $250 million. In the case of a successful drug, this investment can be recovered during several years of patent protection. But why spend a fortune to prove that echinacea can shorten colds when this herb cannot be patented? Under the current federal rules (specifically the Dietary Supplement Health and Education Act of 1994), an herb or supplement need not run the FDA's gauntlet for approval as long as a specific disease treatment claim is not being made. More importantly, major drug manufacturers have an important name recognition advantage, at least among physicians, and the resources to ensure quality control. As a result, Warner Lambert, a major pharmaceutical house, has issued a number of herbal products (including St. John's wort, ginkgo biloba and saw palmetto) under its new Quanterra label and dispatched sales representatives to promote them to doctors with an attention-grabbing message: if your patients are going to use these products, it is important to know that they can expect consistency and quality. Centrum, a familiar multivitamin label manufactured by Whitehall-Robins (makers of Advil, among many other products), has also introduced several herbal products. Ditto for the herbal products from One-a-Day Vitamins, which are made by Bayer (as in aspirin).

The Good, the Bad and the Natural

What's good about the widespread promotion and use of herbal therapies?

☐ There are no doubt a significant number of remedies from the herbal realm—many yet to be discovered—that can help prevent disease, relieve symptoms and effectively treat illness.

☐ Herbal remedies may prove to be useful adjuncts to conventional treatments, or even be superior to them in some cases.

☐ Herbal treatments may affect health problems through biological mechanisms that are not currently addressed by conventional medications.

☐ A person's interest in using herbs may lead to a more proactive approach to health.

☐ Herbal preparations are generally less pharmacologically potent than their counterparts on the drug shelf (whether prescription or over-the-counter) and thus are less likely to cause toxic or fatal effects.

These assets of herbal therapies are not at all trivial, and undoubtedly during the coming decade we will see even more widespread use of herbs. But there are nevertheless some problems inherent in the current widespread promotion and use of herbal remedies. They are, as a matter of fact, the same kinds of problems that are inherent in the widespread promotion and use of *all* drugs, both prescription and nonprescription.

Safety issues. A widespread but unrealistic assumption regarding herbs and supplements holds that they are "natural" and thus cannot be harmful. As Socrates could attest, the natural herbs commonly known as hemlock *(Conium maculatum* and *Cicuta maculata)* can definitely prove fatal if ingested. Whenever one or more biologically active compounds are concentrated or otherwise compiled into a pill, tonic or other concoction, they should be looked upon as a medication, with both benefits and hazards to be considered. Like any other drug, an herbal preparation may provoke an allergic response or have direct toxic effects, depending upon the dose, duration of use and sensitivity of the individual taking it. The preparation most commonly cited in this regard is ephedra (or *ma huang*), which contains various quantities of ephedrine, a drug once commonly included in oral asthma medications. Ephedra has been included in a variety of products marketed as decongestants, energy boosters and athletic performance enhancers.[5] While ephedrine does indeed dilate airways, it is also notorious for provoking a host of stimulant side effects: tremors, palpitations (a feeling that the heart is pounding), nervousness, elevated blood pressure or even more serious events—heart attack, stroke and seizures.

The other side effect issue is the potential for adverse interactions between herbal preparations and other drugs. For example, ginkgo biloba contains ingredients that inhibit the action of platelets (the component of blood that initiates clotting), which may lead to spontaneous bleeding episodes. These may be particularly hazardous when one is already taking coagulation inhibitors such as Coumadin or aspirin. The Eisenberg alternative medicine study from November 1998 noted that "nearly 1 in 5 individuals taking prescription medication also was taking herbs, high-dose vitamin supplements, or both. Extrapolations to the total US population suggest that an estimated 15 million adults are at risk for potential adverse interactions involving prescription medications and herbs or high-dose vitamin supplements. This figure includes nearly 3 million adults aged 65 years or older." Unfortunately, the vast majority of adverse interactions are unlikely to be reported, even if they are recognized as such by patient or physician. The same article pointed out that "no adequate mechanism currently is in place to collect relevant surveillance data to document the extent to which the potential for drug-herb and drug-vitamin interaction is real or imaginary."[6]

In all fairness it could be reasonably argued that drug-herb interactions would be less of a problem if our population used far more herbs and far fewer drugs. When it comes to adverse effects and fatalities, herbal remedies (at least for now) are not even in the same league with conventional medications. Perhaps the most alarming estimate of this problem was published in the April 15, 1998, issue of *JAMA*. Over three decades University of Toronto researchers analyzed the data from thirty-nine separate U.S. studies of adverse drug reactions either causing hospitalization or occurring in hospitalized patients. Extrapolating their results to the year 1994, they estimated that approximately 2.2 million people experienced serious reactions (resulting in hospitalization, permanent disability or death) and that some 106,000 were fatal.[7] What was more sobering was that these reactions were not the result of noncompliance, overdose, drug abuse, therapeutic failure or errors (such as wrong drug, wrong dose, wrong time or wrong patient) made by hospital personnel. This statistic would place adverse drug reactions as the fourth leading cause of death in the United States, after coronary artery disease, cancer and stroke.

Not surprisingly, the Toronto study results were widely disseminated in the media, especially among websites and periodicals promoting alternative therapies. However, an editorial published in the same edition of *JAMA* pointed out that the statistics might be inflated because all of the studies analyzed were from teaching hospitals, where patients' cases are more complicated, and the patients are generally sicker than their counterparts in community hospitals. Another factor that escaped the notice of the press is that the lead researcher in the study, Bruce Pomeranz, Ph.D., is the author of numerous studies and books on acupuncture and is admittedly fascinated by alternative medicine. In a 1996 interview for the journal *Alternative Therapies in Health and Medicine,* Dr. Pomeranz referenced his yet-to-be-published drug reaction study and concluded, "I believe that the side effects of drugs are the raison d'être [the reason for being] for alternative medicine."[8]

Nevertheless, even if the calculations in this article were two or three times too high, the order of magnitude of serious reactions to medications, even when properly used, is still breathtaking. Without question, one of the strongest potential benefits of the rise of alternative medicine in this generation may be a more measured approach to the use of potent medications, whether initiated by patients or by their physicians.

The hype factor. We have already described in chapter two an all-too-common practice among promoters of supplements of all types (herbs, vitamins and blends of various ingredients): their tendency to proclaim that their products are literally "good for what ails you." If one believes their books, brochures, infomercials and testimonials, a host of "completely natural" products can improve an equally impressive list of symptoms with miraculous speed and a complete lack of side effects. Very often the explanations for these feats stretch credibility to the breaking point, using vague concepts such as "detoxifying the body," "cleansing the colon" and "building up the immune system." In so doing, they disseminate distortions and general misinformation regarding the human body and how it functions. But as long as there is no claim to treat a specific disease, these promotions remain within the bounds of the 1994 Dietary Supplement Health and Education Act (DSHEA). Even so, the boundary between a "health support" and a disease treatment claim often becomes hazy, especially during testimonials when an enthusiastic satisfied customer describes how her rheumatoid arthritis subsided or her ulcerative colitis disappeared after she took the product.

Critics of conventional medicine often correctly point out that the pharmaceutical industry unleashes vast sums to sell their products to physicians and the general public. With annual expenditures on prescriptions in the United States reaching the $80 billion level, and with the cost of bringing a new medication to the marketplace typically in the $200 million range, medications are definitely big business. A *New York Times* article noted that in 1998 drug companies spent more than $5 billion in sending an army of some fifty-six thousand representatives into doctors' offices and hospitals, then spent another billion on a variety of marketing events for physicians. Critics also note that doctors frequently learn about the products they prescribe primarily through drug company representatives and literature, including prescribing information compiled each year in the *Physicians' Desk Reference* (or *PDR*, as it is commonly called). Isn't this just another form of hype, only on a grander scale?

In one sense, yes. Drug companies are determined to portray their products in the best possible light, especially in comparison with similar medications from their competitors. The difference is that the claims that may be made by ads and representatives are tightly regulated by the FDA based upon the evidence presented to it, and serious penalties are imposed if anyone strays outside agreed-upon boundaries. Even the *PDR*, which some misconstrue as a giant compendium of drug advertisements, contains product information that is nothing more or less than that demanded by the FDA. If any manufacturer claimed that one of its products "cleanses the body of toxins," for example, there would be hell (and the FDA) to pay.

Nevertheless, even though the marketing claims made by drug companies are highly constrained, physicians all too often base their prescribing habits on this information rather than on evenhanded analysis from unbiased sources. As a result, they are prone to prescribe the "latest and greatest" products, which also happen to be the ones the companies are most anxious to disseminate widely (and thus recoup their development costs). Unfortunately, these may not be the most economical for the patient, let alone the optimal choice. In the case of antibiotics, what's newest is also frequently more potent and widely effective than older products (the good news) but also more likely to be overused (the bad news). As a result, common bacteria such as the pneumococcus, which for decades was noted for its willingness to roll over and play dead in the presence of plain penicillin, now are dangerously resistant to a broad range of antibiotics.

Quality control. One of the greatest challenges for the supplement industry (and to some degree, alternative medicine in general) has been that of addressing shortcomings in the content, potency, purity and general quality of many products now flooding the shelves. For herbal products the problem begins with the number of variables that affect what eventually enters the intestinal tract. The type of plant, where and how it was grown, when it was harvested, how it has been concentrated and in what form it is selected by the consumer—tincture, tablet, tea, by itself or combined with other compounds—all impact what it may or may not accomplish. And those variables also don't reflect how carefully the manufacturer controls and standardizes its flow of products, nor whether the label accurately reflects what sits inside the container.

A classic example of this problem was described in a series of articles published by the *Los Angeles Times* in September 1998. The *Times* commissioned an independent laboratory to test samples of St. John's wort from ten different companies, comparing the potency of the active ingredient (hypericum) in the pill with what was listed on the label. The results were eye-opening: the potency ranged from 20 percent to 140 percent of the amount stated on the label, and half of the brands tested contained less than 80 percent.[9]

The problem of accuracy in labeling has been more complicated by the availability of herbs in formats that offer intensely variable concentrations. One *Consumer Reports* study of ginseng products, for example, found a fifty-eightfold difference among brands in the active ingredients present.[10] To make matters more hazardous for the consumer, there are case reports of preparations, especially Chinese herbal or *ayurvedic* mixtures, altered by the presence of adulterants (such as pesticides), drugs (such as diazepam, the generic form of Valium) and substitutions of key ingredients. Herbal expert Varro Tyler, one of the most widely respected authorities on the subject and author of *The Honest Herbal,* has pointed out that many side effects attributed to ginseng have probably been caused by adulteration or substituted ingredients.[11]

Needless to say, the herb and supplement boom has come to resemble a combination of the California Gold Rush and Dodge City—a lot of new money to be made, an army of prospectors jumping into the field and no sheriff in sight. Indeed in many respects this situation is not unlike the state of affairs one hundred years ago, when patent medicines and nostrums were widely marketed to a willing public, claims were spectacular, proof consisted of testimonials from satisfied customers, and the bottles sold at the medicine show contained who knew what. Today some twenty thousand dietary supplement products are sold in the United States. Unlike prescription and nonprescription drugs, which are tightly regulated by the FDA, no organization, governmental or otherwise, is directly responsible for ensuring the efficacy, quality and safety of herbs and supplements. Proposals that the FDA more strictly regulate dietary supplements have been greeted with strong resistance from manufacturers and consumers and with little enthusiasm from Congress. At present the FDA can remove a product from the market only when it has been clearly shown to be hazardous to the public.

Many critics of our current system have contrasted it with European, and especially German, management of herbal products. In 1978 the German Federal Health Agency authorized an organization called Commission E to gather information from a variety of sources and formulate reports on the safety and efficacy of plant and herbal products. (More than three hundred of these monographs have been translated into English and are available in the United States.)[12] Based on Commission E findings, products are characterized as "Approved" or "Unapproved," tested and regulated under government auspices, and sold only in standardized forms. In addition, German physicians receive formal instruction in the appropriate use of herbal remedies—a practice especially valuable in light of the fact that 80 percent of German doctors prescribe or dispense herbs, accounting for more than 10 percent of all prescriptions.[13] Some have argued that the Commission E materials could be the basis for regulating dietary supplements in the United States. But others have raised concerns that the German criteria for approving a substance are not as rigorous as those imposed by the FDA on drugs to be marketed here. However, compared with our current Wild West environment, adopting the German approach appears entirely sensible and would represent a vast improvement.

The "pill for every ill" mentality. One of the most important criticisms of conventional practitioners is that they often work like carpenters whose only tool is a hammer: they can be very effective as long as the problem involves a nail. A combination of training, personal experience, time pressure, the concerted efforts of drug companies and, very significantly, the expectations of patients has resulted in a widespread tendency for medication to be the first line of treatment for almost every problem or symptom. (Contrary to the opinions of some, this is not driven by the profit motive on the physician's part. Few doctors dispense prescription drugs from their office, and no one receives a kickback or bonus from manufacturers for prescribing one brand over another.) Medications are simply much easier (and more importantly, much quicker) solutions for all concerned. It takes a lot less time for the doctor to prescribe a sleeping medication than to explore all of the reasons why sleep might be delayed or interrupted. It also takes a lot less effort for the patient to swallow a tablet than to do relaxation techniques, resolve some persistent conflicts or reconfigure his or her entire lifestyle. The same observation holds for a multitude of other concerns: headaches, obesity, elevated blood cholesterol levels and anxiety, to name but a few.

But the proliferation and promotion of dietary supplements of all types can easily fuel the same tendency. A quip in one article regarding herbal remedies says it all: "Name an ailment. Any ailment. Somewhere in the world there's an herbal remedy suggested for it."[14] One need only listen to the weekly parade of infomercials on many Christian radio stations every weekend to confirm this suspicion. One after another features either a single product that resolves almost every ailment or else an alternative practitioner who quickly diagnoses callers' complaints and then offers a sure-fire recipe of "natural" products that are conveniently available through the practitioner's clinic or toll-free number.

Needless to say, the desire to find the quick and easy solution to a problem is not unique to those who visit the conventional doctor's office. Many patients find it much easier to manage their symptoms with "all natural" remedies that they can swallow rather than change habits and deal with the issues of life. Those who seek help at many alternative clinics may walk out not with a handful of prescriptions to be filled but instead with enough supplements to fill a tackle box. These might include combinations for general "nutritional support" as well as several individual remedies for specific problems. Often these products are sold out of the office (and thus paid for directly out of pocket rather than through insurance coverage), and their ongoing use—to the tune of one or two hundred dollars per month or even more—is strongly encouraged by the practitioner and his or her staff.

Dubious necessity ("How did we ever live without X?"). Closely related to the "pill for every ill" orientation is the conviction that a reasonable amount and variety of food is not adequate for the average individual to remain healthy. Despite the unprecedented availability of foods from all nutritional groups in most Western nations over the past few decades, some would have us believe that we cannot thrive (or survive) without handfuls of daily vitamins and supplements. The usual explanation for this apparent shortfall is that modern foods are of poorer quality and more likely to contain toxins, hormones and other threats to life and limb, compared with their counterparts in the "good old days."

Yet in spite of these dire warnings and the vast sums spent every year to ward off dietary deficiencies, mainstream scientific organizations continue to take a very conservative posture regarding the use of supplements. For example, in its statement on dietary supplements, the Food and Nutrition Science Alliance (FANSA)—a partnership of four professional societies, including the American Dietetic Association—notes without fanfare that "a daily multivitamin may help some people meet their nutritional needs."[15] Pregnant women, for example, are usually given prenatal vitamins that contain enough folic acid to prevent a congenital deformity called a neural tube defect in the newborn. Supplemental calcium may help elderly women reduce the risk of osteoporosis (thinning of bone). Women with heavy menstrual flow may need additional iron to prevent anemia. But professional organizations that analyze peer-reviewed research and address nutritional issues without financial or ideological agendas have been consistent in advocating sound food choices, and not the wholesale use of supplements, for the general population to attain nutritional health.

Sanctified products ("God's pharmacy"). Among evangelical Christians it is not at all unusual for the use of herbs and dietary supplements to be given some degree of spiritual significance. A product or formula is often described as "God-given," and its dissemination may be characterized as a ministry for restoring health to the body of Christ, not to mention the general public. The old adage that "Nature has a remedy" is often adjusted for Christian audiences by referring to supplements and herbs as "God's pharmacy." Such remedies are said to be preferred over medications created by human effort because they are based in nature (God's creation) and are not harmful. Some even suggest that God has provided specific treatments for any and all human disease, if we would only put forth the effort to find and utilize them.

It is indeed true that a wide variety of vegetables, fruits and grains growing on our planet (not to mention animal products) are capable of keeping us alive and well when consumed in appropriate amounts. In addition, a number of plant products contain compounds that improve certain disorders. Perhaps the most frequently cited of these is foxglove, which was identified generations ago as helpful for treating what was once called "dropsy"—fluid retention caused by congestive heart failure, which swelled legs and impaired breathing. Eventually the compound digitalis was isolated as the ingredient in foxglove that improved heart function, and its mechanism of action was identified. More precise and predictable formulations took a great deal of guesswork out of treating many heart conditions. It is certainly appropriate to offer thanks to God for creating the foxglove plant, but it would also be unwise to insist that foxglove should displace digitalis in the intensive care unit. God has given us not only the raw materials of his creation but also the curiosity and intellect to work with them in ways that can vastly improve our lives. As a result, we wear fabrics instead of animal skins and fig leaves, we live in homes and apartments rather than caves, and we also use medications—and herbal preparations—that are the result either of modifying and manipulating raw materials or of designing compounds from scratch.

It is naive to assume that every product of modern science is a marvelous breakthrough without drawbacks or risks, and it is equally naive to assume that remedies derived from plant products are not only healthful but uniformly superior to those fashioned by human effort. The latter view fails to acknowledge the fact that we live in a fallen world. Presumably such a perspective would have applied before the events described in the third chapter of the book of Genesis. But humanity's willful rebellion against the Creator has not only tainted every person born on this planet (with one very important exception) but also resulted in a world that is not uniformly friendly to human beings. In the book of Romans the apostle Paul states plainly that in the wake of this rebellion "the creation was subjected to frustration" and "the whole creation has been groaning as in the pains of childbirth right up to the present time" (Romans 8:20, 22).

Eight Keys to the Wise Use of Supplements, Herbs and Other "Natural" Medicines

For the most part, the keys for using "natural" medicines wisely are the same as those for the wise use of any medicine, with a generous dose of common sense added. Please note that in this section we are focused primarily on dietary supplements, herbs and other products that are taken internally or applied to the skin. Many other alternative therapies—acupuncture, relaxation techniques, massage and so forth, which are discussed in other sections of this book—are also commonly billed as "natural," but the term is most commonly applied to the materials we have been considering here.

1. Do not assume that everything promoted as "natural" is necessarily safe or even beneficial for your particular need. Some supplements and herbs can have toxic effects, especially in large doses, and a number of them interact with medications (and each other). Similarly, both prescription and nonprescription drugs can have toxic effects and interactions with one another, even when they have been deemed safe and effective by the FDA and appropriately recommended by a competent practitioner.

2. Weigh the sources of information about anything you are thinking about using. All too often, such a decision is based solely on the advice or recommendation of a friend, a relative, a radio program or even a teenage sales clerk. The personal testimony of others, especially those we trust, can be compelling, but the fact that a certain remedy worked for someone else does not mean that it will work for you—or that it works at all. A particular symptom or disease can change for the better for many reasons, including (most importantly) the body's own healing capabilities, with or without supplements, medications or anything else. To assume that a specific treatment resulted in the healing is known as the post hoc fallacy— the assumption that if one event follows another, the first caused the second.

So who and what might be a reliable source of information?

☐ Books that provide a balanced view of the benefits and potential risks of using various supplements. Examples include *The American Pharmaceutical Association Practical Guide to Natural Medicines* as well as Varro Tyler's evenhanded books, *The Honest Herbal* and *Herbs of Choice: The Therapeutic Use of Phytomedicinals.* A newer book, *Alternative Medicine: The Christian Handbook,* includes an evidence-based review of the use of herbs and supplements.[16]

☐ Websites with balanced and responsible information. Examples include <www.herbalgram.org> and <www.NaturalDatabase.com>.

☐ A pharmacist or a physician (ideally one who knows your medical history) who has at least some knowledge and an open mind about the use of supplements and herbs. As already noted, there are a number of potential interactions between herbs and drugs, and it is a bad idea to make a solo foray into the realm of supplements if you have a number of medical problems.

Whom (and what) should you specifically avoid as a source of information?

☐ A retailer, website, radio program, friend or relative who appears bent on selling one or more products, especially if they are promoted as cure-alls.

☐ A practitioner who diagnoses a variety of deficiencies (especially by dubious methods, such as arm-pulling techniques or mysterious devices) and then happens to have all of the remedies you need for sale at his or her office.

☐ Anyone who claims to have a "secret formula" that no one else knows about. If the individual also claims to be persecuted by the AMA, the FDA or any other organization, head for the exit as quickly as possible.

☐ A conventional physician who will not listen to you and answer your questions, or one who maintains a "My way or the highway" philosophy of practice. If the response to your inquiries—on any subject—is a dismissive shrug or a rapid termination of the visit, you may need to find another doctor.

3. Inform any health care professional who is caring for you—whether your personal physician, an emergency room doctor, the surgeon and anesthesiologist if you are having a procedure done, even your pharmacist—what types of nutritional supplements you are taking. Even if a conventional doctor is not particularly interested in this type of approach, he or she still needs this information. A number of medical conditions and the effects of many drugs may be altered by the presence of certain herbs in the system. Similarly, be sure to speak with your pediatrician or family practitioner before giving your child a supplement or herbal preparation. If you are pregnant, the same goes for any product you might consider taking (in this case, check with whoever is providing your prenatal care). In general, the risks and benefits of using *any* drug or supplement in an infant younger than two years of age, or during pregnancy, should be weighed very carefully. When there is little reliable data available for the substance, the better part of valor usually is to refrain from using it.[17] (By the way, make sure that dietary supplements, like any medication around the house, are completely inaccessible to children.)

4. Beware of the age-old fallacy that "if a little is good, more must be better." Anything—even water, the most "natural" substance on earth—can cause problems if enough of it is swallowed in a short period of time.

5. Find out whether the preparation you are using is intended for short-term or long-term use. For example, Germany's Commission E consensus statement on echinacea (used, among other things, for shortening the duration of colds) has recommended that this herb not be taken for longer than eight successive weeks. This is a common source of misunderstanding with conventional medications as well. Drugs (such as pain relievers) that are intended to be used as symptom-relieving "fire extinguishers" for an immediate problem (such as a headache) can become a permanent fixture in a person's life or even a habit that is difficult to break. Medications that are supposed to be taken routinely to manage a chronic problem (such as drugs to normalize elevated blood pressure) may mistakenly be used sporadically ("I take it when I feel like my blood pressure is up").

6. Be aware of the many factors, including overall quality, that can influence the effect of a product (especially herbs). Fortunately, many of the most popular herbs sold in the United States now come in standardized preparations. In 1998 the *United States Pharmacopeia (USP)*, the official listing of drugs in the U.S., included nine botanical monographs in its *Ninth Supplement* to the *USP National Formulary.* These contained standards for such widely used herbs as chamomile, feverfew, St. John's wort and saw palmetto. According to a November 2, 1998, press release, the *USP* has "identified 21 dietary supplement, botanical and herbal products, that constitute more than 80 percent of the market for such products in the United States, for which it will direct its efforts to maximize the public health impact of the work of its expert volunteers."[18] In general, it is wise to use products from manufacturers who not only use standardized extracts but also provide appropriate information on their labels: the ingredients (including scientific names of herbs), exact amounts present, a batch or lot number, expiration date and name and address of the manufacturer (including a number to call for further information). As we have already noted, a number of mainstream pharmaceutical companies have introduced lines of herbal products, and some of these feature standardized extracts that have been used in multiple studies.

7. *Be wise about possible adverse reactions to any medication or supplement.* Most people assume that a negative response occurring within a few hours or days after starting a new drug or herb must somehow be related to it. In many cases such a connection is in fact likely, while in others the problem is coincidental. Needless to say, it is often difficult to determine whether there is a cause-and-effect relationship between what we take and how we feel later on. When in doubt, it is nearly always appropriate to stop using the product in question, although for a prescription drug the physician who ordered it should be consulted for further input. If it does indeed appear that you have suffered an adverse drug reaction, especially one that requires additional evaluation and treatment, at some point consider reporting the problem to the FDA at 800-332-1088.

8. *Do not assume that the length of time a particular remedy has been in use is a guarantee of its usefulness.* For example, a claim that a particular herb "has been used by the Chinese to treat X for hundreds of years" may be true, but it does not prove that the product actually does anything for that particular problem. More rigorous research methods than "It worked for me" are needed to state with any degree of certainty that a given substance is actually likely to make a meaningful difference in recovery or prevention. The same process, we might add, is worth applying to some "tried and true" conventional remedies as well. For example, recent research has suggested that common cold remedies (containing various combinations of decongestants and antihistamines) that have been used for decades are probably of little benefit in young children. In many cases, the primary effect is that of sedating the infant or child rather than decreasing the amount of nasal drainage. But to the weary parent this may appear to be a major improvement.

8

ANDREW WEIL
Natural Medicine & the Natural Mind

The character of Tom Bombadil appears in the classic J. R. R. Tolkien trilogy The Lord of the Rings. He is a mystery of sorts, in that Tolkien never fully explains Tom's background or place in the fictitious world of Middle-Earth. In many respects Bombadil is a "Father Nature," a kind of master of his domain (the Old Forest) who seemingly possesses a unique communion with the natural world.

So, it would seem, does Andrew Weil, M.D. With his distinctive balding scalp, bushy beard and smiling countenance, he is the most recognizable, and arguably the most widely respected, apologist for alternative medicine in the United States. More important, to the millions who have bought his books, watched his PBS specials and visited his website, he appears to be firmly grounded in, and readily conversant with, both conventional and alternative medicine.

Despite being described in the prestigious *Encyclopaedia Britannica* as a "guru of alternative medicine" (a title he would probably find amusing), Weil does not speak with the ethereal lilt of a saffron-robed mystic or the muddled enthusiasm of a middle-aged flower child. He received his M.D. in 1968 from Harvard Medical School and, in keeping with this distinguished academic pedigree, writes and speaks in a manner that sounds both thoughtful and reasonable. He has spent more than three decades studying phytomedicinals (medications derived from plants) and possesses considerable expertise in that field. He has written nine books since

1972, seven of which (including bestsellers *Spontaneous Healing, Eight Weeks to Optimum Health* and *Eating Well for Optimum Health*) focus primarily on health and healing, and has endorsed or written forewords for countless others. He has appeared on several magazine covers, including *Time,* and his website receives millions of visits every month.[1] He currently serves as director of the program in integrative medicine at the University of Arizona, where he pursues his passion for training physicians to use both conventional and alternative therapies in daily practice.

The task of integrating medicine, of bridging the gap between ancient healing traditions and modern science, is one that Weil not only embraces but feels well suited to carry out. When asked in an interview whether he felt torn between his Harvard medical training and his interest in alternative medicine, he stated, "I really think I'm in the middle. Sometimes I'm attacking traditional medicine, sometimes I'm defending it; sometimes I'm defending alternative medicine and sometimes attacking it, so I think I'm pretty even-handed in my criticism. I'm unique in that I'm not aligned with any one school of thought."[2]

While an exhaustive study of his writings and discourses is beyond the scope of this book, a review of his favorite themes would suggest that Dr. Weil may not be quite as evenhanded as he portrays himself to be. His strongest agendas do not spring from a typical medical career his track has been anything but conventional—but rather from a lifelong interest in altered states of consciousness. He notes in one interview, "I can recall that as I child . . . I was very interested in hypnosis as soon as I read about it. It just fascinated me, and everything that had to do with the mind, and how in changed mental states there was changed physiology, changed body functions—that always interested me terrifically."[3]

In the early 1960s, as a Harvard University undergraduate and journalist for the *Harvard Crimson,* he investigated rumors that certain professors and their students were experimenting with mind-altering drugs. As it turned out, the rumors were true. The drug turned out to be LSD, and as part of the fallout from Weil's articles, two professors lost their jobs. They were none other than Timothy Leary, who ultimately put LSD and the motto "Tune in, turn on and drop out" on the cultural map, and Richard Alpert, who became a major proponent of altered consciousness and New Age thinking under the name Ram Dass. Ironically, at that time Weil was hardly a crusader against mind-altering drugs—and neither is he now.

From Straightland to Stonesville

After graduating from medical school, he spent a year of medical internship in San

Francisco, followed by another at the National Institute of Mental Health (NIMH) in Washington, D.C. Neither of these were banner years for his relationship with conventional medicine. In *Spontaneous Healing* he describes his mindset after completing his internship:

> In 1969, when I finished my basic clinical training, I made a conscious decision not to practice the kind of medicine I had just learned. I did so for two reasons, one emotional and one logical. The first was simply a gut feeling that if I were sick, I would not want to be treated the way I had been taught to treat others, unless there were no alternative. That made me uncomfortable about treating others. The logical reason was that most of the treatments I had learned in four years at Harvard Medical School and one in internship did not get to the root of disease processes. . . . I had learned almost nothing about health and its maintenance, about how to prevent illness.[4]

The year following internship was not much better. His medical school research on the effects of marijuana, which had been published in medical journals in 1968 and 1969 and generated considerable publicity in the press, proved to be a continuing source of conflict within NIMH. He ultimately resigned halfway through a two-year assignment and then sojourned in South Dakota with a Sioux medicine man in order to learn about herbal medicine and methods to alter consciousness without drugs. "On the reservation," he notes, "I participated in sweat lodge ceremonies, grew a beard, and 'dropped out.' " A year later, upon returning home to Virginia and learning that he had been granted conscientious objector status, he was free to pursue a variety of interests: "Suddenly and unexpectedly, I had no obligations and nothing but free time. Over the next year (1970–1971), I started to practice yoga, experiment with vegetarianism, and learn to meditate. I also reflected on events of the recent past and began to write."[5]

The product of this effort was *The Natural Mind,* a forceful manifesto regarding altered states of consciousness and mind-altering drugs. In it Weil proposes that the desire to spend time in states other than normal waking consciousness is deeply ingrained within human beings and that the widespread use of drugs to induce such states (whether alcohol, marijuana, LSD, heroin or anything else that rapidly brings on this effect) is virtually inevitable. Furthermore, he maintains that efforts to suppress drug use through criminalizing it are futile. The book does not so much press for legalization of illicit drugs as call for a complete reorientation of cultural attitudes toward altered consciousness. The pivotal presentation of this idea occurs in two chapters entitled "The Topography of Straightland" and "A Trip to Stonesville." These are not only the centerpiece of *The Natural Mind* but they also set forth Dr. Weil's perspectives on health and medicine, which reverberate through his subsequent books. They are must reading for anyone seeking insight into Weil's philosophical orientation as well as that of much of the alternative medicine movement. They would also be illuminating for anyone who views him as a mainstream adviser on health care, whether personal or societal.

Weil introduces "straight thinking" as ordinary thinking.

> It is what all of us do most of the time with our minds when we are normally alert and functioning in the world. It is what our conventional educational systems reward us for doing well. It is the kind of thinking that predominates in most of the institutions of our society at the present time. We are so used to it that many of us do not suspect the existence of another way of interpreting our perceptions of the world around us.[6]

Straight thinking tends to acquire knowledge through the intellect rather than direct experience. But the intellect is "merely the thought producer of the mind and . . . thoughts are not realities. In order to perceive reality directly, one must sooner or later learn how to abandon the intellect and disengage oneself from the thoughts it produces incessantly."[7] Straight thinking is also tied to the senses, which bring it information about external reality. Not only does this interfere with accessing the "inner reality," whose contents are no less real, but it also leads toward materialism, whose essence is "the attribution of causality to external, physical reality. . . . The problem with formulations of this kind," Weil states, "is simply that they do not work."[8] Furthermore, straight thinking is prone to perceive differences rather than similarities, as distinct from the common experience in altered states of consciousness of the essential unity of all things. Finally, it is Weil's conviction that straight thinking ultimately ends in negativity, pessimism and despair.

In contrast, altered states of consciousness—what Weil likes to call "stoned thinking," whether brought about by mind-altering drugs, meditation, hypnosis, rituals or any other means—are the gateway to benefits beyond measure.

> Stoned thinking is the mirror image of straight thinking. When we step into nonordinary reality even for a moment, we experience things directly, see inner contents rather than external forms, and suddenly find ourselves able to participate in changing things for the better. This other way of interpreting perceptions comes first as episodic flashes, unpredictable, discontinuous. But the more flashes of it one has, the easier it becomes to maintain.[9]

Stoned thinking relies on intuition rather than on intellect alone. In fact, intuition, once trusted, can be fed to the intellect as premises for "very interesting and very useful ideas to guide us." It also allows us to accept the coexistence of opposites that appear to be mutually antagonistic.

The idea that reality manifests itself to us in the guise of pairs of opposites is a very old one. It appears frequently in Oriental philosophies and religions, and in the Western tradition is traceable back to the Garden of Eden, where it takes the form of the Tree of Knowledge of Good and Evil. . . . The problem is not that things have this ambivalent nature, but that our ordinary consciousness cannot accept it. Stoned consciousness, however, is perfectly capable of substituting a both/and formulation for the either/or of the ego. In fact, in altered states of consciousness people often experience pairs of opposites simultaneously and find the experience very worth-while.[10]

Before elaborating on Dr. Weil's applications of straight versus stoned thinking to the world of medicine, it is worth pondering whether these proposals, however artfully set forth, suggest the musings of a very bright but possibly overreaching young medical school graduate. With the passage of nearly three decades, presumably laden with life- and worldview-shaping experiences, one might wonder whether the Dr. Weil who at midlife advises the nation about alternative health care has adjusted any of these youthful viewpoints. His preface to the 1998 edition of *The Natural Mind* speaks for itself:

When I am interviewed by the media on these subjects, reporters frequently ask pointed questions about my earlier work, thinking that I might wish to disown *The Natural Mind* and the two books which followed it. Far from it. The philosophy of my first book is the same philosophy that underlies my writing about health. Just as *The Natural Mind* argues that highs originate within the human nervous system and are elicited or triggered by drugs, so my later works propose that healing responses originate within us and can be elicited or triggered by treatments applied. In fact, the seed of my thinking about conventional and alternative medicine can be found in chapter 7 ["A Trip to Stonesville"] of this book.[11]

As advertised, several themes set forth in *The Natural Mind* reverberate through-out Weil's later (and current) work. Indeed familiarity with these presuppositions helps one to make at least some sense out of the breadth of his opinions about health and healing, many of which sound well reasoned, while others seem enig-matic or even incoherent. When dealing with many everyday aspects of health on the purely physical level, he can be practical and insightful, if at times leaning toward the eccentric. Undoubtedly, it is this side of Weil's material—especially as it is distilled into recommendations such as are found in *Spontaneous Healing* and, in more detailed form, in *Eight Weeks to Optimum Health*—that draws many who might be less inclined to alternative therapies.

Dr. Weil's Health Advisories
Weil's dietary advice is generally straightforward: fewer calories, saturated fats and

transfatty acids (as in margarine, vegetable shortening and common vegetable oils); increased intake of omega-3 fatty acids; more fish and soy foods instead of animal protein; more fruits and vegetables; and more whole-grain products. He rightly rejects the ideologies of "food fascists" who insist that their dietary advice must be strictly followed—or else. He also skillfully debunks fads such as the increasingly popular diet that links nutritional health to one's blood type (A, B, AB or O).[12]

He is worried about the cumulative effects of toxins and pollutants in air, water and food, and he offers several measures—most of them reasonable—that one might take to limit exposure to, or the effects from, these substances. He also warns against exposure to ionizing and ultraviolet radiation, whose risks are well established. In addition, he cautions that the electromagnetic fields generated by familiar appliances such as electric blankets and clock radios may interfere with healing. While the latter are not widely acknowledged as health hazards, at least Weil is addressing possible biochemical changes in tissue and not disturbances in mystical "universal energy."

When dealing with questions about botanical remedies (an area of expertise for him), his approaches are generally straightforward. He is certainly an enthusiastic advocate of their use, especially as an alternative to more potent (and thus potentially more risky) pharmaceuticals. He is particularly interested in "tonics"—substances such as garlic, ginger, green tea and ginseng. These are said to have generalized beneficial effects on bodily functions such as digestion and immunity as well as to help an individual "resist the effects of toxins, stress, and aging on your healing system."[13] Like the vague but promising "function" statements that are currently allowed on the labels of herbal products, Weil's claims for his favorite tonics sound a little too good to be true, but none demand fanciful or mystical mechanisms that represent a departure from known biological mechanisms. Their widespread acceptance among conventional practitioners, however, may require a more convincing body of evidence.

He advocates undertaking a sensible, walking-based exercise program and making room in one's life for flowers, music and art, which are edifying and uplifting. He also recommends regular "news fasts"—a few days (or more) of deliberate isolation from the adrenaline-jolting and attitude-sinking flow of the daily news, most of which is discouraging or overtly alarming. He points out that it is virtually impossible *not* to hear about any truly significant news development that might occur while one is taking one of these time-outs.

Although he has made his mark primarily as a writer rather than as a full-time provider of patient care, Weil quite eloquently identifies many of the pressures of contemporary medical practice and the pitfalls of all too many conventional practitioners: time pressure, which hampers interactions and trusting relationships with patients; overreliance on high-powered and expensive technology (often carried out as "defensive medicine" to prevent a potential lawsuit); skyrocketing costs and the tendency to resort to potent medications or surgery when less drastic approaches might be just as effective.

He defines himself as an "open-minded skeptic" when assessing various alternative therapies, although "selective skeptic" might be a more accurate characterization. For example, his book *Natural Health, Natural Medicine* contains an eloquent and concise refutation of the theory that a host of human ailments are brought on by the common organism *Candida albicans.* Yet while finding the "yeast connection" to be a far-fetched idea, he appears to have no difficulty accepting the length and breadth of traditional Chinese medicine, including tongue and pulse diagnosis, meridians and the manipulation of *chi.*

Weil is generally less impressed with chiropractic than with classical osteopathy. He complains that chiropractors "still take too many X-rays and are too likely to have patients commit to long and costly treatment regimes." He also takes a very conservative view of the scope of chiropractic, clearly not buying the claims of "straight" chiropractors that they can successfully treat all manner of bodily illnesses through manipulation of the spine. In *Spontaneous Healing* he notes, "Chiropractic treatment can be helpful in cases of acute musculoskeletal pain, tension headaches, and recovery from trauma; it is less effective with chronic pain syndromes."[14]

In contrast, he speaks highly of classical osteopathy, as conceived by its nineteenth-century founder, Andrew Taylor Still, and practiced by only a small number of present-day D.O.s (doctors of osteopathy). (He criticizes the majority of D.O.s, whose practice of medicine is virtually indistinguishable from that of conventional M.D.s, for having "sold out" and abandoned their heritage.) He has particularly high regard for an obscure osteopathic practice called "craniosacral therapy," which, as we will describe momentarily, is at least as far-fetched as the straight chiropractor's claim that the key to health is the unimpaired flow of the Innate through the branches of the spinal cord.

Last, Dr. Weil gives at least some credit where it is due by acknowledging conventional medicine's prowess in dealing with acute illness and trauma. "If you have a medical crisis, you go to an allopathic emergency room," he notes in one interview. "If I were in a major car accident, I would not want to be taken to a chiropractor or a shaman."[15] But he is quick to add an opinion that conventional medicine tends to be far less effective, and potentially more toxic, when it deals with many chronic ailments.

Consciousness: The Root of Illness and Healing

At face value these viewpoints about medicine give the impression that Weil is basically a well-trained and open-minded conventional physician who is exploring some new ways to help his patients. However, further reading into *The Natural Mind* confirms that his passion for altered states of consciousness and the perspectives they generate is the foundation upon which his understanding of illness and health (and the means to impact them) are built. For example, Weil uses conventional medicine as a prime example of straight thinking. He sees it as driven by intellect rather than intuition, materialistic, obsessed with treating what it sees (the symptoms) rather than the true causes of illness below the surface and blind to the role of the mind in creating health and sickness. He consistently uses the mildly pejorative term "allopathic medicine" to denote conventional practice, and he states that he rejects allopathy as a theoretical system. "My retrospective impression of allopathy is that it is unable to control well the phenomena of health and illness and that it is often unwittingly productive of methods that intensify manifestations of illness rather than ameliorate them."[16]

Strictly speaking, allopathy is the philosophy of treating illness by counteracting its symptoms, as opposed to homeopathy, which purports to treat illness by giving minute doses of substances that create the same symptoms when given in larger amounts. This narrow definition is in fact an inaccurate characterization of the length and breadth of contemporary medical treatment. Conventional medicine does indeed treat symptoms, but it does so most often for the purpose of providing some relief and comfort to those who are not feeling well. It also treats manifestations of complex processes—for example, hypertension (high blood pressure), which can be the product of a host of physiological factors—that increase the risks for serious consequences if left alone over time.[17]

In attacking what he sees as conventional medicine's wrong-headed focus on the symptoms and manifestations of disease, he declares no less than a comprehensive explanation for the cause of all disease:

> My experiences in allopathic medicine, both as a patient and as a practitioner, have led me to conclude that all illness is psychosomatic. I do not use the word in the sense of "unreal" or "phony," as many allopaths do. Rather, I mean that all illness has both psychic and physical components, and it seems to me that the physical manifestations of illness (including the appearance of germs in tissues) are always effects, while the causes always lie within the realm of the mind, albeit the unconscious mind. In other words, the disease process seems to me to be initiated often by changes in consciousness.[18]

As if to throw down a rhetorical gauntlet before the medical establishment, he applies this insight to infectious disease. According to Weil, microorganisms do not really cause any disease—this is one of the fallacies of straight thinking—but rather merely appear in tissues when there has been a "breakdown in the normal, harmonious balance between the body and the microorganisms surrounding it." He ridicules Koch's Postulates, which were a milestone in understanding the association between infectious agents and specific diseases, as "materialistic nonsense."[19]

While it is true that the state of one's general health and immunity play a significant role in resisting infection, these—and certainly not consciousness alone—are not the only factors that determine who does and does not become ill. Those of us who are not currently afflicted with smallpox, polio, diphtheria and a host of other plagues can only be grateful that the efforts of infectious disease researchers from the nineteenth century onward were not constrained by the dictates of *The Natural Mind*. In a footnote Weil retreats briefly on this subject, noting, "As an example of an area of my own ignorance, I might mention that I have no ready explanation for serious infectious illness in infants and young children," but he finishes the sentence by returning to his prior stance: "which is to say that I do not fully understand the development and workings of the unconscious mind."[20] He could add to his list of problem areas the phenomenon of infectious disease in animals and plants. What sort of consciousness change brings on Dutch elm disease?

If illness is primarily a problem of consciousness, then it would follow that altering it could lead to healing—and much more. These themes have in fact been widely proclaimed in alternative medicine since the days of the holistic health movement and before. Weil offers this insight into the true causes of disease and the nature of "nonallopathic" healing: "My intuitions about disease are: first, that its physical manifestations are mostly caused by nonmaterial factors, in particular by unnatural restraints placed on the unconscious mind; and second, that the limits of what human consciousness can cause in the physical body are far beyond where most of us imagine them."[21]

When viewed through this grid, many of Weil's seemingly contradictory opinions begin to line up more consistently. When a conventional or alternative practice appears to be dealing strictly on the physical level, one generally hears from him a relatively straightforward, and frequently insightful, assessment not only of its risks and benefits but also its reasonableness. But if a practice appears to involve nonmaterial factors in any way, shape or form, especially the impact of the mind on the body, his critical faculties seem to be disengaged.

Some noteworthy examples of this inconsistency may be found in his most recent book, *Eating Well for Optimum Health*.[22] The book consists primarily of relatively straightforward "natural" nutritional guidelines and a number of recipes, seasoned with some noteworthy digressions. For example, Weil makes some pointed and accurate comments about the fantastic, too-good-to-be-true claims made by certain weight loss products:

> The most outrageous of these ads, and I'm sure the most effective at promoting sales, are frequent scenes of lean, attractive people helping themselves to enormous servings of high-fat foods—pizza, cheesy casseroles, cream pies, cakes—and stuffing themselves, comfortable in the knowledge that Fat Trapper is protecting them from absorbing the calories and gaining weight. And, if you order now, you get the companion product to use along with it—Exercise-in-a-Bottle—that will spare you the need of engaging in annoying physical activity. P. T. Barnum would be proud.[23]

He has equally astute comments to offer about the pharmaceutical industry's efforts to create useful drugs to curb appetite.

> Desperate people want magical solutions: a magic formula for eating or, most of all, a magic pill that will yield the desired result without effort or sacrifice. The pharmaceutical industry is well aware that if it could come up with such a product, it would be the best-selling drug of all time. Unfortunately, the track record of the industry in the area of weight loss is not impressive. The drugs it has brought to the market either do not work or work very modestly; those that work best are toxic, causing such problems as addiction, cataracts, and heart damage.[24]

Yet in the same book with these thoughtful comments lies a curious appendix section entitled "The Possibility of Surviving Without Eating." Weil notes, "Shortly after I finished my medical training, I read a delightful book that awakened in me an interest in yoga and Indian religious philosophies: *Autobiography of a Yogi* by Paramahansa Yogananda (1893–1952)." The book contains a photograph of a woman who had allegedly mastered the ability to survive without food, with the following caption: "She employs a certain yogic technique to recharge her body with cosmic energy from the ether, sun, and air." Weil expands on this peculiar claim: "In my own research I have not encountered this technique or any direct evidence of its existence. . . . But there is spectacular, large-scale revival of claims for living without food by the mostly Chinese followers of modern *qigong* master, Yan Xin."[25]

Later in this appendix Weil shares an anecdote about a woman who supposedly abstained from food for eight years through an application of *qi gong* called *bigu*. Rather than stating the obvious—that this story must be mistaken or fabricated (or that the woman was eating while no one was looking!)—Weil proceeds with a surprisingly credulous disclaimer:

> Please bear in mind that I am simply reporting secondhand information here, that I have no direct experience of *bigu,* and cannot vouch for the veracity of any of this

material. I would very much like to know if the studies done by Yan Xin's followers can be replicated by disinterested Western scientists and whether the *bigu* state is real. If so, it is, at least, an anomaly not explainable by prevailing scientific and medical paradigms.[26]

One can only ponder why Weil would entertain such a fanciful idea in an otherwise serious book about nutrition. Presumably his willingness to do so arises from his comfort level with Eastern mysticism and his convictions regarding the mind's untapped capacity to control bodily functions.

He is, as might be expected, keenly interested in the placebo effect. He repeatedly stresses the importance of the observation that at least 30 percent of patients respond to inert substances during controlled experiments, and he argues that this is not an aberration to be rooted out of scientific experiments. Rather, he views the placebo effect as a true healing event arising from the patient's belief and expectations. He thus quite rightly calls for conventional doctors to harness rather than dismiss it, using a trusting relationship to help elicit healing responses from their patients. In a debate with Arnold Relman, M.D., former editor of the *New England Journal of Medicine,* he elaborated on this possibility:

> It seems to me that the ideal treatment is to give the least invasive measure possible, and get the maximal placebo response in return. And rather than worrying about trying to rule out placebo responses, we should be figuring out how to make them happen more of the time. . . . This is in the realm of what I'd call the art of medicine rather than the science of medicine, and I think this is something we were better at teaching in former years than we are now. I think this is an area that really needs to be stressed again in medical education—that there is an art of communicating, of listening, of using suggestion, that the way in which we present a treatment to a patient can increase or decrease its therapeutic efficacy.[27]

This is an important insight into the value of the physician-patient relationship. But Weil notes that a shaman in the jungle can accomplish the same goal by convincing the sick person that he has made the appropriate intervention within the spirit world. In one interview he states:

> Shamans are often master psychotherapists. They are very skilled at intuitively sensing the nature of a person's belief system, and impacting that belief system in a way to maximize the possibility of activating healing mechanisms. That aspect of treatment, to my mind, is crucial. I think it goes on all the time. I think any time a patient visits a doctor, there is an interaction on that level of belief, since people have enormous projections of belief onto medical doctors.[28]

In this and many other statements it is clear that in Dr. Weil's economy the primary measure of the validity of a treatment is whether it can provoke the placebo healing response within the patient. Any other biological effect is at best of secondary importance.

Unlike many prominent voices in alternative medicine, Weil has not built his career on the concept of optimizing the flow of "universal life energy." For the most part, his books do not focus a great deal of attention on the idea that health depends on the proper balance of *chi, prana* or invisible energy by any other name. But he is clearly comfortable with these ideas and expresses no particular concern that invoking them represents a radical departure from fundamental principles of biology and physics. We have already noted his esteem for traditional Chinese medicine, and this is but one of many energy-based systems he endorses or at least considers viable.

In *Spontaneous Healing,* for example, he describes Therapeutic Touch—an extraordinarily subjective and overtly mystical practice—as "a form of energy healing taught and practiced mostly by nurses" and "a learnable skill of great utility. It can relieve pain without the side effects of drugs, can speed healing from injury, and can identify and dissipate energy blockages that may be impeding the healing system."[29] Homeopathy is described in *Spontaneous Healing* as having a "distinguished two-hundred-year history." In one audiocassette interview he elaborates on the issues raised by homeopathy's use of substances that have been diluted so extensively in water that none of the original molecules remain in the solution:

[Homeopathy is] . . . very interesting as an intellectual challenge—if homeopathy really works, and there certainly is abundant evidence that it does, I think it really forces us to try to come up with a new model of how treatments interact with the body, because this is something that may be working on an energetic level, rather than on a physical level, that we don't now understand.[30]

As we will describe later in this book, both Therapeutic Touch and homeopathy represent profound departures from well-established principles of biology and physics.

Weil's intense interest in the healing process has launched a number of sojourns, including some arduous adventures in far-off lands, to see and experience a wide variety of healing techniques. Some of these proved to be more fruitful than others, but perhaps the most pivotal encounter took place in his own "back yard" in Tucson, Arizona. There, at the request of a colleague, he met an elderly osteopath, Dr. Robert Fulford, whom he has repeatedly characterized as one of the most effective healers he has ever encountered. Dr. Fulford is one of a small number of osteopaths who practice craniosacral therapy, which is based on an obscure notion of a subtle rhythmic expansion and contraction of the central nervous system called "primary respiration" (as opposed to the familiar exchange of gases in the lungs, which is downgraded as "secondary respiration"). Craniosacral therapists claim to be able to detect subtle movement (or lack thereof) in the bones of the skull and through hands-on manipulation to restore normal movement, which is considered essential to good health.

The osteopath's apparent successes with a variety of medical problems and his simple, seemingly homespun approach to people and their ailments clearly made a impact on Weil, as evidenced both by an entire chapter devoted to him in *Spontaneous Healing* and by glowing comments in other materials. They also seem to have disarmed a good deal of his scientific training. For when Dr. Fulford speaks for himself, rather than through Weil's smooth and selective prose, it is readily apparent that his healing philosophy hinges on vitalism. In his book *Dr. Fulford's Touch of Life,* which is both endorsed by Weil[31] and promoted on his website, Dr. Fulford repeatedly contends that the flow of the "natural life force" through the body is the key to health and that his hands-on techniques are specifically manipulating that flow.

> Besides the systems and processes well-known to everyone, the body is also composed of a complex and interflowing stream of moving energy. When these energy streams become blocked or constricted, we lose the physical, emotional and mental fluidity potentially available to us. If the blockage lasts long enough or is great enough, the result is pain, discomfort, illness and distress. My goal as a doctor is to help my patient open these energy blockages, for once the energy is unrestricted, the body can begin its own healing process. . . . Unfortunately, most doctors don't believe this. As a result, contemporary medicine is facing a crisis. It insists on considering a human being merely as an object of science.[32]

A recurring theme in Weil's books, especially those that contain advisories for optimizing health, is the importance of breathing. This is not merely a matter of sitting up straight and expanding the diaphragm, as a vocal student might be taught, but a full-blown spiritual exercise. He draws both from ancient traditions and from Dr. Fulford's teachings, both of which insist that during proper breathing one inhales not merely oxygen but also the "life force." Two of the five breathing exercises that Weil recommends require that the tip of the tongue be positioned just above the back side of the upper front teeth—a yogic practice that supposedly "closes an energy circuit in the body, preventing dissipation of *prana* during breathing practice." These exercises are nothing less than "formal breathing techniques from *pranayama,* the ancient Indian science of breath control that forms a part of yoga. *Prana* is a term for universal energy, of which breath is the bodily expression, and *pranayama* practice is intended to harmonize body energies and attune them with cosmic energy."[33]

In what is perhaps his most overt endorsement of vitalism, the book *Spontaneous Healing* states in no uncertain terms what breathing exercises are meant to accomplish:

> As I said earlier, this is genuine spiritual practice, not just a method of improving health. The science of conscious breathing is not taught in medical schools. Throughout history it has been an esoteric subject, mostly passed on as oral tradition, and even today remarkably few books about it are available.
>
> The energy that you can feel in your body after doing the bellows breath is the energy that Chinese doctors call qi (chi), their term for universal life energy. Most people experience it as warmth or tingling or subtle vibration. With practice you can learn to feel it more, move it about the body, and even transmit it to another person. Many healing systems from both East and West make use of energy transmission, usually through the hands, with or without touch contact between giver and recipient. . . . It is useful to try to feel, send and receive this subtle energy. Not only can this practice relieve pain and accelerate healing; it directs attention toward the spiritual pole of existence, away from the material pole. The more you can experience yourself as energy, the easier it is not to identify yourself with your physical body.[34]

Here Weil adopts the language and optimism of the "materialist magician," mentioned by C. S. Lewis in *The Screwtape Letters*, the practitioner/priest who does not (at least in his writing and speaking) acknowledge a sovereign Creator, except perhaps to mention the concept briefly in a discussion of faith healing. Instead he affirms that energies of the spiritual realm are waiting to be manipulated for our benefit, if we only learn the proper techniques. It should be noted that Weil never treats breathing techniques as a matter of faith or religious conviction, which may be embraced or declined depending on one's personal understanding of God or spirituality. He never suggests that a time of daily prayer might be considered as an alternative to the breathing exercises for those who don't accept the idea of *prana* or *chi* on spiritual (let alone scientific) grounds. Instead he insists that they are as integral a part of optimal health as drinking clean water and avoiding cigarette smoking.

Finally, it is worth returning to the original premise of *The Natural Mind* to note that while Weil issues numerous warning about the risks of using cigarettes, excessive alcohol (he calls it "the hardest drug"), coffee and most pharmaceuticals, he hedges a bit on marijuana and quite a lot on hallucinogens. In his economy the latter represent an important steppingstone into altered states of consciousness and hold significant potential for personal growth if used properly. In an audiotape interview entitled "A New Approach to Medicine," he states:

> The psychedelic drugs—the true psychedelics—I think have enormous potential by
> working on the mental sphere to change very dramatically, with one exposure, habit
> patterns that people have built up of perceiving their bodies in certain ways. . . . This
> is such a neglected area of medicine, despite the fact that these drugs, whether it's
> LSD or psilocybin or mescaline or MDA or MDMA or any of these synthetics—
> their toxicity is so low relative to most medical drugs that we use (that is, physical
> toxicity on the body). Their main risks are psychological, and those are manageable
> by arranging the setting properly. . . .
>
> So maybe we'll hear in the coming years of more therapeutic uses of psychedelic
> drugs under supervision, I hope for medical purposes, not just psychological pur-
> poses.[35]

In this passage one can hear the echoes of Aldous Huxley, who, while best
known for his works of fiction (particularly *Brave New World*), undertook some
serious explorations of the world of psychedelic drugs.[36] Advocating the deliberate
use of drugs to disconnect from reality—a state in which one is essentially incapacitated for several hours or perhaps much longer—is a controversial position at best
and a reckless one at worst, even allowing for the possibility of "controlled" therapeutic settings for this activity. Surprisingly, in *The Natural Mind* he makes an even
more startling claim for the possibility of "positive psychosis."

> Psychotics are persons whose nonordinary experience is exceptionally strong. If they
> have not integrated this experience into conscious awareness (or so repressed it that it
> causes physical illness), it takes very negative mental forms. But every psychotic is a
> potential sage or healer and to the extent that negative psychotics are burdens to
> society, to that extent can positive psychotics be assets. (In American Indian societies,
> what we might call psychotic experience in adolescence is a sign that the individual
> is chosen as a future shaman.) To effect this transformation we must remove obstacles
> to the change (such as antipsychotic drugs and most institutional psychiatry) and
> bring patients into contact with healed compatriots—that is, with persons who have
> themselves made the transformation. Such people exist; we simply must allow psy-
> chotics to seek them out and learn from them.[37]

For anyone who has dealt with psychosis, whether professionally or personally,
this notion is both extreme and patently foolish. This condition routinely brings
some degree of disruption and distress (frequently extreme) to the individual, and
it nearly always brings a significant burden of care to family, health care providers
and the community at large. If Weil has found one or more individuals who are
having "positive" psychotic experiences or who function in any meaningful way as
"sages and seers" while in this condition, he is in very rare company. Referring to
an impaired sense of reality or overt delusions of psychosis as "exceptionally strong
nonordinary experience" is specious wordplay, much on the order of calling a

bank robbery a "precipitous monetary relocation." Not surprisingly, this idea has not been featured in his subsequent books dealing with health and healing.

What Is—and What Isn't—Natural?

As we draw this chapter to a close, it is important to consider why we have reviewed Dr. Weil's views on conventional and alternative medicine at some length. Aren't there other voices to be heard on these topics? There are indeed, but Weil's opinions are worth particular attention for a number of reasons:

☐ He is articulate, highly visible, frequently quoted in the media and generally perceived as a source of reasonable (or even conservative) information about alternative therapies. Whether one agrees with him or not, there is considerable breadth and depth to his knowledge. He can hold his own in any discussion about this subject, as witnessed by his able defense of his views in a 1999 debate with Arnold Relman, M.D. (a fervent critic of alternative medicine), at the University of Arizona.[38]

☐ He is a passionate advocate for his ideas and ideals, but he is not a profiteer. He has scrupulously avoided jumping on alternative medicine's commercial bandwagon, even when he could no doubt become wealthy by marketing a line of products and services bearing his name.

☐ He has advocated his case not only in the public square, where the vast majority of alternative practitioners normally hold court, but also among medical professionals. In particular he has established a training program in integrative medicine for physicians at the University of Arizona in Tucson.

☐ Perhaps most important, he is the public figure most commonly identified with "natural medicine," which is arguably the most common portal into the world of alternative therapies for the average citizen.

Weil's preeminence as one who not merely promotes but in essence defines the precepts of natural medicine is both instructive and problematic. In many ways he brings us full circle, back to the questions raised at the beginning of the previous chapter regarding what might or might not be considered "natural" in promoting health and healing.

Clearly the strongest selling point for any treatment billing itself as natural is that it might help the body function optimally or repair itself quickly when something goes wrong. Weil has certainly done well by focusing on the "healing system"—his general term for the wondrous array of maintenance and reparative mechanisms with which our bodies are equipped. He rightly reminds us that the best medicine removes impediments to the proper function of these mechanisms and does not impair them.

Weil also correctly takes conventional medicine to task for often failing to give the body's healing processes the credit they deserve, instead focusing on aggressive interventions that are somehow perceived as superior to them. One might wonder whether such headstrong confidence might arise, even subconsciously, from the prevailing doctrine of the scientific establishment that we are the product of billions of years of molecular accidents and natural selection. While a critique of evolutionary ideology is well beyond the scope and purpose of this book, it would not be unreasonable to propose that its true believers would view deliberate human interventions as an improvement over biological mechanisms that were created by pure chance.

If, on the other hand, our bodies are actually "fearfully and wonderfully made" by a Creator whose ways and wisdom are far beyond our intelligence and comprehension (see Psalm 139), then simple respect—and common sense—should lead us to honor and conserve what he has designed. If God himself has fashioned our defenses against infection and our ability to repair injuries, for example, then our primary goal in responding to these problems should be to remove any impediments to their proper function and then allow them to do their work. Any and all health care interventions that do any good—whether a vitamin supplement, a high-powered antibiotic, a major surgery or simply going to bed and getting some much-needed rest—could be considered "natural" therapies in the sense that they only work to the degree that they cooperate with the body's fundamental design.

Herein lies a point of tension and a major reality checkpoint for all practitioners—conventional and alternative, Christian and atheist, mystical and agnostic. All must acknowledge and account for two profound and seemingly contradictory truths. For centuries scientists and poets alike have rightly praised the human body as a marvel, a work of art, an engineering masterpiece, even a mystery. Yet this same body, for all of its wondrous intricacy, has a meter running. Our self-repair and defense systems are neither invulnerable nor permanent. Eventually, inevitably, something always goes wrong. Even people who eat prudently, exercise regularly, manage their stress and avoid risky behavior grow tumors, suffer strokes, become infected, lose their eyesight. They may have an accident or suffer injury at the hands of another person. At some point all of their systems shut down and cease functioning. Like it or not, no lifestyle can keep anyone alive for 150 years. Furthermore, the physical and biological world around us, for all of its diversity and splendor, is not a realm of Edenic perfection. Animals (many of whom eat or parasitize one another) as well as plants can suffer illness, and all inevitably die. And while the plant and animal kingdoms provide both nourishment and all manner of remedies for the human race, there is no shortage of toxic or lethal compounds in the world that are not synthetic. What is (and will no doubt continue to be) an ongoing risk for practitioners of all stripes is that of losing sight of this "big picture"—especially when one is committed to a specific worldview.

Those who adopt the materialistic, Carl Sagan-esque, "nature is all there is" vantage point may be tempted to believe that "if it can be done, it should be done." (Why wait for evolution to move things along when we can do it ourselves?) Genetic engineering, fetal experimentation, and exotic biologic tamperings without regard for consequences (or ethics) are driven by this perspective. So is, to some degree, the aggressive, invasive, impatient element of conventional medicine. (Why wait for a patient to resolve a health problem on his or her own when we can jump all over it with our latest drug or surgery or technology?)

Those who believe that "Nature, with a capital 'N,' is all there is" may be drawn in the opposite direction. The true believers have traded the quaint symbol of Mother Nature for Gaia, the living, breathing, conscious Earth, who does not particularly appreciate the byproducts of human enterprise. A few suggest that Gaia turns loose a plague or two when we mistreat our home planet. They would argue that humans, who are on par with every other animal, have no right to manipulate biology to save their own hides. A less extreme ideology is far more pervasive: "Nature has a remedy." Whatever we need to get and stay well is already out there among the animals, vegetables and minerals and is inherently superior to anything that human effort might design.

Christians are at risk for adapting their theology to the thinking of either of the above camps. At one extreme is the notion that God gave humanity dominion over the earth, according to Genesis 1, and so by all means we should have our way with it. While such a sentiment is not voiced often in our environmentally sensitive day, it is not a major leap from this vantage point to a presumptuous opinion of our technological prowess and an inclination to use it in medical and other applications with few holds barred. At the other extreme is the conviction that the world around us contains "God's pharmacy," whose products are automatically deemed superior to any manipulated or synthesized by human effort. Those of this persuasion tend to be more doctrinaire than informative when sharing their viewpoints.[39]

The Scriptures, not surprisingly, provide a clear-eyed understanding of the wondrous but flawed body (and world) in which we live, and we will take a closer look at their insights later in this book. For now, we would like to conclude this chapter with a few important questions about the natural medicine movement and

its practitioners. Is their vision of "allowing the body to heal itself" entirely coher-
ent and consistent? Consider the following:

*Given the abundant supply and variety of foods available to most citizens in developed
nations, do all of us truly need supplements—whether a few or a tackle box full of them—to
thrive?* Is there a fundamental design problem with the normal human body? How
did the race ever survive before the birth of the food supplement industry? In this
arena, mainstream dietary associations are clearly more conservative and less
"interventional" than their alternative counterparts. The Food and Nutrition Science Alliance, for example, makes the conservative statement that "a daily multivitamin may help some people meet their nutritional needs. For example, a balanced diet alone may not suffice to meet the greater nutritional needs of pregnant
women."[40] But what about Dr. Weil's "tonics" or high doses of vitamins C and E
and beta carotene? What about bee pollen, royal jelly, green tea, growth hormone,
oregano, natural progesterone and DHEA? How can we make it to a ripe old age
without the support of these and other products, which are apparently necessities
of life?

The standard explanation for the need for supplements is that our current food
supply is contaminated with toxins or short on basic nutrients because of modern
agricultural practices. The first issue is not trivial—none of us wants to accumulate
heavy metals, pesticides or other poisons from our dinner. But it is also more a
matter of public safety than of supplementation. (In other words, if your tuna cas-
serole is contaminated with mercury, swallowing a handful of vitamins will not
necessarily prevent its toxic effects.) The second issue is much more suspect. Are
we to believe that an apple taken home from the supermarket today is drastically
different from one pulled off the fruit stand one hundred years ago? And if toma-
toes brought directly from the garden to the serving tray taste better than those in
the produce section, is the difference between them remedied by taking a supplement?

The problem for most citizens of developed countries, in fact, is not so much
that nourishing food is scarce but rather that our eating decisions tend to be driven
by runaway taste buds, convenience, clever marketing or even overt addictions
rather than by reason, planning and self-discipline. As a result, our most prevalent
national nutritional problem is not a shortage of vitamins but rather an excess of
calories that are usually less than ideally distributed among the basic food groups.
Once again, however, corrective action for this problem rarely involves taking supplements but rather a more careful and disciplined selection of foods every day.
(Ironically, marketers for many "all natural" products that are supposed to "melt
away excessive fat" are tapping into the same desire for shortcuts that fueled the

"fen-phen" phenomenon of the late 1990s.) Obviously there is a need for supplements in certain specific conditions—iron deficiency caused by blood loss, for example, or pernicious anemia (resulting from an inadequate supply of vitamin B_{12} to the body's cells). But the idea that it is somehow "natural" for a well-fed individual to ingest a dozen different supplements every day seems not only paradoxical but also more the product of a sales pitch than of solid research.

Once a compound of any type, whether derived from animal, vegetable or mineral, is concentrated into a pill or tonic, is it truly natural? Are such preparations really foods, or are they merely drugs by another name? This is a particularly important question when one is taking formulas that are purported to have specific benefits—saw palmetto for prostate enlargement, for example, or St. John's wort for depression. We would propose a simple but important distinction. If it is bought in the produce, meat, grain and dairy aisles at the store, and then prepared in the kitchen, it is a food. Otherwise, if a particular substance is deliberately concentrated in order to bring about a particular effect, it is a drug, regardless of what one calls it. This is not to say that the compound might not be useful. By all means, if a compound is safe and effective for preventing or treating disease, let its proper uses be proclaimed throughout the land. But calling it "all natural" or labeling it a type of food as a marketing ploy is little more than verbal sleight of hand.

Even if a supplement has little risk of causing harm, how do we determine whether it is at all useful or effective for a given health problem? And if it does in fact carry some risk, how will we find out about it? Many health professionals have complained that the 1994 Dietary Supplement Health and Education Act (DSHEA) gave supplement manufacturers too much latitude in making health claims without any requirement that they be supported by evidence. (A regional administrator for the California Health Services Department's Food and Drug Branch dubbed DSHEA the "Food Fraud Facilitation Act.")[41] Furthermore, while drug manufacturers must first demonstrate to the FDA that their products are safe and effective—an expensive and arduous process—before they can be sold, the reverse situation exists for supplements. The FDA must prove that a herb or supplement is harmful before it can be removed from the market.

Does the average individual need to practice special breathing techniques in order to attain optimal health? The human body, under normal circumstances, elegantly regulates breathing to supply oxygen to tissues and expel carbon dioxide. This is certainly one of our most "natural" functions, a system whose day-to-day operation would seem to be a genuine example of the concept "If it ain't broke, don't fix it." It may be appropriate on occasion to override one's automatic breathing pattern for a specific purpose—as a relaxation technique, for example, or to counteract hyperventilation during a panic episode. But Dr. Weil, his mentor Dr. Fulford and many others in alternative medicine (especially those involved in yogic practices) imply not only that normal breathing is somehow inadequate but also that daily practice of their contrived breathing exercises is somehow necessary for both physical and spiritual health. If these exercises seem meaningful to them as a form of religious practice, they are certainly entitled to promote them in those terms. But since there is no credible evidence that they actually improve normal respiratory function, nor any that *prana* or *chi* (the invisible energies supposedly affected by these exercises) exist, labeling them as a necessary component of natural health and healing once again seems to be a semantic ploy—and a deceptive one at that.

In the face of a worldwide epidemic of sexually transmitted diseases (STDs), why does the alternative medicine movement in general and Dr. Weil in particular say nothing about the most foolproof and truly natural way to avoid them? STDs are in fact problematic for alternative medicine in numerous ways. Their causative agents, and the manner in which they are spread, are indisputable. The illnesses that they bring about cannot be explained away as "imbalances of life energy." No one in his right mind entrusts his infection with gonorrhea, syphilis or any other treatable STD to an herbalist, acupuncturist or homeopath, nor would a rational person risk a sexual encounter with someone who had in fact done so. More importantly, for all of its interest in healthy lifestyles, alternative medicine as a whole does not promote the completely natural approach to preventing STDs: preserving sexual activity for a "closed system" within marriage. It has, in fact, offered little on this subject except for an occasional echo of conventional medicine's ongoing reliance on condoms and "safe sex." Weil's website <www.askdrweil.com>, for example, links visitors who click on the term "safe sex" to a lengthy and highly explicit explanation at the website of the Seattle-based Society for Human Sexuality, which is overtly committed to "sex-positive" material. For this organization—and presumably for those who direct others to it—"doing what comes naturally" in the realm of sex means literally whatever, whenever, with whomever, as long as it is consensual and measures are taken to avoid the spread of infection.

Without a doubt natural medicine, especially the use of herbs and supplements for maintaining health and treating disease, is the aspect of alternative health care that shares the most common ground with conventional medicine. Practitioners from all segments of the alternative-conventional spectrum are interested in expanding the number of treatment options for their patients, and each perspective has a significant contribution to make to this process. Conventional medicine could take some cues from alternative practitioners who are intentional about engaging the patient's own healing resources and who are striving to use remedies that are gentler to body and mind. Alternative health care could benefit from adopting conventional medicine's evenhanded rules of evidence for declaring a substance useful for a given purpose. It could also learn to tone down the sales-pitch rhetoric that so often accompanies its product promotion.

The widespread dissemination of information about common herbal products among conventional physicians is certainly a step in the right direction, although it remains to be seen how often this will translate into heartfelt recommendations for their patients. The expanding number and scope of well-designed studies of herbs and supplements is likewise a promising development. But the issues raised in the preceding paragraphs highlight a number of problem areas in the natural medicine movement that show no sign of fading away. Helping the body heal itself is a wonderful goal—provided that the methods used for this purpose are safe and effective not only for the body but for the mind and spirit as well.

9

DEEPAK CHOPRA

The "Think System" &
the Revival of Ayurveda

MARIAN (THE LIBRARIAN): I've been wanting to talk to you about
Winthrop's cornet.
PROFESSOR HAROLD HILL: His cornet? Mother-of-pearl keys.
MARIAN: I'm sure it's fine. But you see he never touches it. Oh, the first week or so,
he made a few—ah—experimental—blats? I guess you'd say?
HAROLD: Yes—yes, blats.
MARIAN: And he sings the "Minuet in G" almost constantly. . . . But he never touches
the cornet.
HAROLD: Well, you see—
MARIAN: He says you told him it wasn't necessary.
HAROLD: Well.
MARIAN: He tells me about some "Think System." If he *thinks* the "Minuet in G,"
he won't have to bother with the notes. Now Professor—
HAROLD: Miss Marian. The Think System is a revolutionary method, I'll admit.
So was Galileo's conception of the Heavens, Columbus' conception of the egg—
ah—globe, Bach's conception of the Well-Tempered Clavichord. Hmm?
Now I cannot discuss these things here in public. But if you'll allow me to call . . .
(*THE MUSIC MAN*, ACT II, SCENE 1)[1]

Most alternative health care systems have a flagship therapy for which
they are most well known. Traditional Chinese medicine, for example, is usually
associated with acupuncture. Chiropractic is most noted for its spinal manipulation. And homeopathy is known for its extremely dilute concoctions through

which "like cures like." Mention the traditional East Indian system *ayurveda*, however, and for most people no specific practice immediately comes to mind. Does it center on diet and herbs? Meditative postures? Breathing techniques? In fact, all of these and more are part of the total package. But at its core *ayurveda* is, like Professor Harold Hill's "Think System" for playing band instruments, geared toward the idea that overhauling our thoughts trumps any other activity when we want to alter our physical (and spiritual) reality.

Of all the alternative approaches we will review in this book, *ayurveda* is arguably the most enmeshed with a specific religious tradition: Vedism, from which Hinduism is derived. Ironically, it is two health-related pursuits—*ayurveda* in the 1990s, especially as it has been promoted by bestselling author Deepak Chopra, M.D., and Transcendental Meditation two decades earlier—that have had the most visible success at infusing the mindset and practices of Vedism into Western culture. Still, few Westerners, especially Americans, are conversant with India's mystical vocabulary: the average person's list rarely extends beyond *yoga, mantra* and perhaps the sexually charged *tantra*. Fewer are familiar with, let alone attentive to, Hinduism's pantheon of gods and goddesses. But mention reducing stress, slowing the aging process (an emerging priority among the post-fifty baby boomers), enhancing personal wealth and power, and especially boosting sexual performance, and Western hearts and minds are likely to snap wide open.

Ayurveda has been promoted most actively in the West by two men: Maharishi Mahesh Yogi, who put Transcendental Meditation on the map a quarter century ago, and Deepak Chopra, who was at one time a protégé of the Maharishi. Yet despite the long-standing visibility of its champions, *ayurveda* as a health practice has been slow to catch on in America. It was conspicuously absent from the list of therapies mentioned in the landmark 1993 and 1998 studies by David Eisenberg, M.D., that surveyed the alternative landscape in the United States.[2] Even now *ayurveda* has not gained anything close to the widespread interest and acceptance of traditional Chinese medicine. One reason for this is that *ayurveda* lacks a specific, signature treatment (such as acupuncture) that Westerners might find intriguing. But a more obvious reason becomes apparent when one takes a look at the fundamental precepts of *ayurveda*. From all appearances this East India import would seem to be remarkably out of step with contemporary science.

India's Ancient Medicine

Ayurveda's proponents, as might be expected, put a positive spin on its ancientness. One practitioner describes it as "the oldest existing medical system," which "began in ancient India at least 5,000 years ago."[3] A 1995 article extolling *ayurveda* in the journal *Alternative and Complementary Therapies* notes that

> Ayur-Veda is said to be as old as humanity. It is knowledge that is inherent in the
> laws that govern life throughout the universe. It is a branch of a complete body of
> knowledge known as the "Vedas." This science of health was founded by the great
> seers of ancient India. Through their deep insight into the depths of nature's func-
> tioning, they came to know the laws that govern our health and lifespan.[4]

Deepak Chopra, in his book *Ageless Body, Timeless Mind,* describes the origin of
the word *ayurveda:*

> In India, longevity was traditionally assigned to a branch of learning called *Ayurveda,*
> derived from two Sanskrit roots, *Ayus,* or "life," and *Veda,* meaning "science" or
> "knowledge." This ancient "science of life" is usually referred to as India's traditional
> medicine, but there is a deeper spiritual basis for Ayurveda. The most famous verse
> from the ancient Ayurvedic texts says, *Ayurveda amritanam* ("Ayurveda is for immor-
> tality"). The meaning is twofold: Ayurveda is for promoting longevity without limit,
> and it does this from a belief that life essentially is immortal.[5]

As these quotes only begin to demonstrate, current-day proponents of *ayurveda* are
not at all reserved about its spiritual origins, nor do they shy away from the
detailed applications of its cosmic worldview to the human body. They do, however, tend to downplay some of *ayurveda*'s more exotic holdovers from ancient
times, such as its belief that gods, demons, stars and planets play a role in health
and illness.

Like traditional Chinese medicine, *ayurveda* postulates that all of nature, including human beings, is derived from five primal elements: "ether" (or "space"), air,
fire, water and earth. The five elements are said to govern the five senses and manifest themselves in the body in a variety of ways. Fire, for example, is represented
in body temperature, metabolism and digestion, while air is associated with respiration and heartbeat. The elements also combine to form three *doshas,* which are
variously described as "biological humors," "basic forces" and "physiological principles." Their names: *vata, pitta* and *kapha.*

Each *dosha* is said to regulate a major component of bodily structure and function. *Vata* (the combination of ether and air) deals with anything related to movement, such as neurological and muscular functions, circulation and respiration.
Pitta (fire and water) oversees metabolism and digestion, while *kapha* (water and
earth) governs structure and the overall cohesion of the body. The three *doshas* are
said to be present in varying combination in every organ, tissue and cell. Furthermore, each of us is supposed to be born with a unique *prakriti,* a basic tempera-
ment derived from the dominance of one or two of the *doshas* within us (or, in

some people, an equal balance of all three).The *doshas* combine to create ten basic types of individuals (for example, *vata-pitta* or *kapha* dominant), with typical physical characteristics, personality types, behavior patterns and vulnerabilities to disease. For example, the popular handbook *Alternative Medicine for Dummies* describes *pitta* types as "intense, quick to anger, sharp-witted, enterprising, impatient, commanding, orderly and critical.They tend to have medium and muscular builds, fair or reddish complexions, warm skin and large appetites, and are prone to heartburn, gallbladder and liver disorders, skin problems, ulcers and hemorrhoids."[6]

There are, in addition, *subdoshas* in various locations of the body; seven *dhatus,* or tissues (plasma, blood, muscle, fat, bone, nerve and reproductive); three *malas,* or wastes (feces, urine and sweat); and *agni,* the energy of metabolism. And connecting all of these dots, so to speak, is the flow of *prana,* the East Indian universal life energy. *Prana* is said to enter the body with air, water, food and sunlight, travel through invisible channels called *nadis* and congregate in energy centers called *chakras.* Disease is said to occur when there is disharmony in any of these arenas, usually involving a disturbance in the flow of *prana* or an imbalance of the *doshas* in a specific organ or throughout the body.[7] Such imbalances can arise from emotional states, congenital factors, diet, trauma, personal habits, seasons and supernatural factors, among others.

If you recall the main points of our discussion on universal energy and traditional Chinese medicine, some of this may sound familiar.The Chinese also postulated five elements (including wood and metal rather than ether and air.) They conceived of health in terms of balance and harmony between inner and outer environments, and they assumed the existence of a universal life energy *(chi)* whose orderly flow was necessary for well-being.There are some similar themes in diagnosis and treatment as well. *Ayurvedic* physicians, like their traditional Chinese counterparts, seek clues through a detailed history of a person's complaints, diet, work, sleep and other personal details.They also claim to be able to assess a person's health status not only by his or her physical characteristics but also by careful assessment of the radial (wrist) pulses—six on each side, three superficial and three deep, each associated with a specific organ. And like the Chinese, *ayurvedic* physicians pay careful attention to the appearance of the tongue, on which the status of individual organs is supposedly displayed in specific areas. The lungs, for example, are said to be projected onto the upper-forward surface, the left lung affecting the right side of the tongue, and the right lung affecting the left side of the tongue. The urine may also be examined, apparently yielding a wealth of information not available to today's conventional practitioner. Not only does its color and clarity reflect the state of the *doshas* but also the behavior of a drop of sesame oil placed into the sample is said to yield a wealth of information:

> If the drop spreads immediately, the physical disorder is probably easy to cure. If the drop sinks to the middle of the urine sample, the illness is more difficult to cure. If the drop sinks to the bottom, the illness may be very difficult to cure. If the drop spreads on the surface in wave-like movements, this indicates a *vata* disorder. If the drop spreads on the surface with multiple colors visible like a rainbow, this indicates a *pitta* disorder. If the drop breaks up into pearl-like droplets on the surface of the urine, this indicates a *kapha* disorder.[8]

Once the specific imbalance is identified, the *ayurvedic* physician has a wealth of treatment options at his or her disposal. Again, broad similarities to traditional Chinese medicine are noteworthy. Most significant of these is the notion that each patient's diagnosis and treatment are unique—a concept that modern apologists might call "physiologic individuality." *Ayurvedic* practitioners, like their traditional Chinese counterparts, are primarily concerned about the specific underlying imbalances in *doshas* and *prana* that they claim are ultimately responsible for a person's illness, rather than the actual identification and classification of disease manifestations and mechanisms. Because foods are said to have specific effects on the *doshas,* dietary and herbal recommendations tend to be very detailed. Contemporary alternative medicine promoters who may not promote the entire *ayurvedic* package are often enthusiastic about its herbal remedies. For example, Andrew Weil, M.D., whose expertise in botanical therapies we have already noted, extols this aspect of *ayurveda*:

> Ayurvedic remedies are primarily herbal, drawing on the vast botanical wealth of the Indian subcontinent, but may include animal and mineral ingredients, even powdered gemstones. . . . Although Ayurvedic herbs are little known outside India and few have been studied by modern methods, many may have great therapeutic value. For example, guggul *(Commiphora mukul),* a plant indicated traditionally for control of obesity, has been shown to lower cholesterol in a manner similar to pharmaceutical drugs used for that purpose, but with much less risk.[9]

But present-day apologists for *ayurveda* rarely mention some of the more exotic and stomach-churning remedies that would no doubt prove to be a stumbling block to modern audiences. In his excellent and comprehensive history of medicine, *The Greatest Benefit to Mankind,* British social historian Roy Porter describes the remedies listed in the *Caraka Samhita,* one of the two huge compendia that he identifies as forming the cornerstone of *ayurveda:*

> For dealing with the 200 diseases and 150 other conditions mentioned, the *Caraka*

Samhita refers to 177 materials of animal derivation, including snake dung, the milk, flesh, fat, blood, dung or urine of such animals as the horse, goat, elephant, camel, cow and sheep, the eggs of the sparrow, peahen and crocodile, beeswax and honey, and various soups; 341 items of vegetable origin (seeds, flowers, fruit, tree-bark and leaves) and 64 substances of mineral origin (assorted gems, gold, silver, copper, salt, clay, tin, lead and sulphur). The use of dung and urine are standard; since the cow is a holy animal to orthodox Hindus, all its products are purifying. Cow dung was judged to possess disinfectant properties and was prescribed for external use, including fumigation; urine was to be applied externally in many recipes.[10]

Ayurvedic physicians may also prescribe a rigorous regime of purification called *panchakarma,* which is intended to rid the body of toxins and impurities. In this area *ayurveda* resembles the harsh regimes of bleeding and purging used by eighteenth-century Western physicians. The *panchakarma* regime may involve a mixture of herbal sweat treatments, steam baths, laxatives, enemas, vomiting and even bloodletting. Deepak Chopra's most detailed celebration of *ayurveda,* his book *Perfect Health: The Complete Mind/Body Guide,* recommends that everyone over the age of twelve experience at least a week of *panchakarma* every year.[11]

Ayurveda also recognizes more than one hundred points called *marmas* at which *prana* is claimed to interact with the outside world. Pressing or massaging the appropriate *marmas* is said to help balance the *doshas,* just as acupressure and acupuncture are supposed to normalize the flow of *chi.* Breathing exercises called *pranayama,* which are an integral part of yoga, are reputed to improve the flow of *prana.* And speaking of yoga, the physical and meditative exercises of its various schools are likely to be included in an *ayurvedic* healing program. Above all, proponents of *ayurveda* stress the importance of overhauling one's basic understanding of oneself and the universe. A summary of *ayurveda* by the National Institutes of Health (in its publication *Alternative Medicine: Expanding Medical Horizons*) mentions this in passing: "Ayurvedic theory states that all imbalance and disease in the body begin with imbalance or stress in the awareness, or consciousness, of the individual."[12] A more elaborate statement by an *ayurvedic* practitioner, Walter W. Mills, M.D., is more revealing:

> In Ayurveda, the body is viewed as the physical expression of an underlying abstract field of intelligence. Ayurvedic physicians identify this underlying field as consciousness, and they emphasize consciousness as the basis of physiology, rather than an epiphenomenon of the nervous system. In keeping with this view, Ayurvedic physicians use mental techniques to treat diseases, to reduce stress and to develop each patient's consciousness.[13]

From the vantage point of the twenty-first century, *ayurveda* seems like a com-

plex relic from a time when there was little comprehension of how the body actually works. For all of its complicated diagnostics and formularies, it is medicine at
its most primal level—a complete enmeshment of religion and primitive therapeu-
tics. Its foundational notion of five elements and three *doshas* that govern body
type, personality and risk of disease sounds much like beliefs in body humors
(blood, phlegm, choler and black bile) and personality types (sanguine, phleg-
matic, choleric and bilious) that were discarded generations ago in the West. Invisible energy flows, pulse and tongue diagnosis, astrology and even ceremonies to
appease Hindu gods are integral to *ayurvedic* tradition and practice but are thoroughly out of step with contemporary understandings of biology that have been
validated around the world for decades. *Ayurveda's* validity appears even more
dubious when one considers how much (or how little) it has actually contributed
to the well-being of its country of origin. Tal Brooke, a one-time devotee of
Transcendental Meditation and its founder, Maharishi Mahesh Yogi, has written a
particularly unflattering assessment of *ayurveda's* efficacy in India:

> A large part of the immense culture shock that I underwent during my first weeks in
> India, many months before I became a resident and became used to it all, was the
> unspeakable poverty and disease that was everywhere. The land literally groaned.
> Even the fact that I had traveled in the Middle East as a teenager in no way prepared
> me for the stark poverty and disease that I saw in India. When I went to Rishikesh to
> meet Maharishi during that time, I became attuned to the pervasive reality of India's
> ancient Ayurveda side by side with sickness and disease of every kind. Everywhere,
> ashrams and stores were selling the land's ancient Ayurveda's non-material cures
> (which involves *asanas* (yogic postures), *mantras, yajnas* (rites to deities), astrology,
> precious gems, physiology and body types and much more.) Yet everywhere I
> looked, I saw disease. What hit me in the gut was that none of this stuff really
> worked, or if it worked at all, it was never effective enough.
>
> I wondered in those days, "Why is India wracked in poverty and sickness when
> the realm of Vedanta and Ayurveda are supposed to banish these things?"[14]

Deepak Chopra and the Popularization of a Movement

All things considered, one might wonder why there would now be a flowering of
interest in *ayurveda* in the West. In chapter four we outlined several reasons for the
rise of alternative medicine's popularity in Western countries over the past two
decades. For *ayurveda* we can add one critical factor: the impact of one man,
Deepak Chopra, M.D. Chopra is founder and CEO of the Chopra Center for
Well Being in La Jolla, California, a fourteen-thousand-square-foot facility where
one can "experience the healing traditions of ayurveda." He is also the author of
twenty-five books, which have been translated into thirty-five languages, a speaker

on more than one hundred audio- and videotape series, a perennial favorite on the Public Broadcasting System, a globetrotting speaker and a health adviser to movie stars and other luminaries. According to the biography on his official website, he is "acknowledged as a world leader in establishing a new life-giving paradigm that has revolutionized common wisdom about the crucial connection between mind, body, spirit and healing. He has transformed our understanding of the meaning of health."[15] That's quite a claim, even for website hyperbole. But there is no disputing that he has blazed significant new trails for *ayurveda* and Eastern mysticism into American culture.

Chopra is somewhat reserved about his birth date, perhaps because of his recurring claim that the aging process is not inevitable—at least theoretically. According to two sources, he was born in New Delhi, India, in 1947.[16] His father was a Western-trained physician, and Chopra followed in his footsteps, earning a medical degree at the All India Institute of Medical Sciences in 1968. He then moved to the United States, where he trained at the Lahey Clinic and the University of Virginia, ultimately achieving board certification in internal medicine and endocrinology. By the age of thirty-five, he was elected chief of staff at New England Memorial Hospital and had established a sizable practice. But in spite of these accomplishments, he was, by his own account, experiencing a general lack of fulfillment, wondering whether he was doing enough for his patients and seeking solace in the regular use of tobacco and whiskey.

A monumental change in direction occurred in the early 1980s, when he was reintroduced to the medical and spiritual traditions of his homeland. While visiting New Delhi in 1981, he met Dr. Brihaspati Dev Triguna, a prominent *ayurvedic* physician. According to Chopra's book *Return of the Rishi,* Triguna is a master pulse diagnostician, one who can discern someone's "whole medical history— past, present and future" simply by putting three fingers on his or her wrist. Triguna applied the technique to Chopra, whom he declared was "thinking too many unnecessary thoughts" and needed to learn how to meditate. While he was at first resistant to this advice, sometime later he began reading about Transcendental Meditation (or TM as it is commonly abbreviated) and its founder, Maharishi Mahesh Yogi. TM's relative simplicity and the scientific research that appeared to show its utility in managing stress struck a responsive chord, and he became a regular meditator. He claims that within two weeks he had quit smoking and drinking.[17] This was but the beginning of a journey deep into the medical and spiritual traditions of his homeland.

Chopra's conversion to the metaphysics of TM proved to be no little significance to the maharishi as well. In the 1970s the guru had succeeded in packaging a centuries-old meditation technique in a format that could be easily accessed and accepted by materialistic Westerners. The key was presenting it as "nonreligious," as a simple, even scientific technique to help manage stress and improve overall health. For a nominal fee (around $100), interested parties were instructed in a simple process of sitting quietly and repeating a secret word, or "mantra," over and over for twenty minutes twice daily. The mantra was supposedly chosen specifically for the individual meditator by the trainer and imparted during an initiation ceremony that also included an invitation to pay homage to the maharishi's departed teacher, Guru Dev. Medical studies demonstrating that meditation seemed to produce favorable physiological responses were widely publicized, as were testimonials from celebrities such as the Beatles and Mia Farrow.

By the mid-1970s, Americans by the thousands were being initiated, and TM was poised to be taught in schools, prisons and other institutions. But skeptical researchers discovered that the mantras were none other than the names of Hindu deities—a fact that did not sit well with governmental bodies concerned about separation of church (or gurus) and state. Furthermore, investigators such as Harvard cardiologist Herbert Benson, M.D., determined that there was nothing magical about the TM mantras for inducing physiological relaxation and that any word or phrase that sat well with an individual could be used in a simple relaxation technique.

Despite these setbacks, TM continued to be taught and practiced around the world. In the 1980s the maharishi shifted gears with an endeavor to package *ayurveda* for the masses, just as he had done with meditation. *Ayurveda* needed to be seen not merely as folk medicine but as a comprehensive science of life, health and consciousness. According to one promoter, the maharishi's efforts represented nothing less than the revival of a vast but nearly lost treasure:

> During centuries of foreign rule in India, Ayur-Vedic institutions declined, and much of the Ayur-Vedic knowledge was misunderstood, fragmented, or lost. . . . Maharishi assembled hundreds of Ayur-Vedic physicians in India to evaluate the direction of the practice of Ayur-Veda in modern India. He inspired them to join their efforts to ensure that Ayur-Veda is once again practiced as the holistic system of health care envisioned by the great rishis who founded this comprehensive health science. Thus, the term *Maharishi Ayur-Veda* was given to this holistic natural science of health in order to recognize its source (*maha* meaning great, and *rishi* meaning a person who has deep insight into the wisdom of life).[18]

The transformation of the word *ayurveda* into *Ayur-Veda* (or, as the quote above proclaims, into *Maharishi Ayur-Veda*) paralleled the conversion of *meditation* into *Transcendental Meditation*. Both represent an apparent determination of the maharishi to convert a generic practice into a recognizable, brand-name product. But gaining widespread acceptance in the West for such an intensely foreign approach to health and illness would require more than an adjustment in its name. Whether *ayurveda* or *Ayur-Veda,* it needed a face and a voice that would be credible and that could smooth over some of those prickly ancient concepts—or even make them sound like cutting-edge science.

Enter Deepak Chopra, M.D.

The embrace of TM by this bright, articulate, successful Western-trained endocrinologist undoubtedly produced a serious blip on the radar among the movement's leadership, and by 1985 Chopra was enjoying audiences with the maharishi himself. In his book *Quantum Healing: Exploring the Frontiers of Mind/Body Medicine* Chopra describes being summoned to meet privately with the guru while visiting his settlement near New Delhi in 1987. He was somewhat surprised by this invitation, but he arrived at the maharishi's room the next morning with mind and heart wide open:

> He beckoned me in, and we sat together quietly. Then he said very simply, "I have been waiting a long time to bring out some special techniques. I believe they will become the medicine of the future. They were known in the distant past but were lost in the confusion of time; now I want you to learn them, and at the same time I want you to explain, clearly and scientifically, how they work."
>
> Over the course of the next few hours he taught me a series of mental techniques, including those he called "primordial sounds." The way they are used is related to meditation, but they are prescribed for specific illnesses, including those we consider incurable in the West, such as cancer. Maharishi explicitly told me that these were the strongest healing therapies in *Ayurveda,* the ancient tradition of Indian medicine. He taught them to me quite simply, and I had no difficulty learning what I was to do when I got home to my patients. At the same time, I realized that he was asking me to step far beyond the physician's role as it is known in the West.[19]

If learning the maharishi's techniques, including the "primordial sounds" (which continue to be taught at the Chopra Center), was straightforward, the second assignment—explaining them "clearly and scientifically"—was another matter. How would this set with his Western-trained colleagues? "I had to laugh thinking about their reactions," he mused, well aware of his own disregard of *ayurveda* up to that point. But his encounters with TM and the maharishi changed this perspective in a decisive way:

> Before meeting Maharishi, I assumed that Ayurveda was folk medicine, because all I saw of it were folkways—the herbs, diets, exercises, and incredibly intricate rules for

daily life that are just "in the air" when one grows up in India.

Maharishi's interest, however, centered on the lost Ayurveda and its ability to cure patients through non-material means. Now that he had given me those means, he also expected me to tell people how they worked.[20]

As the next decade would bear out, Chopra was more than up to the task—at least from the standpoint of telling a convincing story to the general public. His success, like that of many of cultural icons, has been the direct result of his savvy use of popular media, his communication skills and his mastery of presentation. He is very good with an audience and, more importantly, he presents very favorably on TV. He is warm, personable and seemingly guileless. His informal lectures and books blend an engaging flow of personal anecdotes, scientific propositions, hard-core Eastern metaphysics, boundless optimism and practical applications. All of them stress transformation of consciousness, of the way we understand and experience the "true" nature of the universe and ourselves, as the key to health, wealth, success and happiness. The spiritual emphasis has been so intense, in fact, that Chopra has been dubbed the poet laureate of the alternative medicine movement—and now could reasonably be considered its theologian as well. The spring of 2000 saw the release of his book *How to Know God,* a title one might expect from a Christian evangelist or pastor, from a Billy Graham or a Charles Swindoll. But it is, in fact, not at all inconsistent with the cosmic scale on which Chopra routinely paints his murals of health, wealth and happiness.

During the waning years of the 1980s, Chopra effectively worked to put Maharishi Ayur-Veda, and himself, on the map. He founded the American Association for Ayurvedic Medicine and became medical director of the Maharishi Ayurveda Health Center for Stress Management and Behavioral Medicine in Lancaster, Massachusetts. He wrote a series of books bearing dedications to the Maharishi, all of which promoted *ayurveda,* meditation and intensely metaphysical themes. One in particular, *Quantum Healing: Exploring the Frontiers of Mind/Body Medicine,* garnered plaudits from reviewers in mainstream publications (*The New England Journal of Medicine*[21] and the *Washington Post,* for example), as well as promoters of New Age ideologies (such as Marilyn Ferguson, Elisabeth Kübler-Ross and Larry Dossey), and became a national bestseller.

The string of successes during those years, however, was not unbroken. Chopra, along with his New Delhi *ayurveda* mentor Brihaspati Dev Triguna and Ohio State University pathology professor Hari M. Sharma, coauthored an article about Maharishi Ayur-Veda that was published in the May 22/29, 1991, edition of the *Journal of the American Medical Association (JAMA).* This was not a formal scientific study but rather a general-interest piece (identified as a "Letter from New

Delhi") for a theme issue dealing with international health. Bearing the title "Maharishi Ayur-Veda: Modern Insights into Ancient Medicine," the article extolled the benefits of TM and discussed research studies of *ayurvedic* herbal treatments. It was undoubtedly intended to introduce conventional physicians to this traditional healing system in a manner that would inform, generate curiosity and hopefully build a bridge to the mainstream medical community. Instead the article provoked some blistering criticism within *JAMA*'s normally placid pages over the next several months.[22]

Furthermore, before the ill-fated "Letter from New Delhi" was even published, Chopra had parted company with the TM movement on somewhat awkward terms. In a candid conversation with John M. Knapp, an ex-Transcendental Meditator who runs a website called Trancenet (<www.trancenet.org>), Chopra described an uncomfortable private meeting with the maharishi in 1990, during an observance called the "Guru Purnima." Knapp describes how Chopra revealed the presence of some friction among TM's international staff at that time:

> Dr. Chopra talked about how they struggled among themselves and with him for the Maharishi's attention and leadership of the Movement. Dr. Chopra indicated he was never comfortable in this atmosphere. . . .
>
> "On this Guru Purnima in Holland, Maharishi asked everyone to leave the room except me. Maharishi said to me, 'Everyone tells me you are competing with me.'"
>
> Dr. Chopra said he was stricken. He told the Maharishi, "I would never do that," and after a minute added, "Probably it would be best for me to leave the Movement."
>
> "Maharishi was very sweet then; he said, 'Whatever decision would be best for you.' The whole thing lasted two minutes. So I left the Movement. I had lost my practice. I didn't know where to turn. . . ."
>
> Dr. Chopra said he went home to Boston immediately and sought his family and friends. "Later I got a call from [the Maharishi] in Boston. He told me that I could be a great spiritual leader. That everyone would follow me. He said that he would put me in charge of the whole Movement. But I said, 'I don't want to be a spiritual leader. I am a very regular guy—with a wife and kids. I just have the gift of gab.' He seemed perplexed, but in the end he was very sweet. 'Whatever decision you make will be the best for you.' "[23]

Without a doubt (and the *JAMA* fallout notwithstanding), Chopra's decision to part company with TM was indeed "the best" for him. In his absence Hari Sharma, M.D., one of the coauthors of the "Letter from New Delhi," picked up the standard for Maharishi Ayur-Veda and continues to promote it in relative obscurity. Bogged down with TM's grandiosity, marketing tactics and pricey product line, Maharishi Ayur-Veda has failed to win respect even among alternative medicine promoters. Andrew Weil, for example, warns readers who might be interested in *ayurveda* that "finding a good Ayurvedic doctor takes some effort."

> Many practitioners in the West are members of the international religious organiza-
> tion of Maharishi Mahesh Yogi, the Holland-based billionaire, whose promotion of
> Ayurveda is definitely a for-profit endeavor. (In India Ayurveda is medicine of the
> people, an inexpensive alternative to allopathic treatment. Maharishi Ayurveda is
> anything but inexpensive.) This group offers training programs for physicians that
> certify them to be Ayurvedic practitioners after minimal exposure to the philosophy
> and methods of the system. I recommend seeking out practitioners who are inde-
> pendent of this organization.[24]

But before long Chopra, no longer encumbered with TM's baggage, was well
on his way to fame, fortune and extraordinary public recognition. In 1993, after a
television appearance with Oprah Winfrey, he became an overnight celebrity. His
newest book at the time, *Ageless Body, Timeless Mind,* reportedly sold more than
130,000 copies in one day after the program aired.[25] That year he moved to La
Jolla, California, where he accepted the position of executive director of the Sharp
Institute for Human Potential and Mind-Body Medicine. This organization was an
affiliate of Sharp HealthCare, a conglomerate of seven hospitals, twenty-three
clinics and three medical groups. However, following a change in ownership of
Sharp HealthCare, he departed to establish the Chopra Center for Well Being.

While no longer engaged in clinical practice, he has made ample use of nearly
all forms of contemporary media to disseminate his views to millions of apprecia-
tive seekers of health and enlightenment, including a number of celebrities:
former Beatle George Harrison (no surprise, considering Harrison's past involvement with the maharishi and fascination with things Eastern), Demi Moore,
Michael Jackson, Elizabeth Taylor, Naomi Judd, Prince Charles and the late Dr.
Benjamin Spock, to name a few. In addition to overseeing the Chopra Center and
producing a continuous flow of high-profile books, Chopra also appears on CD-
ROM *(Deepak Chopra's The Wisdom Within),* publishes a monthly newsletter, pursues an active global lecture schedule, markets a line of herbal supplement and
maintains a popular website (<www.chopra.com>). He has also written numerous
magazine columns, usually for alternative medicine or New Age–themed publications, a novel, song lyrics and even a script for a yet-unproduced movie. More
recently his accomplishments were acknowledged by President Clinton at a state
dinner held in India on March 21, 2000: "My country has been enriched by the
contributions of more than a million Indian Americans, which includes Dr.
Deepak Chopra, the pioneer of alternative medicine."[26]

When asked about his success, Chopra has generally downplayed his own acumen and resisted any mantle of spiritual leadership: "I happened to be at the right

time for a lot of people obviously interested in this stuff," he explained in one interview. "So I come along, and if I didn't come along, somebody else would have. We're all just blips on the ocean of consciousness."[27] Given the visibility, celebrity status and cash flow of his particular blip, however, not all of the attention he has drawn has been flattering. A *Los Angeles Times Magazine* lead article featured Chopra's picture with the superimposed title "NIRVANA INC" on the cover, referring to him as a "One-Man Multimedia Empire."[28] *Newsweek* playfully introduced him as follows:

> Deepak Chopra, M.D.—educator, author, lecturer, endocrinologist, Hollywood guru and scribe of the *Playboy* essay "Does God Have Orgasms?"—is, by his own metaphysical lexicon, a manifestation of our collective conscious. In a culture that craves a spiritual, mind-body fix, he is a fixer: handsome, charismatic, an erudite amalgam of hard science and celestial seasonings, drawn selectively from the Vedic texts of ancient India. To his critics, he is a dabbler with an M.D., making millions by conflating sound medicine with New Age hoo-ha. But to the growing legions inside his tent, dissatisfied with the parental shadow of both mainstream religion and medicine, he is a gift: the Buddha as benevolent technocrat [29]

We should make it clear that it is not our goal to "expose" Chopra or in some way assault his character. The fact that he has been highly successful does not at all imply that he is unscrupulous or disreputable. We do, however, have some serious concerns about the content of his teachings. Given his high profile in our culture and around the world, those teachings should not be immune to scrutiny and, when appropriate, challenge.

The Universe According to Deepak Chopra

So what do the books, columns, website, audio and video materials have to say? While he certainly promotes the practice of *ayurveda,* even a casual perusal of Chopra's output makes it abundantly clear that his primary concern is the grand scheme of things: the nature of reality, the universe, consciousness and, above all, "God," though definitely not the Creator described in the pages of the Bible. And while he puts his own spin on these topics, including a generous flow of anecdotes and quotes to illustrate his ideas, his primary thrust is stating and restating the basic principles of a Vedic, monistic worldview.

1. All is one. Chopra entitles chapter thirty-seven of his book *Creating Health* "One Is All, and All Is One," and he certainly is not shy about this declaration of monism. As we already noted (and will discuss in more depth later), his recent book *How to Know God* goes to some length to attach the term *God* to this impersonal, all-encompassing "oneness" of the universe. In his previous books, however, he avoided overtly religious terminology by using phrases such as the "field of all possibilities," "pure consciousness," "pure potentiality" and a "field of energy and information" as synonyms for the infinite One. He also appropriated quantum physics as an all-purpose explanation and rationale for concepts that might not otherwise set well with Western readers.

In his early bestseller *Quantum Healing: Exploring the Frontiers of Mind/Body Medicine*, Chopra used the term *quantum* with two primary meanings. One is that of a dramatic shift or change—a quantum leap, as it were—in consciousness or awareness, which brings about healing or at least a significant improvement in one's condition. Chopra refers to such events as "quantum healing," hence the title of his book. But his more pervasive use of the term attempts to use quantum physics as a rationale for monism and, more importantly, to bolster his energetic promotion of the idea that we can alter the physical world by changing the way we think about it.

2. We are, at our core, perfect and divine. "Our essential nature is one of pure potentiality," Chopra writes in *The Seven Spiritual Laws of Success*. We are no less than the universe itself:

> Your body is not separate from the universe, because at quantum mechanical levels there are no well-defined edges. . . . The larger quantum field—the universe—is your extended body.
>
> The physical universe is nothing other than the Self curving back within Itself to experience Itself as spirit, mind, and physical matter. In other words, all processes of creation are processes through which the Self or divinity expresses itself. . . . These three components of reality—spirit, mind, and the body, or observer, the process of observing and the observed—are all essentially the same thing. . . . The physical laws of the universe are actually this whole process of divinity in motion, or consciousness in motion.[30]

Chopra's interactive CD-ROM *The Wisdom Within: Your Personal Program for Total Well-Being* includes a number of affirmations that are intended to help the user grasp this idea:

> I am a field of pure potentiality.
> I have the power within me to heal myself.
> I'm awakening to the wisdom within me.
> Freedom, love and bliss are my natural states of being.
> The infinite flow of the universe is within me.
> My body is ageless, timeless and boundless.
> I am in touch with my divine nature every day.
> My spirit soars, my spirit dives deep—I am space, I am the earth.

My body is a concentration of the energy in the universe.

The knowledge of the universe is within me.

I am no longer seeing myself as separate from the consciousness of the universe.

My body is part of the universal body.

The creative power within me can give birth to a shooting star.[31]

3. We must become enlightened regarding the unity of all things and regarding our true, perfect nature. If everyday experience does not exactly validate the notion that all is one and that we are perfect, how might we gain this perspective? Chopra strongly promotes meditation, and the altered states of consciousness it might induce, for this purpose. In his interactive CD-ROM Chopra declares:

> If you could bring only one ayurvedic technique into your life, meditation should unquestionably be your choice. Though it's often represented as a relaxation method, a kind of self-hypnosis for getting your mind off your troubles, this is an entirely incomplete picture of meditation in the ayurvedic sense. . . . The ancient sages of India were already quite relaxed by the time they began to meditate. Their intention was really something much more profound. And yours can be also. Through the practice of meditation . . . you can create an internal reference point of spirit rather than ego. You can enter the silent spaces between your thoughts.[32]

In his book *Journey into Healing* he adds:

> The practice of meditation takes our awareness from the disturbed state of conscious-ness in the mind and the world of physical objects to the silent, undisturbed state of consciousness in the realm of soul and spirit. Through regular practice we gain access to the infinite storehouse of knowledge—the ultimate reality of creation. We have the experience of who we really are—pure unbounded consciousness.[33]

4. Enlightenment leads to healing and other major benefits. Rather than withdrawing from the material world, Chopra proposes instead that we tap into the "field of pure potentiality" in order to generate whatever version of reality we desire. Not only does optimal health beckon to those who grasp these ideas (and also pursue wellness through *ayurveda*), but in addition the aging process itself—an "illusion" that a sizable number of baby boomers, including Chopra, all happen to be expe-riencing at the present time—can be slowed down or even brought to a halt. His bestseller *Ageless Body, Timeless Mind* plants this flag boldly in its first paragraph:

> I would like you to join me on a voyage of discovery. We will explore a place where the rules of everyday existence do not apply. These rules explicitly state that to grow old, become frail, and die is the ultimate destiny of all. And so it has been for century after century. However, I want you to suspend your assumptions about what we call reality so that we can become pioneers in a land where youthful vigor, renewal, creativity, joy, ful-

fillment, and timelessness are the common experience of everyday life, where old age, senility, infirmity and death do not exist and are not even entertained as a philosophy.[34]

While we are avoiding the aging process, we can also draw to ourselves a bountiful flow of the goods and experiences commonly associated with "the good life" on our nonexistent planet. In *The Seven Spiritual Laws of Success* Chopra is particularly enthusiastic about the benefits of affluence:

> You can think of your physical body as a device for controlling energy: It can generate, store and expend energy. If you know how to generate, store and expend energy in an efficient way, then you can create any amount of wealth.
>
> True wealth consciousness is the ability to have anything you want, anytime you want, and with the least effort. . . .
>
> There are many aspects to success; material wealth is only one component. Moreover, success is a journey, not a destination. Material abundance, in all its expressions, happens to be one of those things that make the journey more enjoyable. But success also includes good health, energy and enthusiasm for life, fulfilling relationships, creative freedom, emotional and psychological stability, a sense of well-being, and peace of mind.[35]

In the same book he makes a specific connection between the flow of invisible life energy and the flow of cold, hard cash:

> The word affluence comes from the root word "affluere," which means "to flow to." The word affluence means "to flow in abundance." Money is really a symbol of the life energy we exchange and the life energy we use as a result of the service we provide to the universe. Another word for money is "currency," which also reflects the flowing nature of energy. The word currency comes from the Latin word "currere," which means "to run" or to flow.
>
> Therefore, if we stop the circulation of money—if our only intention is to hold on to our money and hoard it—since it is life energy, we will stop its circulation back into our lives as well. In order to keep that energy coming to us, we have to keep the energy circulating.[36]

Indeed the titles and subtitles of Chopra's books are a series of irresistible promises. Note the well-written enticement in each of the following:

☐ *Ageless Body, Timeless Mind: The Quantum Alternative to Growing Old*

☐ *The Seven Spiritual Laws of Success: A Practical Guide to the Fulfillment of Your Dreams*

☐ *The Seven Spiritual Laws of Success for Parents: Guiding Your Children to Success and Fulfillment*

☐ *Boundless Energy: The Complete Mind/Body Program for Overcoming Chronic Fatigue*

☐ *Creating Affluence: Wealth Consciousness in the Field of All Possibilities*
☐ *Creating Health: How to Wake Up the Body's Intelligence*
☐ *Healing the Heart: A Spiritual Approach to Reversing Coronary Artery Disease*
☐ *Perfect Digestion: The Key to Balanced Living*
☐ *Perfect Weight: The Complete Mind/Body Program for Achieving and Maintaining Your Ideal Weight*
☐ *Restful Sleep: The Complete Mind/Body Program for Overcoming Insomnia*
☐ *Unconditional Life: Discovering the Power to Fulfill Your Dreams*
☐ *The Way of the Wizard: Twenty Spiritual Lessons for Creating the Life You Want*

Similar titles beckon the curious to participate in Chopra's workshops and seminars, most of which are held at the Chopra Center in La Jolla (although Chopra himself teaches only a limited number of them). These are undoubtedly all-encompassing experiences, far more so than reading a book or clicking a mouse to activate the contents of a CD-ROM. Some have been accredited by the National Board of Certified Counselors for continuing education credit.[37] Offerings include the following:

☐ Seduction of Spirit ("Seven days of spiritual awakening that will transform your life forever")
☐ Return to Wholeness ("Supports the integration of the best of holistic and Western scientific approaches to cancer")
☐ Vital Energy ("For people facing chronic fatigue and low energy")
☐ Creating Health Program ("The core component of the Center's teachings and treatments to reduce stress and make healthier lifestyle choices")
☐ SynchroDestiny ("Spontaneous fulfillment of desire")
☐ Sacred Sexuality ("Traditional Chinese medicine and ancient sages teach how to convert sex from a pastime into a holy art form")[38]

Who would not be interested in perfect health, boundless energy, restful sleep, ideal weight, successful children, vibrant sex, indefinite youth, boundless affluence and fulfillment of all of one's dreams? Furthermore, what society would not benefit from having a large number of its populace living in bliss and harmony? In a passage that is reminiscent of the expansive optimism of Maharishi Mahesh Yogi (who has envisioned himself and Transcendental Meditation as agents for massive social change in the world), Chopra predicts the following as more and more people experience a "rise in consciousness":

> Because of a rise in consciousness, we will witness a steady decline in the number of deaths from today's common diseases—cancer, stroke, hypertension, heart disease—and fewer fatalities from accidents of all kinds. . . . People will live longer and health-

ier lives. . . . Spontaneous right action will become commonplace as a normal trait.
. . . Groups of people who have learned the process of transcending will activate the
field of consciousness more and more deeply, and with more and more benefit to
themselves. . . . As the dynamics of group consciousness are further explored, they
will be applied successfully to solve social problems on the widest possible scale. . . .
Crime and social deviance will dramatically decrease. . . . Prosperity and progress
will be dramatically advanced. . . . World peace will become a practical possibility. . . .
What the mind of man conceives, it will find the power to accomplish."[39]

Enlightening our children is a priority as well: "If a critical mass of our children
are raised to practice the Seven Spiritual Laws, our whole civilization will be
transformed."[40]

One can almost hear Professor Harold Hill's exuberant patter in these claims
as Chopra clicks through this marvelous checklist of benefits from his "Think
System." ("If a critical mass of River City's children join the boys' band, we can
avoid Trouble with a capital 'T'!") Why bother with the tedious process of scientific research and development (practicing the cornet), when all we need do in
order to rid the world of disease is to "raise our consciousness" (think the Minuet in G)?

What's Wrong with This Picture?
No one can fault Deepak Chopra for wanting to help people feel better and live
more abundant lives, nor for pursuing the fulfillment of his personal and spiritual
dreams. No one can argue that he is not good at what he does—disseminating his
vision of health, wealth and enlightenment through all of the vehicles available to
him. But the gospel he preaches, in our opinion (and we are hardly alone), leads
the masses who follow him in several wrong directions—logically, scientifically,
medically, spiritually and possibly morally as well. We wish to register the following objections.

The Permanent Problem of Object Permanence
In chapter four we noted that neither our everyday experience nor the exercise of
normal waking consciousness validates the notion that all is one in the universe,
that the world around us is illusory, that there is no objective reality, that there in
fact are no real distinctions among me, you, a tree, a bug, a rock and the Milky
Way. But Chopra insists that we accept these ideas if we are going to experience
true health and happiness. He presses relentlessly on this point throughout his
writings, but perhaps nowhere as forcefully as in the opening paragraphs of *Ageless
Body, Timeless Mind.* What perpetuates aging and death, he proclaims, is "our con-

ditioning, our current collective worldview that we were taught by our parents, teachers and society."

> The way of seeing things—the old paradigm—has aptly been called "the hypnosis of social conditioning," an induced fiction in which we have collectively agreed to participate.
>
> Your body is aging beyond your control because it has been programmed to live out the rules of that collective conditioning. If there is anything natural and inevitable about the aging process, it cannot be known until the chains of our old beliefs are broken. In order to create the experience of ageless body and timeless mind, which is the promise of this book, you must discard ten assumptions about who you are and what the true nature of the mind and body is. These assumptions form the bedrock of our shared worldview.[41]

The first assumption that Chopra invites us to toss out is the belief that there is "an objective world independent of the observer, and our bodies are an aspect of this objective world."[42]

On the contrary, gaining comprehension that there is an "objective world independent of the observer" is a critical developmental passage from infancy to childhood and beyond. One of its earliest manifestations is the acquisition of what is called "object permanence." This is demonstrated when an infant watches someone cover a toy with a blanket and then the baby pulls the blanket away because she knows the toy is still there. But object permanence does not just apply to babies and blankets, nor is it the product of a "current collective worldview" or "social conditioning." It arises from the fact that there really *is* an objective world around us, that it exists independently of our personal or collective observations and that dealing intelligently with it is a necessary developmental milestone for an infant—and for a civilization. Without this understanding we remain stuck in perpetual infancy, in primitive helplessness.

Here are a few Zenlike—but actually biblical—questions for any proponent of monism: Were there oceans and jungles and continents teeming with life before any of us were around to collectively create them,? Who created the North Pole, the Grand Canyon and the Hawaiian Islands before the first human being saw them, and why did they look essentially the same (aside from changes brought about by climate, erosion or other natural processes) to the next human who came along? Whose consciousness determined that Halley's comet would be visible from the earth every seventy-five to seventy-nine years? Who set galaxies in place millions of light-years away from our planet before we had telescopes to see them?

In the book of Job, God posed similar questions to the title character:

Where were you when I laid the earth's foundation?
    Tell me, if you understand.
Who marked off its dimensions? Surely you know! . . .
Have you journeyed to the springs of the sea
    or walked in the recesses of the deep? . . .
Have you comprehended the vast expanses of the earth?
    Tell me, if you know all this. . . .
Can you raise your voice to the clouds
    and cover yourself with a flood of water?
Do you send the lightning bolts on their way?
    Do they report to you, "Here we are"?
Who endowed the heart with wisdom
    or gave understanding to the mind? (Job 38:4-5, 16, 18, 34-36)

Someone who has embraced the core teachings of Chopra's books might be tempted to answer, "I, the Self curving back within Itself, the pure unbounded consciousness, the field of infinite potentiality, have indeed done and know all of these things."

On a day-to-day level, monism raises some eminently practical questions. If the world around us is not real, why is there any consistency to it? If we are generating all of this in some sort of shared illusion, how is it that we can follow a map to a place where we have never been? If monism is true, why get out of bed, bathe, go to school or attempt to accumulate knowledge of anything except whatever emerges while in an altered state of consciousness? If aging is an illusion, what shall we say when wrinkles appear on our faces, when our eyes refuse to focus the way they used to, when our joints stiffen, when our intestinal tract slows down? Will we exclaim, like the Wizard of Oz when Toto pulled away the curtain, "Pay no attention to the man with the graying temples"? Are we to maintain till the moment of death that our impending demise is not actually going to happen but that we're having a little trouble resisting the "collective worldview"? The ultimate demonstration of the futility of monism is the fact that no one who proclaims it can actually live as if it were true.

The Hijacking of Quantum Mechanics

While a detailed account of quantum theory is beyond the scope of this discussion, it is important to understand a few of its broad strokes in order to assess how Chopra, and others who think along similar lines, have misappropriated it.

In the early twentieth century the theory of quantum mechanics was born in an effort to account for certain phenomena that could not be adequately explained using classical Newtonian physics. Three components are of particular significance, and their rather mysterious nature has provided abundant food for mystical and New Age thought:

☐ The seemingly paradoxical wave-particle duality of light and subatomic particles. Light, usually considered to be a wave phenomenon, also behaves as if it occurs in small, discrete bundles of energy called photons. And electrons, which had been conceived of as extremely tiny particles, were found to have wavelike properties.

☐ The Heisenberg uncertainty principle, which states that at the subatomic level certain measurements, such as position and momentum, cannot be made simultaneously with absolute precision. In experiments in the subatomic realm one can predict certain results only with probabilities rather than with total certainty.

☐ The observer effect, which states that the act of observing events at the subatomic level has an effect on what is being observed.

We noted in chapter four that Einstein's equation $E = mc^2$, which describes the conversion of matter into energy under very specific conditions, has been misunderstood by alternative therapists and wrongly applied to human physiology. Our bodies are not atomic reactors, and this equation has no relevance to health, disease or any biological process. Chopra repeatedly makes the same mistake with quantum mechanical events on the subatomic level, not only misinterpreting them but also generously misapplying them to suit his rhetorical purposes. He is fascinated, for example, with the observation that the configuration of atoms includes a considerable amount of empty space. Combining this idea with the equivalence of matter and energy, and stirring them vigorously, he redefines the "One" of monism as "energy and information."

> Energy and information exist everywhere in nature. In fact, at the level of the quantum field, there is nothing other than energy and information. The quantum field is just another label for the field of pure consciousness or pure potentiality. And this quantum field is influenced by intention and desire. . . . Your body is not separate from the universe, because at quantum mechanical levels there are no well-defined edges. . . . The larger quantum field—the universe—is your extended body.[43]

He frequently refers to the "energy and information" surrounding us as "quantum soup" and insists that quantum theory proves that our belief in the physical reality of ourselves, or anything else, is an illusion.

> The basic conclusion of quantum field theorists is that the raw material of the world is non-material; the essential stuff of the universe is nonstuff. All of our technology is based on this fact. And this is the climactic overthrow of the superstition of materialism today.[44]
>
> Reality exists only because we agree on it. Whenever reality shifts, the agreement has been changed.[45]

In *Ageless Body, Timeless Mind* he sets forth ten assumptions of the "new paradigm," a "more complete and expanded version of the truth." These include the following:

☐ "The physical world, including our bodies, is a response of the observer. We create our bodies as we create the experience of our world."

☐ "In their essential state, our bodies are composed of energy and information, not solid matter. This energy and information is an outcropping of infinite fields of energy and information spanning the universe."

☐ "The biochemistry of the body is a product of awareness. Beliefs, thoughts, and emotions create the chemical reactions that uphold life in every cell. An aging cell is the end product of awareness that has forgotten how to remain new."

☐ "Although each person seems separate and independent, all of us are connected to patterns of intelligence that govern the whole cosmos. Our bodies are part of a universal body, our minds an aspect of a universal mind."

☐ "Each of us inhabits a reality lying beyond all change. Deep inside us, unknown to the five senses, is an innermost core of being, a field of non-change that creates personality, ego and body. This being is our essential state—it is who we are."

☐ "We are not victims of aging, sickness, and death. These are part of the scenery, not the seer, who is immune to any form of change. This seer is the spirit, the expression of eternal being."[46]

In order to back up this expansive manifesto, he repeatedly introduces quantum physics into the conversation. Chopra frequently invokes the Heisenberg uncertainty principle and the observer effect, which he mistakenly applies to our daily experience.

> These are vast assumptions, the making of a new reality, yet all are grounded in the discoveries of quantum physics made almost a hundred years ago. The seeds of this new paradigm were planted by Einstein, Bohr, Heisenberg, and the other pioneers of quantum physics, who realized that the accepted way of viewing the physical world was false. Although things "out there" appear to be real, there is no proof of reality apart from the observer. No two people share exactly the same universe. Every worldview creates its own world.[47]

It is true that, at the subatomic level, the process of observing changes what is being observed. A crude analogy would be that of using a finger to determine the location of grains of sand on the sidewalk. It is very difficult to touch one of the grains without moving it, and in so doing we change what we were trying to determine. In subatomic experiments it is the apparatus involved in the measurements that causes the change. But Chopra and others who are enamored with things quantum wreak havoc with this idea by claiming that it is our mind, our consciousness, that provokes changes—not only in quantum physics experiments but in everyday experience as well. He takes this notion even farther out on a limb by claiming that quantum mechanics supports the postmodern view that reality is defined solely by the observer.

Physicists have generally taken a dim view of this sort of foray into their domain, and some have applied rhetorical saws rather vigorously to the limb where Chopra has chosen to perch. Victor Stenger, professor of physics and astronomy at the University of Hawaii, has written extensively about what he has dubbed "Quantum Quackery." His conclusions about misappropriations of quantum mechanics are blunt:

> Quantum mechanics, the centerpiece of modern physics, is misinterpreted as implying that the human mind controls reality and that the universe is one connected whole that cannot be understood by the usual reduction to parts. However, no compelling argument or evidence requires that quantum mechanics plays a central role in human consciousness or provides instantaneous, holistic connections across the universe. Modern physics, including quantum mechanics, remains completely materialistic and reductionistic while being consistent with all scientific observations.[48]

Another pointed critique of Chopra's quantum reasoning, published in the magazine *Skeptic,* notes that he "finds connections where there may be none, and recklessly superimposes the laws of one level of reality on the matter of another." Summarizing Chopra's questionable logic, this 1998 article by author Phil Molé continued:

> Chopra's plea for a paradigm shift, ironically, seems to stem from the very dichotomous thinking abhorred by mystics for centuries. If classical physics has been proven to be limited, he reasons, then it must not contain any "real" truth. Modern physics, with all of its new laws and insights, must therefore represent the deeper reality. But this "either/or" business of choosing paradigms is patently absurd, because modern and Newtonian physics are both perfectly valid theories in their own rights and within their own applications. The classical model is a perfectly good description of macroscopic objects moving at relatively low velocities—it only breaks down when matter approaches subatomic size, or when it travels at velocities near the speed of light. Quantum mechanics also has its breaking point: at sizes somewhat bigger than that of a single atom, quantum effects such as wave-particle duality are no longer observed. It would be just as valid, from Chopra's narrow viewpoint, to point to this limitation of quantum mechanics as proof that classical physics is the one true model of reality. For our bodies, the classical view is clearly the most accurate, since we're well beyond the size limit of quantum mechanical nature.[49]

We have pressed our argument against Chopra's use of quantum theory because he invokes it so liberally to support his viewpoint. Unfortunately, even a well-educated reader may be intimidated by these rather mysterious concepts of modern physics and Chopra's apparent command of them, and may come to the conclusion that physical scientists around the world stand behind his proclamations about consciousness, healing, energy fields and the rest. This, of course, is not at all true. More than anything, the quantum arguments serve a variety of rhetorical rather than logical purposes throughout Chopra's works. An accurate and amusing depiction of this state of affairs appeared on the cover of the *Skeptic* magazine in which the above-quoted article appeared. Next to a delicate drawing of Chopra contemplating a flower there stands an old-fashioned patent medicine bottle bearing, in elaborate nineteenth-century typeface, the following inscription:

Elixir of Quantum Mechanics

☐ Generates awe
☐ Eliminates hand waving
☐ Patches spotty arguments
☐ Easily explains the inexplicable
☐ More profound than relativity
☐ More satisfying than "vibrates on a higher frequency"
Add a dash to any argument.

An excellent example of adding a dash of quantum mechanics to bolster an argument may be found in one of Chopra's more recent discussions of meditation. He describes a variety of meditative techniques and exercises throughout his books, although he frequently showcases the use of "primordial sounds, the basic sounds of nature." This form of meditation is not the quiet reflection, contemplation of one's life and relationships or focusing on God's precepts as described frequently in the Psalms. Rather it is the repetition of a mantra, one of several words or phrases said to have unique power and significance in the universe. In the Vedic traditions that he embraces they are viewed as having direct ties to Hindu gods and goddesses. For example, an introductory guide to yoga for the beginning meditator (not written by Chopra) notes that

> mantras are Sanskrit syllables, words or phrases which, when repeated in meditation, will bring the individual to a higher state of consciousness. They are sounds or energies that have always existed in the universe and can neither be created nor destroyed. There are six qualities common to any true mantra: it was originally revealed to and handed on by a sage who attained self-realization through it; it has a certain meter and a presiding deity; it has a "bija" or seed at its essence which invests it with special power; it has divine cosmic energy or shakti; and lastly it has a key

which must be unlocked through constant repetition before pure consciousness is revealed.[50]

Chopra hedges his bet on the significance of mantras in his book *How to Know God*. He clearly does not promote the biblical notion of contemplating the attributes of the God who is "out there," since that would contradict his conviction that God is within and that we are all divine. But this is a book for Western readers, who are not likely to connect with the idea of doing spiritual business with "presiding deities" from the Hindu pantheon. He is also not willing to accept the premise of the "relaxation response" described by Herbert Benson, who concluded that the particular word one repeats during meditation does not matter, as long as it is agreeable or meaningful to the individual doing so.[51] In order to maintain his ties with Vedism while sounding reasonable, he invokes, as an all-purpose rhetorical tool, quantum theory. Commenting on Dr. Benson's approach to relaxation, he notes:

> He removed the mantra, replacing it with any neutral word that could be repeated mentally while slowly breathing in and out (he suggested the word *one*). Others, including myself, have disagreed with this approach and based our approach on the central value of a mantra as a means of unfolding deeper spiritual levels inside the mind. To us, the recited word has to be connected to God.
>
> The spiritual properties of mantras have two bases. Some orthodox Hindus would say that every mantra is a version of God's name, while others would claim and this is very close to quantum physics—that the vibration of the mantra is the key. The word *vibration* means the frequency of brain activity in the cerebral cortex. The mantra forms a feedback loop as the brain produces the sound, listens to it, and then responds with a deeper level of attention. Mysticism isn't involved.[52]

This is clever but misleading wordplay. He repeatedly mentions *God,* the word to which nearly all Western readers will have some sort of connection, even if merely cultural (for example, "In God we trust"), when he is actually referring to Hindu deities. (If orthodox Hindus say that "every mantra is a version of God's name," they are not exactly thinking of Jehovah.) Furthermore, mantras, vibrations, brain activity, feedback loops and quantum physics may be somehow related in Chopra's discourse, but not in contemporary science. Passages such as this may impart a sense of importance and substance to the subject at hand and, more importantly, help convince people that practices such as repeating a magical word over and over are not superstitious and primitive. But they are, in fact, incoherent.

How to Know Whom?

In the spring of 2000 Chopra released a book that appeared to break new ground, shifting from health and wealth, *ayurveda* and quantum physics to a full-blown exposition of theology. Actually, this was not as much of a stretch as one might imagine, since all of his previous books were primarily concerned with promulgating an all-encompassing worldview. They were undercover theological works, using a variety of aliases for God such as "pure consciousness" and "the field of energy and information." In *How to Know God: The Soul's Journey into the Mystery of Mysteries,* however, Chopra approached the subject of ultimate reality head-on. Judging by the endorsements that fill several pages in the front of the book, one might wonder whether Chopra had entered the rarefied company of St. Augustine, Carl Jung, Lao-tzu or even Jesus himself. His well-wishers include, among many others, religious leaders (the Dalai Lama), former heads of state (Mikhail Gorbachev, Oscar Arias), professors, scholars, alternative medicine promoters (Drs. Andrew Weil, Larry Dossey, Bernie Siegel) and celebrities (Shirley MacLaine, Larry King, Uri Geller). Not surprisingly, conservative biblical teachers or scholars—evangelical, Catholic or Jewish—are not represented.

Chopra's deft, almost elegant writing—arguably the best of any of his books— appears to draw liberally from the wisdom and insights of a number of faiths: Hinduism, Buddhism, Judaism, Christianity, Islam and others, mixed with an ample dose of Chopra's trademark "quantum" verbiage. He also seems, at face value, to be courteous and generous to all of the traditions from which he draws. But a closer look reveals a tendency to reinterpret, or even reinvent, ideas that have been taught for centuries, in order to mold them to his purposes. Ultimately his drive to the goal line of the book's title involves deconstructing any religious teaching or doctrine that might stand in the way of our embracing monism and thus experiencing ourselves as God. Readers who navigate through the entire book will encounter some vivid descriptions of becoming "one with everything" in the cosmos. They will also encounter a jarring paradox of monism: when we finally arrive at that supposedly blissful point, we cease to exist. In becoming God we become nothing.

> If God has a home, it has to be in the void. Otherwise, he would be limited. Can we really know such a boundless deity? In stage seven two impossible things must converge. The person has to be reduced to the merest point, a speck of identity closing the last minuscule gap between himself and God. At the same time, just when separation is healed, the tiny point has to expand to infinity. The mystics describe this as "the One becomes All."[53]

Prospective readers should mark well the language of one of this book's most ringing, and revealing, endorsements:

Deepak Chopra has blessed the world by spreading the light of vedic knowledge and the timeless teachings on nonduality. Vedanta has inspired and transformed the lives of seekers for thousands of years. However, every age needs a voice that can articulate ancient Wisdom in a contemporary framework. Dr. Chopra has given the seekers of self-knowledge a clear and scientific road map to understand and realize the ultimate reality. I congratulate him for his brilliant work.

His Holiness Vasudevanand Saraswati,
Jagad Guru Shankracharya of
Jyotirmath World Headquarters
established by Adi Shankara
(sage-philosopher of India, A.D. 686–718)[54]

A good portion of *How to Know God* takes the reader through "Seven Stages of God," seven "versions" of God that arise not just from human need but from intrinsic biological responses. In a statement that greets visitors to his How to Know God website (<www.howtoknowgod.com>), Chopra explains:

I have come to the conclusion that all human beings are structured to know God. Our nervous systems are structured to make sense of the world around us, and spirit is essential to our understanding of the forms and phenomena that constitute the material universe. In *How to Know God,* I present a framework of seven stages of human experience—and therefore of God consciousness—through which we respond to the challenges of life. We begin with a survival or "fight or flight" response that yields an all powerful, capricious God, and end with unity consciousness, through which we can experience the divine in all things, living and inert. While formulating these ideas, I became very excited by the recognition that these seven sacred responses apply to everyone, regardless of religion or spiritual tradition. They even explain how those who do not consider themselves religious can have the direct experience of God.[55]

Unfortunately, the passages of this book that draw on the Old and New Testaments feature "insights" and commentaries that demonstrate a lack of understanding, or complete disregard, of biblical interpretation (hermeneutics). For example, Chopra comments on the Old Testament account of Adam and Eve in the context of a discussion of Jehovah as the most primitive understanding of God, a literal projection of our unreasoning "old brain."

The old brain is reflected in a God who seems not to possess much in the way of higher functions. He is primordial and largely unforgiving. He knows who his enemies are; he doesn't come from the school of forgive and forget. If we list his attributes, which many would trace back to the Old Testament, the God of stage one is

Vengeful
Capricious
Quick to anger

Jealous

Judgmental—meting out reward and punishment

Unfathomable

Sometimes merciful

This description doesn't only fit Jehovah, who was also loving and benevolent. Among the Indian gods and on Mount Olympus one encounters the same willful, dangerous behavior. For God is very dangerous in stage one; he uses nature to punish even his most favored children through storms, floods, earthquakes, and disease. The test of the faithful is to see the good side of such a deity, and overwhelmingly the faithful have.[56]

As Chopra describes the Genesis account of the fall of humanity, God is cast as a "capricious and unpredictable parent."

The first man and woman are the ultimate bad children. The sin they commit is to disobey God's dictum not to eat of the tree of knowledge. If we examine this act in symbolic terms, we see a father who is jealous of his adult prerogatives: he knows best, he holds the power, his word is law. To maintain his position, it is necessary that the children remain children, yet they yearn to grow up and have the same knowledge possessed by the father. Usually that is permissible, but God is the only father who was never a child himself. This makes him all the more unsympathetic, for his anger against Adam and Eve is irrational in its harshness.[57]

Chopra completes his commentary on this passage with a chilling observation: "Another irony is at work here. . . . The only character in the episode of Eve and the apple who seems to tell the truth is the serpent."[58] This comment does not appear to be sarcastic. Chopra literally sees the serpent's temptation—that "when you eat of it your eyes will be opened, and you will be like God, knowing good and evil"—as not only true but also desirable. "The serpent is holding out a world of awareness, independence, and decision making. All these things follow when you have knowledge. In other words, the serpent is advising God's children to grow up, and of course this is a temptation they cannot resist."[59]

As startling as this apparent sympathy for the devil might seem, the serpent's invitation to become a god really *is* the primary quest of monism. We have already noted that this worldview does not acknowledge the existence of evil as distinct from good, and so the idea that yielding to the temptation might be wrong, let alone that it might be advanced by a nonmaterial being with evil intentions, would not be taken seriously in Chopra's spiritual economy. What he fails to acknowledge, however, is that the serpent really *did* lie. Adam and Eve (and everyone born after them) died as a result of their rebellion, despite the tempter's bold claim to the contrary. And no one has yet become a god, although for thousands of years many individuals have thought otherwise.

Chopra goes on to say that we should not be too hard on the "God of stage one," because he was born out of the primal human need to survive in harsh surroundings. Nevertheless, this God is also "a permanent legacy that everyone confronts before inner growth can be achieved."[60] His proposition is that the decision of human beings to disobey their Creator in exchange for a promise of godhood was a merely an attempt to "grow up" and acquire "independence and awareness."

Chopra offers a particularly imaginative take on John 1:1, one of the most familiar and profound statements in the New Testament: "In the beginning was the Word, and the Word was with God, and the Word was God." Within a few verses, John the apostle explained what—or more precisely, whom—he was talking about: "The Word became flesh and made his dwelling among us. We have seen his glory, the glory of the One and Only, who came from the Father, full of grace and truth" (John 1:14). A straightforward reading of the first chapter of the Gospel of John makes it indisputably clear that "the Word" is Jesus, who as God created the universe and who as a man walked upon one of the planets he had created. This is a conclusion that would quickly unravel Chopra's theology.

Rather than taking John's simple but elegant Greek at face value, Chopra offers this interpretation: "Clearly, no ordinary word is implied. Something like the following is meant: Before there was time and space, a faint vibration existed outside the cosmos. This vibration had everything contained in it—all universes, all events, all time and space. The primordial vibration was with God. As far as we can fathom, it *is* God. Divine intelligence was compressed in this 'word,' and when the time came for the universe to be born, the 'word,' transformed itself into energy and matter." He adds another twist when he states, "In India the sound of the divine mother took the name *om*, and it is believed that meditating on this sound will unlock all the mother's secrets. Perhaps *om* is the very word John is referring to."[61] Needless to say, such an esoteric interpretation of the first verse of the Gospel of John is hardly true to its context or the clear intention of its author.

Mystics and monists usually give Jesus special recognition as an "enlightened teacher" or "ascended master" or even "bearer of the Christ consciousness," but they never acknowledge the validity of his audacious claim to be "the way, the truth and the life" (John 14:6). In *How to Know God*, Jesus is actually rather inconspicuous, appearing only now and again to offer quotations that Chopra then adapts freely to his own purposes. For example:

☐ "When Jesus taught his followers that 'the truth will set you free,' he didn't mean a certain set of facts or dogmas but revealed truth. In modern language we might come up with a different translation: seek the knower within and it will set you free."[62]

☐ "In one phrase—'as you sow, so shall you reap'—Jesus stated the law of karma quite succinctly."[63]

☐ "When Jesus said 'I am the light,' he meant 'I'm totally in God's force field.' "[64]

☐ "The story of Jesus reaches its poignant climax in the garden of Gethsemane, when he prays that the cup be taken from his hands. He knows that the Romans are going to capture and kill him, and the prospect gives rise to a terrible moment of doubt. It is one of loneliest and most wrenching moments in the New Testament—and it is utterly imaginary. . . . I think that this last temptation was projected onto him by writers of the gospel. Why? Because they couldn't conceive of his situation except through their own."[65]

The number of ways in which this book tampers with the teachings and sensibilities of major world faiths, especially Judaism and Christianity, as it ushers readers toward Chopra's Vedic version of monism is almost beyond counting. Indeed *How to Know God* could keep a conservative Bible scholar busy for weeks cataloguing and addressing all of its hermeneutical indiscretions. But in closing this segment and transitioning to the next, we want to reiterate what Chopra sees as the ultimate destination for all of us: becoming God and simultaneously becoming nothing.

The Trivializing of Good and Evil

One of the most profound implications of monism is the notion that our identity as the divine Self, the universe, the One means that we are literally without sin. Not surprisingly, to Chopra the concept of offending God is meaningless. In his volume devoted specifically to rearing children—*The Seven Spiritual Laws for Parents: Guiding Your Children to Success and Fulfillment*—he declares that "the seeds of God are inside us."

> When we make the journey of the spirit, we water these divine seeds. . . . In time the flowers of God bloom within and around us, and we begin to witness and know the miracle of the divine wherever we go.
>
> In the eyes of spirit, everyone is innocent, in all senses of the word. Because you are innocent, you have not done anything that merits punishment or divine wrath.
>
> Being in touch with the field of all possibilities means that you experience self-referral—that is, you look within for guidance. . . . Everyone can get in touch with the seed of God that is inside.[66]

Not only are we "innocent, in all senses of the word" but categories such as right and wrong, good and evil, are illusory as well. Expending our time and energy evaluating life events in these terms is therefore counterproductive. In *Creating Affluence* he notes, "When we relinquish our need to constantly classify things as good or bad, right or wrong, then we experience more silence in our consciousness. . . . It is important, therefore, to get away from definitions, labels, descriptions, interpretations, evaluations, analyses, and judgment, for all of these create turbulence in our internal dialogue."[67]

In *The Seven Spiritual Laws of Success* he adds that the aforementioned turbulence also "constricts the flow of energy between you and the field of pure potentiality." He recommends a prayer from the trance-mediated New Age manifesto *A Course in Miracles:* "Today I shall judge nothing that occurs." Chopra notes, "Nonjudgment creates silence in your mind. It is a good idea, therefore, to begin your day with that statement."[68]

In his more recent book *How to Know God* Chopra describes the vantage point of the visionary who is well advanced on his journey toward knowing God:

> He still retains a conception of good. It is the force of evolution that lies behind birth, growth, love, truth and beauty. He also retains a conception of evil. It is the force that opposes evolution—we would call it entropy—leading to decompensation, dissolution, inertia, and "sin" (in the special sense of any action that doesn't help a person's evolution). However, to the visionary these are two sides of the same force. God created both because both are needed; God is in the evil as much as in the good.[69]

In chapter four we raised a strong protest to such lines of thinking, and here we voice it again. Does Chopra really believe that Hitler was "innocent, in all senses of the word" of the deaths of millions of Jews? Are child molesters, rapists, torturers and murderers "innocent, in all senses of the word" for their despicable actions? And are those actions really cut out of the same metaphysical bolt of cloth as kindness and compassion? If we were to take Chopra's statement on innocence at face value, we would need to apologize to all convicts currently incarcerated and release them immediately. All police departments would be declared obsolete, all prisons emptied, all lawyers unemployed—and all hell would break loose.

Chopra moves farther out on this limb as he explains how good and evil are strictly matters of interpretation—apparently even for the victims of abuse, torture, rape and murder:

> Every stage of inner growth is an interpretation, and each interpretation is valid. If you see victims of crimes and heartrending injustice, that is real for you, but the saint, even as he brings untold compassion to such people, may not see victims at all. I am reluctant to go too deeply into this, because the grip of victimization is so powerful. To tell the abused and the abuser that they are locked in the same dance is hard to get across—ask any therapist who works with battered women.[70]

"Hard to get across" indeed. Chopra would no doubt have great difficulty explaining to the parents of a kidnapped, mangled and murdered child that their daughter and her tormentor were "locked in the same dance." Clearly, as a decent and civilized individual, he could not possibly endorse, let alone live with, the full implications of this philosophizing. If abandoning notions of good and bad is so liberating, why does he expend so much energy trying to move us toward what he considers to be a healthier lifestyle? Does he lock his house at night, or his car when it is parked on the street, in order to thwart a thief who has a different (but supposedly just as valid) interpretation of property rights? Even more to the point, on more than one occasion Chopra has taken strong issue with articles that he felt libeled him and has sought remedy by filing lawsuits against those who wrote and published them. That is his right—but it is completely incongruent with his advice to "relinquish our need to classify things as good or bad, right or wrong."

Similarly, what are we to make of Chopra's views about judgment? When Jesus said, "Do not judge, or you too will be judged" (Matthew 7:1), did he really mean that we should practice Chopra's form of nonjudgment? An examination of the passage in question reveals that Jesus was referring to hypocritical judgment. Jesus emphasized his point by reminding us that before commenting about the speck in someone else's eye, we should first remove the plank from our own. But we often read in the New Testament that Jesus did in fact judge others, often in the strongest terms. According to chapter 23 of the Gospel of Matthew, Jesus unabashedly criticized (judged) the hypocritical religious leaders of his day (the Pharisees). In addition, by claiming that he is "the way, the truth and the life" and emphasizing this by stating that "no one comes to the Father [God] but through me," Jesus was in fact passing judgment on all of the world's religions that do not acknowledge his exclusive claim to be the sole means of salvation for humanity (John 14:6).[71] Furthermore, the apostle Paul made it clear that believers in Christ are to "test everything" and to "hold on to the good" (1 Thessalonians 5:21).

Judgment is important and necessary. What would Chopra say to the men and women who serve as judges in our courts of law? Would he tell them to begin their day with the statement that they will judge nothing they hear that day? Clearly there are different types of judgments, and while some are hypocritical and unfair, a great many are not only beneficial but also necessary. When we say that a person is a "good judge of character" or has "good judgment," we are not using the terms *judge* or *judgment* negatively. What we are saying is that such people are discerning—a quality that one would think Chopra might endorse.[72]

If Chopra has passed judgment on judgment and determined that everyone is totally innocent, then the next logical step is to chart life's course by following your heart. It is somewhat humorous to note, in passing, that Chopra's official website contains an area called "Ask Dr. Chopra." Why bother asking, if the response you get will be similar to the following?

> As there are many different situations, it would be hard to give one answer here. The best thing for you to do is to *ask your heart for guidance*. What is it telling you?
>
> There are many paths to enlightenment . . . *listen to your heart and choose which one feels best for you.*[73]
>
> Trust this inner wisdom and all your dreams will come true.[74]

But what if you ask your heart for guidance and it tells you to pay a visit to the nearest fast food restaurant with an automatic weapon in hand? Weren't Eric Harris and Dylan Klebold listening to their hearts when they stormed into Columbine High School on April 20, 1999? These are extreme examples, of course, and obviously Chopra would never condone such behavior, but they are not incompatible with his message taken at face value. Our culture is drowning in problems arising from multitudes of people who are doing what feels right rather than what *is* right, and Chopra's advice is not part of the solution.

The sweeping arc of the Bible is the story of redemption and reconciliation, of a relationship between God and human beings that was lost and can now be restored—not because good and evil are different facets of the same reality but because Jesus, the only person who was truly "innocent, in all senses of the word," willingly took on the most fearsome judgment of all time on our behalf. That message, for two millennia, has been called the gospel, the good news. The fact that Chopra has written twenty-five books that, in so many words, declare that message to be meaningless is ultimately of far greater importance than the logical inconsistencies of *ayurveda* and "quantum healing."

10

POSTMODERNISM & MEDICINE
Escape from Reason, Part 1

Why Are Fire Engines Red?
They have four wheels and eight men;
four plus eight is twelve;
twelve inches makes a ruler;
a ruler is Queen Elizabeth;
Queen Elizabeth sails the seven seas;
the seven seas have fish;
the fish have fins;
the Finns hate the Russians;
the Russians are red;
fire engines are always rushin';
so they're red.[1]

This roundabout explanation is amusing for the absurd logic by which it cobbles together unrelated facts about a familiar sight in any city. It also serves as a lighthearted reminder that pressing forward with mistaken assumptions can lead to some odd conclusions. Unfortunately, for centuries medicine has been no stranger to this type of process. The human race has seen an endless procession of treatments based on misunderstandings about how our bodies work, misinterpretations about the origins of disease, and misplaced logic, especially about cause-and-effect relationships. If someone happens to recover from an illness while receiving a particular therapy, whether a potion, herb, incantation or sophisticated pharmaceutical product, the usual assumption is that the treatment brought about the cure.

Often, however, that assumption is only partially correct or is even completely wrong. Because getting well is such an emotionally charged event, whoever appears to have helped turn the tide will be regarded as a hero, and whatever he or she did will be promoted with evangelical fervor.

But what if the person would have recovered anyway? What if he or she would have made better progress without any treatment at all? The enthusiasm arising from seeing the sick become well again is certainly understandable, but if not tempered by a little clear-headed analysis, it could ultimately send others down the wrong path. The skeptic who suggests, however gently, that perhaps treatment A did not really help resolve disease B (especially when treatment A does not make a lot of sense) had better be ready to face cold stares or even look for a quick exit. But without rigorous investigation that can convince the skeptic that A is a viable treatment for B, our knowledge about health and disease will come to a screeching halt. Furthermore, if we muzzle the skeptic, insist that "how I feel" is the only basis for evaluating any treatment and demand that any and all claims about healing are equally valid, we can bid medical progress farewell.

In the chapters that follow we will take a cautionary look at two popular alternative therapies that vividly illustrate these issues. Homeopathy boasts a two-hundred-year history, a host of enthusiastic promoters around the world and a chain of lapses in logic rivaling that of the fire engine riddle above. Therapeutic Touch, a newer therapy with ancient roots and a unique set of logical inconsistencies, serves as a colorful illustration of the impact of postmodernism, an important cultural movement of the past several decades, on health care. (Postmodernism, as it turns out, also lends considerable support to the advancement of homeopathy.) The fact that both of these therapies are thriving at the beginning of the twenty-first century is unsettling for a number of reasons we will consider later on.

The centuries-old words of Blaise Pascal are more true than ever: "Truth today is so obscure and error so established, that unless we love the truth, we will never know it."[2]

What Is Postmodernism?

Postmodernism is a term that has been applied to a set of assumptions about reality, truth and reason that rose to prominence in Western culture during the second half of the twentieth century. Because it is more of a cultural trend than a formal philosophy or worldview, postmodernism is somewhat difficult to define.[3] It has no founder, preeminent spokesman or primary manifesto. Alan Padgett of Azusa Pacific University has stated:

"Postmodernism" is . . . a diverse cultural movement. In fact, I don't think there is any such thing as postmodernism, as an "ism." Postmodernity has no set of practices and beliefs that gives it the coherence of classical Marxism, say, or logical positivism. Rather, it seems there is a postmodern attitude. This attitude celebrates the demise of King Reason (including linear, "scientific" thinking), the Independent Ego, Absolute Truth and any unifying (or "totalizing") metanarratives.[4]

Perhaps the best way to get a feel for postmodern thinking is to contrast it both with the traditional Judeo-Christian worldview and with modernism. The biblical worldview states without hesitation that the universe has a Ruler: God Almighty, Creator of heaven and earth, by whom all of us were made and to whom all of us are accountable. He is the ultimate source of truth—indeed he *is* the truth—and he is the final authority on what is right and wrong. Furthermore, he has communicated vital information about his character, his expectations and our relationship to him through the writers of the Old and New Testaments, and even more explicitly through Jesus Christ. This grand, overarching story of the fall and redemption of humankind, and of our ultimate destination, is called a *metanarrative*.

In the wake of the Renaissance, Enlightenment and Industrial Revolution, modernism emerged as a prominent worldview in the West. It essentially dethroned God and in his place set humankind as the ultimate arbiter of truth and values. Modernism has its own metanarrative: human reason, unshackled from religious dogma, will expand knowledge and technology, unlock the secrets of the universe and the atom, accelerate the evolution of the human race and lead all of us to untold heights of fulfillment. Postmodernism (no doubt fueled by a century of crumbling moral values and disillusioned about human "progress" in the wake of two world wars) takes modernism's premise—that God is no longer in the picture—to its logical conclusion: there is no absolute truth (from God or anyone else) and no objective reality. There are instead a multitude of descriptions, opinions and preferences, all of which are equally valid. Contradictory ideas may be embraced as true and on an equal footing with each other. Postmodernism unceremoniously dethrones both God and humanity and replaces them with language, which allows each of us to create our own reality and values. There is no metanarrative, and any attempt to create or disseminate one is nothing less than a power play. In *The Universe Next Door* James Sire summarizes postmodern philosophy with the following six points:

1. The first question postmodernism addresses is not what is there or how we know what is there but how language functions to construct meaning itself. In other words, there has been a shift in "first things" from being to knowing to constructing

meaning.

2. The truth about the reality itself is forever hidden from us. All we can do is tell stories.

3. All narratives mask a play for power. Any one narrative used as a metanarrative is oppressive.

4. Human beings make themselves who they are by the languages they construct about themselves.

5. Ethics, like knowledge, is a linguistic construct. Social good is whatever society takes it to be.

6. The cutting edge of culture is literary theory.[5]

If this sounds a little abstract, the following explanation from an insightful article entitled "Mom, What Is 'Postmodernism'?" (not exactly the most common question you will hear over cookies and milk) may be helpful:

A summary of the postmodern worldview would sound something like this:

☐ *What is real?* Reality is what you (or your culture) make it.

☐ *How do we know what is true?* What I like, want and choose are true for me. Whatever works is true. Beyond that, truth does not exist.

☐ *How do we judge right and wrong?* What I like, what I want, and what I choose are not only true for me, but right for me. There are no rules, God's or man's. Sin does not exist, so there is no need to be forgiven. Cultures may make rules, but the rules are only preferences and opinions as to what works in that culture. There is no ultimate reality of goodness and fairness. There is only power. When you communicate, you are just trying to exert your power over another person or group.

☐ *Postmodern password: whatever*—the ultimate in tolerance.[6]

Author Dennis McCallum, who has edited an anthology concerning postmodernism entitled *The Death of Truth,* states it succinctly: "A simple definition for postmodernism is the belief that truth is not discovered, but created."[7]

Postmodernism, Culture and Medical Practice

Even without formal institutions or an established leadership dedicated to promoting it (there is no Worldwide Federation of Postmodernists to our knowledge), postmodernism has made serious inroads into popular culture. Not surprisingly, many of its most vocal critics are worried about its dismantling of morality. If, as a society, we begin to accept the notion that truth is merely a matter of our perceptions and preferences, then it would follow that there is no plumb line for moral standards beyond whatever we decide is agreeable, useful or pleasant. The result, of course, is moral relativism. As Francis J. Beckwith and Gregory Koukl point out in their book *Relativism: Feet Firmly Planted in Mid-Air,* "Moral relativism teaches that when it comes to morals, that which is ethically right or wrong, people do their own thing. Ethical truths depend on the individuals and groups who hold them."[8]

A review of the consequences of this moral free fall over the past few decades—the disintegration of traditional families, sexual anarchy, an epidemic of sexually transmitted infections, unplanned pregnancy and abortion on a monumental scale, acts of random violence in schools and other places once thought to be safe, the coarsening of popular entertainment, the explosive penetration of pornography into all corners of society, the proliferation of legalized gambling and so on—could easily consume the rest of this book. The fallout from these cultural plagues is readily apparent to anyone with eyes to see and ears to hear.

But the impact of postmodernism in the West extends beyond the undermining of moral standards to the repudiation of reason itself. In so doing, matters of truth are lowered to the level of matters of taste. Beckwith and Koukl elaborate on this point:

> Tastes are personal. They're private. They're individual. If you didn't like butter pecan [ice cream] and favored chocolate instead, it would be strange to say that you were wrong. You should not be faulted, it seems, for having different subjective tastes about desserts than someone else.
>
> What if my claim was not about flavors, though, but about numbers? If I say that the sum of two plus two is four, I'm making a different sort of claim than stating my taste in ice cream. As a subject, I'm communicating a belief that I hold about an external, *objective* truth.[9]

What might we expect when truth is confused with taste, when critical analysis is pushed aside in favor of tolerance? A number of trends surface:

☐ The ultimate basis for approval or rejection of any idea is "how it makes me feel."

☐ Style and charisma routinely triumph over substance. Irrational beliefs or absurd logic will not be challenged if they arrive in appealing packaging. Profound insights and carefully constructed arguments will be dismissed if they are not presented with attention-grabbing flair.

☐ Ideas that flatly contradict each other can be embraced as equally valid.

☐ Any attempt to establish the idea that one concept is more truthful or valid than another will be treated with disdain.

One might assume that such ideas would not make much headway in traditional Western science. As James Sire points out, "Most scientists . . . are critical realists. They believe that there is a world external to themselves and that the findings of science describe what the world is like more or less accurately."[10] Interestingly, all of us—even the most diehard postmodernist—suddenly become "critical realists" when a scientific application directly impacts our physical safety. Thus, for example, we would not be happy to hear that the pilot of the jetliner we just boarded is going to shut off the navigational equipment and fly us across the Atlantic Ocean based on what he "feels" is the right direction. And there is no "alternative" school of aeronautics that challenges the physical principles by which Boeing designs and builds aircraft. (If there were, none of us would go near any of their products.)

But in health and disease, where biological systems are immensely complex and where expectation and emotion routinely enter the therapeutic equation, there is enough unpredictability to allow postmodernism a portal of entry into an arena where one would assume scientific methodology and rigorous pursuit of objective truth would reign supreme. Over the past quarter century, that portal has been turned into an expressway, accelerating the widespread acceptance of many alternative medical practices. In his book *The Sensate Culture* Harold O. J. Brown states that "medicine, like engineering or industrial production, is often considered a technique rather than a philosophy or worldview. In fact, however, medicine brings its practitioners into touch with a broad range of human existence; changes in the culture sooner or later must affect medicine, and changes in medicine cannot fail to affect the entire culture."[11]

Like it or not, postmodernism has definitely impacted not just the opinions of the general public about health but medicine as a profession as well. For the past several years Dr. Donal P. O'Mathuna has warned of the rising tide of postmodernism in medicine. In his chapter in the anthology *The Death of Truth,* he notes:

> Postmodernism isn't the source for alternative medical ideas, but it's the Trojan Horse that has brought dubious practices such as alternative medicine to prominence and acceptability on campuses today. . . . However, in the postmodern environment of countless academic institutions, theories like those used in alternative medicine cannot be freely critiqued.
>
> Postmodernism rejects many of the ways by which a worldview—or a medical therapy—can be assessed and judged. Bad research, therefore, carries as much weight as properly structured and controlled studies. Likewise, with the lack of certainty about our ability to discover or know truth, arguments against these therapies may carry no more weight than the cries of one religion against another. Almost anything can gain credibility, *once scientific methodology is declared nothing more than a cultural bias*—namely, that of Western Europe.[12]

We noted in chapter one that the conventional medical establishment has cut alternative medicine a considerable amount of slack. As complementary, alternative and integrative programs have settled themselves comfortably in medical schools, at the National Institutes of Health and in the payment schedules of many insurance plans, only a few voices (such as those of the *New England Journal of Medicine*'s former editors Arnold Relman, M.D., and Marcia Angell, M.D.) have challenged their basic premises and the quality of the research backing them. While some of this apparently conciliatory attitude may arise from healthy (and necessary) self-examination and reevaluation, one can also detect the spirit of post-modernism working relentlessly behind the scenes, wearing the garb of pragmatism:

☐ Among patients: "I don't care what the theory is or how it works—it worked for me, and that's all that matters!"

☐ Among doctors: "I don't understand it, but if you feel okay and don't stop your other medications, go right ahead."

☐ Among insurers: "The people want it, so we need to cover it."

These may sound like practical and open-minded responses to some new ideas. Unfortunately, however, postmodern thinking has the potential to bring as much chaos into medicine as it has already inflicted on our culture's moral standards. But how much irrationality can we accommodate? Is there a point at which the propositions of a particular therapy, no matter how solemnly presented, are too absurd to take with a straight face? With tolerance and inclusiveness reigning as its primary virtues, postmodernism insists that we take even the most far-fetched ideas seriously. Judging by the fervor with which homeopathy and Therapeutic Touch are promoted and practiced in the West, it has succeeded spectacularly.

11

HOMEOPATHY
Escape from Reason, Part 2

In almost every way imaginable homeopathy does *not* appear to be an expression of postmodernism. It is actually more like a two-hundred-year-old religious sect, complete with a venerated (and unquestioned) founder, a metaphysical premise, a fierce claim to having the corner on truth, a set of immutable doctrines, rituals that must be carried out precisely in order to be efficacious, evangelists and testimonials. Its promotional materials are infused with such unbridled fervor that one could almost imagine joining the Church of Homeopathy. None of this fits with the grand "whatever" of postmodernism. But postmodern thinking demands that if people believe that homeopathy works for them, we dare not belittle any of its highly eccentric propositions about health and disease. And so, riding on post-modern coattails, homeopathy continues to be widely promoted and celebrated as a "natural, drug-free" therapy at the dawn of the twenty-first century, even though it was ushered out of the scientific mainstream many decades ago.

Homeopathy: History and Principles
The German physician Samuel Hahnemann (1755–1843) is not only acknowledged but also revered as the discoverer and developer of homeopathy. Fluent in several languages and reportedly respected in his day as a translator of medical books, he was also dismayed—and rightly so—with many of the harsh medical treatments widely used in his day. This was the era of so-called heroic measures,

which compounded the misery of many sick patients. Bleeding, cupping, purging and vomiting were frequently included among the doctor's orders, and in many instances they no doubt ushered people into the grave rather than helping them escape it. George Washington's death from a severe throat infection, for example, was undoubtedly hastened by the relentless bloodletting recommended by his physicians.

In 1789, while translating a medical textbook by Scottish physician William Cullen, Hahnemann disputed Cullen's claim that the well-established benefits of Peruvian or *Cinchona* bark in treating malaria were the result of its distinctly bitter taste. If that were the case, why weren't more bitter substances even more effective at subduing this illness? Hahnemann repeatedly took large doses of *Cinchona* himself and described recurrent symptoms of fever, chills, sweats and weakness that were similar to those of malaria. This observation led him to conclude that a substance that provokes a particular set of symptoms in a large dose would treat the same symptoms in a small one. (As it turned out, Cullen and Hahnemann were both wrong. The reason Peruvian bark helped those with malaria was that it contained the compound quinine, which later would be identified as an effective treatment for this disease.)

Hahnemann conducted similar experiments with a variety of substances, using himself, family, friends and students as test subjects and recording in elaborate detail the symptoms they produced. This process he referred to as "proving," and the catalog of materials and their associated symptoms formed his materia medica, the medicines he administered to patients. We will discuss momentarily the unique manner in which he did so, but suffice it to say that the comprehensive system he devised was a radical departure from the theory and practice of his day. Hahnemann continued collecting his observations and in 1810 published the first edition of his magnum opus, *Organon of Medicine*. Four more editions would appear before his death in 1843, as he continued the process of "proving" new substances and treating an expanding circle of patients.

The system Hahnemann devised, which he called "homeopathy" (from the Greek words for "same" and "suffering"), caught on in Europe and thrived in America as well. On both sides of the Atlantic it was embraced by royalty (including Britain's royal family beginning in 1830) and prominent individuals in politics and the arts. Charles Dickens, William Thackeray, Johann Wolfgang von Goethe and Benjamin Disraeli were counted among homeopathy's European supporters, while Nathaniel Hawthorne, Henry Wadsworth Longfellow, Horace Greeley, William Seward, Harriet Beecher Stowe, Daniel Webster and John D. Rockefeller were prominent advocates in America. Oliver Wendell Holmes, on the other hand, wrote a detailed and biting critique of homeopathy in 1843. By 1900 the United States boasted some twenty-two homeopathic medical schools, one hundred homeopathic hospitals and one thousand homeopathic pharmacies.[1]

Not surprisingly, many among the medical elites of Europe and the United States took a dim view of Hahnemann and his ideas. The fledgling American Medical Association in the late 1800s and early 1900s utilized coercive measures such as "consultation clauses" to prevent its members from consorting with homeopaths and other "nonregular" physicians. Contemporary homeopaths generally attribute this opposition to economic and political factors, and no doubt such motives did enter the equation at least as often as did objections based on scientific grounds. Many patients had figured out that homeopathic remedies were frequently gentler than their conventional counterparts, and thus they may have sought out this alternative for pure self-preservation, or at least to avoid discomfort. Giving credit where it is due, homeopathy undoubtedly saved many lives, especially in the nineteenth and early twentieth centuries, by dispensing inert substances, providing a lot of positive expectation and keeping a large number of patients away from treatments that would have made them worse. Given the substantial number of deaths every year that are attributable to adverse drug reactions, today's homeopaths would argue that this statement still applies. But it is critical to note that homeopathy's life-preserving accomplishment was not attributable to any theoretical or therapeutic superiority but rather to the simple fact that it is easier to get well when no one is harming you. For a multitude of people over the past two hundred years, homeopathy has improved that likelihood.

In all other respects homeopathy remains resolutely planted in the eighteenth century, fixated on a series of doctrines that none of its adherents appear willing to reevaluate. Compared to homeopathy's rigidity, chiropractic's increasing attention to contemporary research (not to mention the widespread willingness of chiropractors to abandon the doctrine that spinal subluxations are the cause of all disease) is a model of adaptability.

Homeopathy's credo contains the following key elements:

Similia similibus curantur, or "Like cures like." This "law of similars" is Samuel Hahnemann's overarching, quintessential and unchallenged healing principle. For a homeopath, questioning this idea would be equivalent to stating disbelief in the law of gravity. Beginning with the legendary encounter with *Cinchona* bark and extending to the present, homeopaths insist that *all* symptoms and illness are subject to this law. It is stated in basic terms by Dana Ullman, one of contemporary homeopathy's most visible and prolific proponents: "Homeopathic medicine is a natural pharmaceutical science in which a practitioner seeks to find a substance that would cause in overdose similar symptoms to those a sick person is experiencing. When the match is made, that substance then is given in very small, safe doses, often with dramatic effects."[2]

In order to validate this idea for contemporary audiences, homeopathic apologists tend to be creative in their use of examples and illustrations. For example, in his book *Discovering Homeopathy: Medicine for the Twenty-First Century* (whose title itself is a bit of a stretch), Ullman discovers proof for the Law of Similars in some unusual places:

☐ He likens homeopathy to immunizations, which he states are based on the principle of similars. But our exposure to a fragment of a virus or bacteria via vaccination induces a well-established and measurable response within the immune system. Homeopathic remedies, as we will note shortly, are said to affect "life energy." They have no consistent, measurable effects on *any* physiological function and in fact are frequently so extremely diluted that not a single molecule of the original substance is present in the remedy. Ironically, many homeopaths are antagonistic to routine vaccinations.[3]

☐ He introduces quotes and examples from such diverse sources as Hippocrates, the Oracle at Delphi, the Trojan hero Telephus and the fifteenth-century alchemist Paracelsus. Hippocrates has long been venerated as the father of modern medicine because of his insistence both that medicine function as a natural science based upon careful observation (rather than superstition) and that doctors behave ethically. He is not famous for any promulgation of a law of similars. Currently no one is seeking medical advice from the Oracle at Delphi; Telephus's healing by a piece of the spear that pierced him is a tale from Greek mythology; and Paracelsus actually believed in the "Doctrine of Signatures," which stated that a remedy physically resembles the organ it treats (so that an orchid shaped like a testicle, for example, would be considered useful in treating venereal disease). These are not convincing references.

☐ He states that conventional medicine at times uses homeopathic principles, citing, as an example, "digitalis for heart conditions (digitalis creates heart conditions)." While in overdoses digitalis does have adverse effects on heart function, so also do dozens of other drugs and toxins that otherwise have no use whatsoever in treating heart conditions.

☐ He even offers quotes from Shakespeare's *Romeo and Juliet* and Goethe's *Faust* ("To like things like, whatever one may ail; there's certain help"). But these towering figures in literature are not necessarily reliable sources of medical information for the twenty-first century.[4]

We might acknowledge that these examples are probably not meant to serve as airtight proofs of the law of similars but merely as illustrations to suggest that the idea is not unique to Hahnemann. But they are nevertheless awkward at best and misleading at worst, a pattern that is repeated throughout not only Ullman's book but homeopathic literature in general. Needless to say, among the vast numbers of substances with which human beings interact, it is certainly likely that some of them will in large doses be toxic to the same organ that they might in small doses help. But the belief that this phenomenon can be generalized to become the supreme principle of healing is unique to homeopathy's sectarian tradition.

The danger of "suppressing" symptoms. Homeopathy rejects the common idea that diseases can be defined, understood and treated on a physical level. Instead it presumes that symptoms represent attempts by the body to "vent" disturbances in some deep inner plane without damaging more vital internal organs. Thus, according to homeopathy, Western medicine's efforts to categorize disease are a colossal waste of time, and any attempts to counteract symptoms (even as simple an act as offering an aspirin for a headache) actually make the patient worse. Homeopathy's message to Western medicine is, in essence, "Everything you know is wrong."

Conventional medicine is frequently referred to as *allopathy,* a term literally meaning "other suffering," in contrast to *homeopathy* as "same suffering." The term *allopathy* is usually pejorative in homeopathic literature, implying that conventional physicians focus on symptoms at face value, seeking only to stamp them out with powerful drugs without considering what they might actually mean. Many homeopaths indict conventional medicine's "suppression" of symptoms as the cause of unnecessary disease and misery in our world. For example, in his book *Let Like Cure Like* Connecticut homeopath Vinton McCabe declares:

> This use of suppressive treatments for the purposes of denial of illness weakens the overall system if used repeatedly. And the stronger the suppression, the greater the overall impact. Therefore, the use of an occasional aspirin is far less toxic to the system than is the use of an occasional antibiotic or steroid. As our society's medical practitioners become more and more liberal in their use of potent allopathic drugs, drugs that mask symptoms but do not heal them, the cost is tremendous. With each generation we become weaker and weaker, both as individuals and as a society, more dependent on these drugs and less resistant to illness as a whole.[5]

Hahnemann taught that generalized propensities toward disease called "miasms" were created by treating skin conditions—the miasm in this case was called "psora," or itch—or by attempting to "suppress" syphilis or gonorrhea. No doubt Hahnemann observed that the remedies available in his day for these sexually transmitted diseases seemed to improve matters for a while, only to allow them to run a more destructive course later. In fact, he was watching their natural course before the antibiotic era: syphilis in particular would appear to improve no matter how it was treated, only to recur later with a vengeance. But clinging to this idea two centuries later is ill-advised. McCabe's book has the dubious distinction of being one of the few works by a modern author to suggest that treatment of syphilis and gonorrhea is a bad idea.

Homeopathic apologists steadfastly promote Hahnemann's teaching that treatments other than those governed by the law of similars drive the illness deeper into the body. Conventional medicine is frequently characterized as seeking only to suppress symptoms, rather than addressing their underlying cause. Even when Western methodologies make a specific diagnosis and successfully resolve a patient's problem, homeopaths commonly claim that this process does not address the *real* cause of disease. In one sense, they are correct: discovering and describing *what* is wrong is often much easier than explaining *why* it occurred. When an otherwise healthy individual develops pneumonia, a wart, cancer, a sinus infection, a stroke or virtually any other ailment, the question "Why did I get this, especially now?" invariably arises. The honest answer is usually "I don't know." This doesn't mean that the answer does not exist. Many health problems have identifiable causative agents or risk factors—the varicella virus for chicken pox, for example, or smoking for emphysema—but determining the precise set of conditions that cause an individual to develop a specific problem at a particular point in time is usually beyond the reach of even the most sophisticated investigation.

Alternative practitioners often claim to understand and identify the "true" cause of a specific illness, which they usually describe as a disturbance in energy flow or some other deep-seated (and unmeasurable) phenomenon. But because they are subjective, speculative and at times fanciful, such explanations cannot be regarded as reasonable or reliable answers to why (let alone the what) questions. If there is a disturbance in the flow of vital energy, how and why did it start? Why did it develop in this person at this particular time? Some practitioners may claim an inside track to such knowledge, and their reassurance may satisfy a deep-seated longing in a person who is ill. Unfortunately, under the current reign of postmodernism, a confident but far-fetched explanation is on equal footing with one that is more uncertain but honest and realistic. As long as the person feels better, the truth doesn't matter.

Homeopaths have one other notion correct—on the surface. They point out that symptoms are not always our enemies. This is an important observation. Ask anyone afflicted with leprosy what he or she would most like, and the answer is likely to be the gift of pain. The damage and disfigurement caused by leprosy is primarily brought about by injuries left unattended because the disease interferes with the perception of pain. Pain tells us when injury has taken place and very often (at least with musculoskeletal injuries) tells us what we should avoid in order to prevent further damage. Coughing is not only a significant symptom but also performs the necessary function of removing mucus and debris from the airway. A person who is so ill that he or she cannot cough is in serious trouble and will be dependent upon others to suction material from the bronchial tubes. Similarly, fever appears to activate the immune system and only rarely causes harm itself. Parents sometimes panic when a child's temperature pushes past 101°, often reaching for the acetaminophen bottle at the same time they reach for the phone to call the doctor. To be sure, a fever is an important sign that something (usually an infection) is going on, but if the cause is determined to be benign, it is almost never medically necessary to take action to reduce it.

But in all of these examples there can also be too much of a good thing. Pain can be disruptive or even agonizing, and while it is important to understand its cause, it is also merciful to offer some relief as well. A cough can become so frequent and severe that sleep is impossible; using an antitussive will definitely not suppress the cough completely but it may allow some much-needed rest. Furthermore, no one has demonstrated that it is harmful to take medication to bring down a fever a degree or two for the sake of comfort. Homeopathy decries the use of "suppressive" drugs, but is it really inappropriate to attempt to relieve another person's suffering? In this arena homeopaths risk sounding like the nineteenth-century fundamentalists who condemned any effort to relieve a woman's pain in childbirth because it would circumvent God's judgment in Genesis 3:16 ("with pain you will give birth to children.")

Interestingly, homeopathy uses a number of "first aid" remedies for many common conditions, ostensibly to offer immediate relief that "cooperates" with the body's efforts rather than suppressing them. But even if one is convinced that these are more effective than conventional pharmaceuticals, herbal remedies or no treatment at all, there is no reasonable way to demonstrate that one type of therapy "suppresses" what the body is doing and that another does not.

The importance of precisely matching remedy to symptoms. Homeopathy's criticism of "allopathic" attention to symptoms is somewhat ironic in light of its own intense focus on them. For like to cure like, one must take an exquisitely detailed inventory of a person's symptoms. Dana Ullman notes:

> Anyone who has gone to a homeopathic practitioner knows that the homeopath asks many questions about the person's chief complaint, minor complaints, and various other physical and psychological symptoms. Homeopaths take pride in their serious

interest and use of the idiosyncratic characteristics of each person. The questions that
homeopaths commonly ask include: Is there a time of day that you feel best or worst
or that any specific symptom occurs? How does weather affect you? How do you
feel at the seashore or in the mountains? Are there any foods that you crave or to
which you feel averse?[6]

The purpose of this detailed questioning is not to address the patient's history logically or to evaluate his or her symptoms systematically in order to arrive at a rational treatment plan. It is done for one reason only: to match this particular
combination of symptoms with those produced by large doses of exactly one substance listed in the homeopathic materia medica. (The "most similar medicine"
for the patient's symptoms is denoted by the term *similimum*.) This approach to
symptoms is surprisingly one-dimensional. By comparison, when one considers
the analysis involved, the most cursory questioning of a patient by a rushed conventional physician seems like a rigorous intellectual exercise.

It is here that homeopathy reveals an important, but extremely shaky, assumption. The constellation of symptoms that a remedy generates—and that is to be
matched precisely to those of the patient—has been carefully identified and cata-
loged through homeopathic "provings," the process of giving substances to normal, healthy individuals and carefully observing what happens. Yet as we will see
momentarily, homeopathy also prides itself on dealing with our unique individuality. No one experiences the flu, for example, in precisely the same way, and
homeopaths would submit that despite basic similarities, my version of the flu
probably has a completely different remedy than yours. So why should we not
expect considerable variation between people who are "proving" the remedies?
Isn't it likely that my responses to belladonna or aconite or nux vomica will vary,
at least in some respects, from yours?

For a vivid illustration of this phenomenon, consider the "adverse effects" section for virtually any drug in the *Physicians' Desk Reference (PDR),* a compendium
of the FDA-approved and mandated information for prescription drugs. Any
symptom reported by any person using the product during clinical trials is
reported, no matter how remote the connection to the drug might be. Usually the
list is so long and laden with diverse symptoms that it is all but useless in everyday
practice. But it casts suspicion on homeopathy's detailed lists of symptoms created
by the "proving" process, which are supposed to be so predictable that one can
choose just the right remedy for an individual with matching symptoms.

Undoubtedly homeopaths will argue that the chaotic adverse effect listings in
the *PDR* result from people taking the medications while ill or otherwise not
"normal." Homeopathic provings, on the other hand, are based upon the meticu-

lous observations of "healthy" people taking the homeopathic substance over sev-eral weeks. But even allowing for an increased degree of reliability under these circumstances, the astonishing detail of the symptoms said to be generated by the substances truly strains credibility. One homeopathic self-help book, *Homeopathic Self-Care: The Quick and Easy Guide for the Whole Family,* lists several treatment options for a series of common illnesses and complaints. The reader is supposed to match his or her complaints as closely as possible to those detailed for each homeopathic substance. But the symptom listings defy common sense. For exam-ple, for the common problem of a sore throat, one might treat with belladonna if there is, among other symptoms, a fever, irritability, tonsillitis on the right side and a "desire for lemons and lemonade." On the other hand, Lachesis might be consid-ered if the pain is worse on the left, the person is "talkative" and "feels tense and pressured," and there is a "desire for oysters and alcohol." Six other remedies are characterized by symptoms as unique as "an abscess that smells like old cheese" with "desire for vinegar" or "bad-smelling perspiration and body odor" with "desire for bread and butter" (treat with mercurius, but use mercurius iodatus ruber if the pain is only on the left side, and mercurius iodatus flavus if it is on the right).[7]

The awesome power of dilution and "succussion." After the law of similars, homeop-athy is most well known for its use of extremely diluted solutions. In an effort to avoid the harsh side effects of the medicines of his time, Hahnemann subjected his remedies to a process of serial dilutions. A tincture of the substance would be diluted ten- or one hundred-fold by adding a small amount to nine (or ninety-nine) times that amount of distilled water in a glass vial. The mixture would then be vigorously shaken in a process called "succussion"—not so much to ensure ade-quate mixing but to "potentiate" the solution. How shaking might increase potency is unclear (various explanations, such as "releasing energy" are typically offered), but this procedure is not to be neglected.

The remedy is then diluted again and again, each time ten- or one hundred-fold, sometimes hundreds of times—and each time with the ritualistic shaking. Homeopathy's law of infinitesimals states that the more diluted the solution, the more potent the remedy. "It is initially startling to learn that medicines that have been diluted so many times have any effect. It is even more surprising to learn that homeopaths for the past 200 years have observed that the more a medicine has been potentized—that is, diluted in this fashion—the longer it generally acts, the deeper it usually heals, and the fewer doses tend to be needed."[8]

One critic of homeopathy playfully referred to these purported benefits as "dilutions of grandeur."[9] But a more serious criticism points out that after twelve hundredfold dilutions or twenty-four tenfold dilutions it becomes likely that there are no longer any molecules of the original substance in the water. Surprisingly, many homeopathic remedies are diluted far beyond this level. Stephen Barrett, M.D., an outspoken critic of many alternative therapies and founder of the website Quackwatch (<www.quackwatch.com>), has described the implications of some of these colossal dilutions. A one-in-ten dilution carried out thirty times (marked "30X" on the remedy's label, using the Roman numeral X for ten) indicates that the original preparation of the remedy has been diluted by a factor represented by the number 1 followed by thirty zeroes (10^{30}). To fathom the size of this number, consider that if the original remedy had the volume of a single drop, it would be diluted by an amount of water that would fill a volume fifty times greater than that of the entire earth. A one-in-one-hundred dilution carried out thirty times (indicated by "30C," using the Roman numeral C for one hundred) is even more mind-boggling, involving dilution by a factor represented by the number 1 followed by sixty zeroes (10^{60}). If one molecule of the original substance were present in a solution of 10^{60} water molecules, this amount of water would fill a container more than 30 billion times the size of the earth.[10] Not only is this number incomprehensible but also it creates a serious dilemma for the manufacturers and prescribers of homeopathic solutions: how could anyone possibly ensure that the water in these highly diluted (and thus supposedly highly potent) solutions is so pure that it doesn't contain a molecule or two of something else? Barrett's article puts this dilemma in perspective:

> Even under the most scrupulously clean conditions, airborne dust in the manufacturing facility must carry thousands of different molecules of biological origin derived from local sources (bacteria, viruses, fungi, respiratory droplets, sloughed skin cells, insect feces) as well as distant ones (pollens, soil particles, products of combustion), along with mineral particles of terrestrial and even extraterrestrial origin (meteor dust). Similarly, the "inert" diluents used in the process must have their own library of microcontaminants. . . . During the step-by-step process, how is the emerging drug preparation supposed to know which of the countless substances in the container is the One that means business? How is it that thousands (millions?) of chemical compounds know that they are required to lay low, to just stand around while the Potent One is anointed to the status of Healer?[11]

Homeopaths appear unfazed by these arguments, and in fact they commonly—indeed often proudly—point out that none of the original substance is likely to be found in highly diluted preparations. This is proof, they say, that homeopathic remedies truly work on a basis vastly different from that of regular medicines. For one thing, they must be affecting a person's (or animal's) "life force." But even allowing for the existence of invisible life energy, how might a vial of repeatedly shaken distilled water, apparently lacking a single molecule of anything else, accomplish so much? A variety of mechanisms have been proposed. Some have suggested that subtle structural changes may be induced in water through dilution and succussion. In the nineteenth century such an explanation might have sounded plausible, but current methods of analyzing the structure of matter—spectroscopy, ultraviolet transmission characteristics and electron microscopy, among others—have failed to detect any specific or consistent changes in homeopathically potentiated water.[12]

The most common explanations, therefore, shift to the suggestion that the diluting water is somehow imprinted with an energy pattern, a magnetic field, a holographic image or a vibrational state that somehow resonates with the person's particular symptom mix. Some even believe that the power of highly diluted solutions extends beyond the walls of the vial in which they are contained. One study claimed to show that homeopathic dilutions of thyroid hormone added to a tank of tadpoles changed their rate of development into frogs. But similar results were obtained when a *sealed* vial of the preparation was added to the tank. Instead of questioning the validity of their experimental design, the researchers concluded that the potentiated water in the vial was somehow transmitting its effects through the glass.[13] This is an extreme, but not unusual, example of straining all incoming information through the grid of one's articles of faith. Evidence to the contrary will either be reinterpreted or simply challenged as untrue.

The dogged commitment to the homeopathic doctrine demonstrated by the tadpole researchers brings to mind an amusing and apropos anecdote. An energetic new psychiatric resident was introduced to a long-term schizophrenic patient who was convinced that he was dead. Years of effort by others to convince him otherwise had been unsuccessful, but this did not dissuade the young physician from trying a bolder approach. "Do dead people bleed?" he asked the patient one day. "Of course not," the patient replied without hesitation. The resident then pulled a sterile needle from his coat pocket and gave one of the patient's fingertips a poke. Blood promptly oozed out of the tiny wound. The patient stared wide-eyed at his finger for several seconds. "Well, what do you know," he announced. "Dead people *do* bleed!"

The critical role of "life energy." If extreme dilutions cannot possibly work on a biochemical level, they must affect something that is not otherwise measurable. Hahnemann believed in the "vital force," and modern homeopaths similarly invoke invisible life energy as the medium through which their therapy functions. Dana Ullman states:

Homeopaths conceptualize a "life force" or "vital force," which they describe as the inherent, underlying interconnective, self-healing process of the organism. This bioenergetic force is similar to what the Chinese call "chi," the Japanese call "ki," yogis call "prana," Russian scientists call "bioplasm," and Star Wars characters call "The Force." Homeopaths theorize that this bioenergetic process is sensitive to the submolecular homeopathic medicines. The resonance of the microdose is thought to affect the resonance of the person's life force.[14]

In their eagerness to reconcile their beliefs with contemporary science, homeopaths have been vulnerable to the same misunderstanding of Einstein's equation $E=mc^2$ that we have observed among other energy therapists. Vinton McCabe's *Let Like Cure Like* provides one example: "As Einstein's discoveries enhance our view of creation, they also enhance our understanding of homeopathy. Einstein gives us this tenet: Matter and energy are essentially interchangeable and their transformations are eternally continuous. All matter, therefore, is energy. . . . You are an energy being."[15]

As we have discussed in chapter five, Einstein's equation describing the conversion of matter to energy applies to unique conditions, such as occur with a nuclear reactor or the core of a star. It does not apply in any way to biological systems, including the human body.

Complete individuality of treatment, with only one remedy at a time. As we have already noted, the practice of homeopathy is built on the notion that each person's set of symptoms is unique and thus has a single appropriate remedy, based solely on its symptom match among the substances in the materia medica. While pharmacies and health food stores may sell homeopathic remedies for specific symptoms such as headache or arthritis, these are not at all consistent with true homeopathic principles. These preparations contain a few of the most popular substances used for that particular acute problem, prepared at "low potency" (that is, few dilutions), hoping that a shotgun approach might include what the purchaser needs. But their use is controversial in homeopathic circles, with some arguing that the effects of one remedy in the combination might negate the effects of another and that their use fosters a symptom-suppressing, one-size-fits-all approach that homeopathy rejects.

In addition to looking at the current symptom picture, many homeopaths believe that each individual falls into one of several "constitutional types" and thus has a "constitutional remedy" that will be useful for a number of different ailments. The types are named for their remedy and are so all-encompassing that it is difficult to understand how exactly the proving process might have identified them. Stephen Barrett summarizes several of these and then adds an important rhetorical question:

The "Ignatia Type," for example, is said to be nervous and often tearful, and to dislike tobacco smoke. The typical "Pulsatilla" is a young woman, with blond or light-brown hair, blue eyes and a delicate complexion, who is gentle, fearful, romantic, emotional, and hyperactive. The "Sulfur Type" likes to be independent. And so on. Does this sound to you like a rational basis for diagnosis and treatment?[16]

Barrett's examples are actually quite abbreviated, and those who explore the length and breadth of homeopathy can find some surprisingly detailed "portraits" of constitutional types. All of these characteristics, along with current symptoms (and perhaps some attention to the presence of one of the "miasms" described earlier), are supposed to be factored into the selection of the single proper remedy for an individual.

Homeopaths correctly point out that no two individuals express an illness in exactly the same way, and most conventional physicians would readily acknowledge that cookbook approaches to caring for human beings (especially those with complex illnesses) are woefully inadequate. But they would also point out that there are patterns to be found among illnesses and that principles can be usefully applied to more than one person with similar problems. Without seeking those patterns and principles, and sorting out which are reproducible and yield consistent results, we would see no medical progress whatsoever.

"Hering's Laws of Cure." Named for Constantine Hering, M.D. (1800–1880), considered to be the father of American homeopathy, these are actually observations, and they do not carry the authority of Hahnemann's doctrines. Nevertheless, they provide explanations for virtually any response to homeopathic treatment and thus are worth mentioning.

First, Hering stated that the body tends to "externalize" disease. That is, it tends to push symptoms literally to the surface (that is, the skin) in order to prevent more serious internal disturbances. So, for example, someone whose asthma is resolving may develop a skin rash. In such a case, attempting to calm the rash could cause the asthma to reactivate.[17]

Hering's second observation is that responses to homeopathic cures tend to occur from the top of the body to the bottom. This is said to be helpful in determining that a true response, as opposed to a placebo effect, has taken place.

His third observation, and perhaps the most useful for explaining an apparent failure to respond to treatment, is that a homeopathic healing progresses in the reverse order from the appearance of the symptoms. As a result, one may reexperience previous symptoms that either were not properly treated or were suppressed by allopathic treatment. This notion is unique to homeopathy and is definitely at odds both with conventional medicine and common experience, which would rarely (if ever) construe a return of symptoms as a sign of improvement.

Unconventional homeopathy. Given homeopathy's significant departures from mainstream scientific thinking, it is interesting to note that more adventurous therapists have taken this practice in some unconventional directions. Combination remedies have already been mentioned as a departure from the original understanding of the law of similars. More exotic approaches to diagnosis attempt to circumvent the long symptom history and laborious review of the materia medica list to find the right remedy. Some therapists measure skin resistance at acupuncture points and then retest points determined to be abnormal while the individual holds bottles containing various homeopathic remedies. The remedy that produces the most "normalized" acupuncture points is deemed the best for the client. A few therapists use a pendulum, an old-fashioned fortunetelling device, to find the right homeopathic remedy. Others use the highly subjective arm-pulling techniques of applied kinesiology to determine the best fit.[18] Needless to say, all of these methodologies take homeopathy's eccentricities to extremes and in so doing compound its discrepancies with contemporary science.

Burdens of Proof

We have gone to some lengths to describe homeopathy's articles of faith and their far-reaching implications. In so doing we have in fact been pursuing a broader and more basic goal, and homeopathy happens to provide a particularly ripe object lesson. Our contention is that a colorful history, an air of respectability, appealing rhetoric, cultural acceptability, optimistic practitioners and satisfied customers do not establish the truthfulness of a therapy's claims. All of these ingredients may be present in a therapy that is utterly mistaken about the workings of human (or animal) bodies in sickness and health. We would also contend that in this realm, as in any other, the truth matters. Postmodernism would counter that truth and reality are a matter of opinion and would object vigorously to our casting doubt on anything that others have found useful or helpful, no matter what reasoning lies behind it. If people feel better and nobody gets hurt, isn't that the ultimate truth?

The problem is that health and illness, suffering and comfort, life and death are extremely important commodities, both for individuals and for society as a whole. Caring for the sick is not a trivial pursuit, a parlor game, a form of entertainment or a philosophical abstraction. It is essential that we pursue an accurate and reliable understanding of how the body truly functions in order to make any progress in relieving suffering and prolonging life. Furthermore, contrary to postmodern thought, if a solid, widely validated body of evidence demonstrates that certain assumptions are true, then it should follow that overtly contradictory assumptions cannot also be true. If well-established scientific knowledge is to be overturned, the burden of proof required to do so must be strong indeed.

Homeopathy and many other alternative systems (including Therapeutic Touch, which we will examine in the next chapter) that are disconnected from mainstream science invariably share a common and fervent defense: "We don't understand how it works—it just does." Commitment to the therapy will thus lead to some predictable responses to any evidence bearing on its validity.

If someone appears to improve following the treatment, the treatment will receive the credit. That person's story may even find its way into an article or book about the treatment, especially if the problem was serious and the improvement significant. This is called anecdotal evidence (or a testimonial, if the individual is praising the treatment for personal or commercial reasons). Anecdotal evidence is not necessarily invalid, and it may in fact suggest useful avenues for future research, but it is not adequate grounds to declare that therapy A helps disease B, because many other people who have disease B may not get better after receiving therapy A. Eventually researchers need to compare people who take therapy A (called the treatment group) with those who take a placebo (the control group). The placebo will be something that looks exactly like therapy A but is completely inert. Furthermore, they need to make that comparison in such a way that neither the person receiving the therapy nor the person giving it knows which is which. This is called a double-blind, placebo-controlled study, and when it is properly executed, it is the gold standard in medical research.

Homeopathy, like many alternative therapies, is so oriented to individualized treatment that anecdotal evidence is likely to be abundant and double-blind, placebo-controlled studies difficult to carry out. Also, homeopaths may be reluctant to identify disease B as a specific entity with definable characteristics. Even if one would focus on a symptom (such as headache) rather than a specific disease, twenty-five people who have the same symptom are likely to receive twenty-five completely different remedies, based on their various ancillary symptoms, constitutional weaknesses and miasms. Insisting that all of them receive the same treatment would defeat the whole purpose and process of homeopathic treatment.

If someone does not get any better following the treatment, it will be assumed that the wrong homeopathic remedy was picked or that the body is still in the process of working out the underlying disturbance in the flow of life energy. If the person's symptoms worsen after the treatment, homeopathy usually has an explanation available via Hering's Laws: the current setback is merely the body reexperiencing prior symptoms, which were suppressed, or perhaps driving more significant inner disturbances to the surface. If a scientific journal publishes a study that appears to support homeopathic treatment of a particular problem, the research will be both praised and publicized. Subsequent criticism of the study will be ignored.[19] Conversely, any study that fails to demonstrate homeopathy's effectiveness can readily be dismissed or criticized as not representative of its basic principles of treatment, especially that of individuality.

The research studies dealing with homeopathy are in fact highly variable both in results and quality, so much so that they are difficult to summarize objectively. This is compounded by an understandable tendency to view results through the grid of one's opinion of the therapy under study or even one's hopes about the way the evidence will turn. For example, a study in the respected scientific journal *Nature* reviewed a year's worth of articles—204 altogether—in four alternative medicine journals and categorized the "bottom line" for each article as either positive, negative or neutral. Overall, nearly two out of three (64 percent) of the articles supported the therapy under study, 35 percent were neutral, and only 1 percent were negative. The authors of the review article concluded that there appeared to be a bias in the alternative journals toward studies that cast therapies in a positive light.[20] Similarly, a skeptic may be more inclined to go over a positive study of an alternative therapy with a fine-toothed comb while accepting without a closer look another that is negative or inconclusive.

One evenhanded review of the reviews from a quartet of authors who are not promoters of alternative medicine summarized six reviews and four "meta-analyses" (studies that combine the data from several studies) dealing with homeopathy in both humans and animals. (Homeopathy has been promoted among veterinarians, and claims for its effectiveness with animals have been cited as proof that its remedies cannot work by a placebo effect.) The authors quoted directly from the studies, most of which offered conclusions such as this: "Despite the large number of comparative trials carried out to date there is no evidence that homeopathy is any more effective than placebo therapy given in identical conditions."[21] The most positive comment, from a 1997 meta-analysis in the British journal *Lancet,* could hardly be construed as an endorsement:

> The results of our meta-analysis are not compatible with the hypothesis that the clinical effects of homeopathy are completely due to placebo. However, we found insufficient evidence from these studies that homeopathy is clearly efficacious for any single clinical condition. Our study has no major implications for clinical practice because we found little evidence for effectiveness of any single homeopathic approach on any single clinical condition.[22]

Most of the reviews made reference to poor methodological quality in many of the studies, especially those involving animals. The authors of the review of the reviews also noted that "no single study of homeopathy showing positive results has been successfully replicated."[23]

An illuminating perspective on the progress of research in mainstream science and the lack thereof for homeopathy appeared in a critical article written by a physicist, a psychologist and two veterinarians. (This analogy could easily be applied to many other alternative therapies built upon doctrine, faith and raw enthusiasm.)

> It is interesting to compare the course of progress between medications such as aspirin and homeopathy. It was known for many hundreds of years that chewing on willow bark helped relieve pain and inflammation. The active component of aspirin, initially called salicin, was isolated in 1823, not long after the advent of homeopathy. In 1899, a derivative of salicin, acetylsalicylic acid, was developed and marketed for the first time. The mechanism of action of aspirin began to be uncovered about fifty years later. From this basic information a proliferation of useful non-steroidal anti-inflammatory drugs developed. . . . This process of development has been advanced through the contributions of innumerable investigators, starting with Bayer and continuing today.
>
> Contrast that situation with that of homeopathy. After over two hundred years, there is no single condition for which homeopathy is proven to be effective. The mechanism of action is unknown. The principles of therapy have remained unchanged since it was discovered by its founder, and individuals who employ the therapy have added little to the original tenets. If homeopathy is science, it appears not to be advancing.[24]

The Ultimate Placebo

A final question must be addressed before we move on. Like many alternative therapies, homeopathy's foundations and basic premises do not conform to any widely accepted or independently verified principles of physics, biochemistry, biology, physiology or pharmacology. Homeopathy has not passed muster in controlled trials for any treatment of any specific condition. So why does it continue to inspire such fervent loyalty among practitioners and users? The answer has been suggested by the review articles mentioned above, and upon a moment's reflection it makes perfect sense: it would be hard to imagine a more ideal placebo.

First, the extreme dilutions virtually rule out any toxic effects from the remedies themselves. Safety has been homeopathy's primary advantage over conventional medicine for two centuries, except, of course, in cases where the use of its remedies delayed more appropriate care for a serious condition. Second, prolonged and detailed attention to an individual's symptoms is not a common event in a conventional medical office (or, for that matter, anywhere else), especially when the list of complaints is long. To have a practitioner listen so intently and attach significance to the remotest details can build great trust in his or her care and make a powerful impact upon one's sense of self-worth. Third, and most important, the remedy is handpicked for the individual, making a powerful therapeutic statement: "I know *exactly* what is going to help you feel better." This can be particularly reassuring when the symptoms have been many and the answers from conventional physicians few. Combine this potent setup for positive expectations with the body's reparative powers, add a pinch of personal autonomy ("I chose this approach, not my HMO") and some out-of-pocket expense to buy in to the treatment, stir with homeopathy's willingness to allow remedies to work over time, and you have a sure-fire recipe for improvement.

Keeping that spirit alive are the eclectic promoters of alternative medicine (Andrew Weil, for example), who have little problem entertaining the possibility that homeopathy might work as advertised. If it does, and if we have to rewrite the textbooks to accommodate it, so be it. And if it really is nothing but a highly effective placebo, that's just as well—in fact, probably better. Whatever provokes the placebo response—whether a highly researched pharmaceutical, an individualized homeopathic remedy, a magnetic hand pass, a shaman's dance in the jungle or bringing a dead cat to the graveyard at midnight—is valid because of the result it yields. Whether the event that brought on the healing is based on truth or fantasy is irrelevant to them.

The problem with this approach, however, is that it is ultimately unethical. If we encourage homeopaths, or any other therapists, to do what they do because it tricks the patient into getting well—even if the weight of evidence and logic says that their technique is in fact bogus—aren't we collaborating in a fraud? If we continue to allow the notion that like cures like and all of homeopathy's other core doctrines to stand unchallenged, we might as well abandon all previous avenues of scientific research and instead focus purely on the arts of persuasion, storytelling and perhaps the creative use of rituals. Indeed, those swayed by postmodernism would argue that this is precisely where our attention should be focused.

12

THERAPEUTIC TOUCH
Escape from Reason, Part 3

As an example of contemporary postmodernism hard at work in medicine, it would be difficult to find a more successful candidate than Therapeutic Touch. Based on mysticism (with ties to some of the darker corners of that realm) and boasting extraordinarily subjective diagnostic and treatment techniques, this practice has nonetheless made significant inroads into conventional health care, primarily among nurses. Therapeutic Touch was conceived by Dolores Krieger, R.N., Ph.D., and birthed into the nursing community in the 1975 article "Therapeutic Touch: The Imprimatur of Nursing" published in the *American Journal of Nursing.* Subsequently hundreds of nurses took Krieger's course at New York University called "Frontiers in Nursing: The Actualization of Potential for Therapeutic Human Field Interaction." In less than a quarter century, according to its proponents, the technique has been taught to more than one hundred thousand people, including forty-three thousand health professionals, in more than one hundred colleges and universities in seventy-five countries.[1]

Therapeutic Touch claims to be a scientific variant of the ancient practice of the laying on of hands—an assertion that has reassured some Christian nurses that this technique need not be off-limits to them. But it bears no resemblance whatsoever, in thought or deed, to the prayerful activities described in the New Testament. Instead the Therapeutic Touch practitioner is said to manipulate a patient's invisible "human energy field" without actually making any physical contact. (The name Therapeutic Touch is thus a misnomer.)

In her book *The Therapeutic Touch* Krieger describes how she became acquainted with the idea of healing through touch while studying Hungarian healer Oskar Estebany. (While a colonel in the Hungarian cavalry, Estebany had discovered an ability to heal animals and humans through the laying on of hands.) Later, under the tutelage of psychic and clairvoyant Dora Kunz, Krieger began to experiment with the "transfer of human energies" and eventually developed a theory for her experiences.

Kunz's role in the evolution of Therapeutic Touch is of no little significance. According to Krieger, Kunz was "born with a unique ability to perceive subtle energies around living beings."[2] She was tutored in her clairvoyant abilities by C. W. Leadbetter, a leader of the theosophical movement in India, and ultimately became both president of the Theosophical Society in America and chair of the Theosophical Publishing House. Therapeutic Touch's primary training site for intensive workshops is a retreat center in Craryville, New York, called Pumpkin Hollow—owned and operated by none other than the Theosophical Society of America. Since 1875 this organization has been dedicated to promoting a blend of ancient religions and occult philosophies, including Buddhism, Taoism, Hinduism, cabalism, Rosicrucianism and spiritualism.

While her academic background was in neurophysiology, Krieger's formulation of Therapeutic Touch was built on the study of yoga, *ayurveda* and traditional Chinese medicine. She concluded that *prana*—the Hindu version of universal energy—is "at the base of the human energy transfer in the healing act."

> Conceive of the healer as an individual whose health gives him access to an over-abundance of prana and whose strong sense of commitment and intention to help ill people gives him or her a certain control over the projection of this vital energy. The act of healing, then, would entail the channeling of this energy flow by the healer for the well-being of the sick individual.[3]

That Eastern mysticism is the cornerstone of Therapeutic Touch was made clear from the outset in Krieger's first book, *The Therapeutic Touch,* and has been evident in other materials promoting this movement for more than two decades. She notes that the idea that "prana may be transferred from one individual to another may not be so readily apparent to us unless we have gotten into the practice and literature of hatha yoga, tantric yoga, or the martial arts of the orient."[4] As we continue to examine Therapeutic Touch, keep in mind that Krieger claims this practice does not have any particular religious orientation.

The widespread acceptance of Therapeutic Touch within nursing academia and mainstream professional organizations (see below) was no doubt facilitated by the late Martha Rogers, former dean of nursing at New York University. Renowned as a nursing theorist, Rogers promoted a variation of an idea already described many times in this book: we are not merely conduits of invisible energy; we *are* bodies of energy, interacting with "environmental fields" around us. Rogers in many ways accomplished for Therapeutic Touch what Deepak Chopra has attempted, with less success, for *ayurveda*. She established its acceptability among academic elites by shifting the descriptive language from religious and mystical to quasi-scientific. Chopra has been far more successful in impacting the general public than the medical profession with his notions of "quantum healing." With Therapeutic Touch, the opposite has generally been the case.

The Four Steps of Therapeutic Touch

The practitioner of Therapeutic Touch is seen not as a generator of energy but as a conduit, one who directs energy where it is needed. (Throughout this discussion we will for convenience refer to the practitioner as "the healer," using a female pronoun, and the recipient of care as "the patient," although Therapeutic Touch literature does not limit this technique to female practitioners, to a medical setting or, for that matter, to human beings. Animals and even plants are said to benefit from being on the receiving end of treatment.) A Therapeutic Touch session entails a four-step process, the first (and most important) of which is called "centering." Here the healer develops a state of inner equilibrium through a meditative process of her choice. Whatever method is used, it is crucial that the practitioner cultivate an intention to heal.

The second step is called "assessment" and involves "scanning" the patient's energy field. The healer places her hands two or three inches from the patient's body and slowly moves them over both front and back surfaces. The object is to perceive subtle sensations such as temperature changes, tingling, pressure or pulsation, all of which are said to reflect variations in the energy field itself. This perception and its interpretation are not considered equivalent to a standard medical diagnosis. Indeed there is no relation between the two:

> Every facet of Therapeutic Touch is concerned with energy flow. . . . From this point of view, one can easily see that a medical diagnosis would be highly inappropriate, since medical diagnoses arise out of a classification system that is unlike the perceptions we are dealing with. The perceptions . . . are at a very direct, perhaps primitive level. Medical diagnosis, on the other hand, is based upon a very complex system of classification that is quite sophisticated, and so there is little relation between the two; indeed there is little reason why there should be, or why there need be.[5]

Step three involves "unruffling the field." When the healer perceives a sense of

pressure while scanning the body, she is said to be literally bumping against stag-
nant energy. The treatment is to "decongest" the energy by making circular
motions over the body with her hands, either moving it to areas of decreased flow
or sweeping it downward and out of the body through the feet. The healer often
shakes her hands vigorously after this process in order to remove any excess energy
that might be clinging to them. This paves the way for transferring energy in the
fourth and final step.

Step four is called "modulation," in which the healer either redirects energy
within the patient or transfers some of her own in a sort of psychic transfusion.
Sensations felt in the hands during step two are used as a guide for treatment. An
area that feels hot will need to be cooled, a cool area warmed, an area of tingling
quieted and so forth. These changes are brought about by creating the desired feeling (cool in place of warm, for example) in her mind and then directing this image
through the hands.

The entire process generally takes from twenty to thirty minutes. The purported beneficial effects for the patient range from calming a colicky infant to
helping raise the dead,[6] although pain and headache relief, generalized relaxation
and an improvement in psychosomatic illnesses are more frequently described. But
given Therapeutic Touch's highly intuitive and meditative nature, changes in
thinking of the healer can assume significance far greater than any effects on the
patient.

Krieger describes two important types of change. First, those who regularly
practice Therapeutic Touch may develop "natural faculties . . . which our culture
allows to lie dormant within us." The most common of these is telepathy—non-
verbal, nonphysical communication. Krieger comments, "If the healer is trying to
get in intuitive touch with another, to learn to react sensitively to that person's
'vibes,' it should not come as a surprise that he or she is going to succeed in developing latent abilities in communication." Second, Krieger writes, the process of
healing through touch can and should lead to the exploration of one's unconscious
mind, the "farther reaches of the psyche." She recommends that her students learn
to tap the subconscious by recording its symbolic expressions, which may be
brought forth through various techniques. "There are several ways of doing this,
but I find that the recording of dreams, the drawing of mandalas, and divination by
means of consulting the I Ching most useful. . . . I find that all three . . . integrate
the search for one's own authentic nature in a unitive manner which can be very
creative as well as enlightening."[7]

Therapeutic Touch epitomizes not only the strong spiritual tide within life
energy therapies but also postmodernism's radical subjectivism and dismissal of

objective truth in favor of a well-told story. A mystical concept is extracted from a distant corner of Eastern metaphysics, recast in Western quasi-scientific terminology and then taught to well-intentioned members of the helping professions who are looking for new ways to relieve suffering. Krieger begins by telling us that we can learn to heal, but before long she has us developing telepathic communication, drawing mandalas (complex visual patterns used to facilitate meditation and alter one's consciousness) and practicing an ancient form of fortunetelling. Whatever its initial appeal, Therapeutic Touch (along with other energy therapies) inevitably beckons the budding healer toward embracing Eastern mystical and New Age worldviews.

It also fosters a supreme regard for subjectivity. The treatment carried out by a Therapeutic Touch practitioner hinges entirely upon the stream of sensations that her palms transmit to her brain during her silent assessment. But a simple demonstration will generate some legitimate doubt about the reliability of this diagnostic method. Spend a few minutes carefully concentrating on the sensations coming from *any* part of the body. Our brain, like a highly competent executive secretary, normally filters out the endless stream of tingles, twitches, itches, jabs and other assorted messages that are normally generated by nerve endings from head to toe, representing a sort of neurologic background noise. But whenever we decide that these sensations have either threat or pay value, we effectively fire the secretary and take all of the assorted incoming calls. Their number and variety at any given time is astonishing, and they can become a major source of worry for one who believes they are harbingers of disease. Consider what is likely to happen, on the other hand, when someone believes that whatever she feels in her palms at some point in time has great significance and concentrates intently upon them. We can guarantee that all sorts of sensations will be experienced, but we propose that they represent random firings from an enormous number of wide-awake nerve endings rather than perceptions of the human energy field.

Even without trying this experiment, a little reflection on the four steps of Therapeutic Touch should raise a few basic but important questions: How does the practitioner know that she is picking up the right signals from the patient's invisible energy field? Will someone else who assesses the patient at the same time get a similar reading? How does one distinguish a skillful practitioner from an incompetent one? Postmodernism, the soil in which Therapeutic Touch flourishes, would say that such questions are oppressive, reductionistic, Western and ultimately irrelevant because each healer essentially generates her own truth about the patient's condition.

Nevertheless, as pervasive as postmodernism has become within our culture, the typical response of an average individual upon first hearing a description of

Therapeutic Touch is usually one of disbelief. Do nurses and their patients really take this seriously?

Indeed they do.

One review of the current status of Therapeutic Touch includes this eye-opening summary of its recognition within the nursing profession:

> The policies and procedures books of some institutions recognize TT [Therapeutic Touch], and it is the only treatment for the "energy-field disturbance" diagnosis recognized by the North American Nursing Diagnosis Association. *RN,* one of the nursing profession's largest periodicals, has published many articles favorable to TT.
>
> Many professional nursing organizations promote TT. In 1987, the 50,000 member Order of Nurses of Quebec endorsed TT as a "bona fide" nursing skill. The National League for Nursing, the credentialing agency for nursing schools in the United States, denies having an official stand on TT but has promoted it through books and videotapes, and the league's executive director and a recent president are prominent advocates. The American Nurses' Association holds TT workshops at its national conventions. Its official journal published the premier articles on TT as well as a recent article designated for continuing education credits. The association's immediate past president has written editorials defending TT against criticism.[8]

Proponents of this practice are indeed very serious about it, responding vigorously to criticism of it—or even to an unimpressive performance in a research study. Several years ago one of us (Paul Reisser) contributed an article critical of Therapeutic Touch to the *Journal of Christian Nursing.* One might have assumed that its readership would have been concerned about TT's overtly Eastern mystical orientation. Instead the Letters to the Editor page in the next issue was filled with epistles staunchly defending this practice. (It should be noted, however, that the *Journal of Christian Nursing,* as well as Nurses Christian Fellowship, which publishes it, have taken a position of strong opposition to the theory and practice of Therapeutic Touch.)

Another notable example of extravagant commitment to Therapeutic Touch was displayed in a 1989 study funded by the National Institutes of Health at the University of Colorado. The effects of "true" Therapeutic Touch versus a mimic procedure were compared in 153 patients in a coronary care unit. The researcher hypothesized that anxiety, blood pressure and heart rate would be significantly lower after the "true" treatment but found instead that there was no difference between it and the sham procedure in producing these effects. Apparently unfazed by the evidence generated by her own study, the author offered a remarkable conclusion:

> Therapeutic Touch continues to be experienced clinically as a uniquely rich and powerful mode of helping/healing which nurses have only just begun to understand from a scientific point of view. There is a need to be cautious and sensitive in con-

ducting this scientific study lest, like the butterfly that is pinned down for closer inspection, the phenomenon is destroyed in the attempt to understand it.[9]

A Child Shall Lead Them

By far the most intense reaction from Therapeutic Touch enthusiasts occurred in response to an experiment devised by a nine-year-old for a fourth-grade science project. Emily Rosa was discussing possible topics for her project with her mother, Linda Rosa, R.N., a long-standing critic of Therapeutic Touch. A tape dealing with Therapeutic Touch was playing in the background, and Emily reportedly heard enough of it to wonder whether the practitioners could actually sense a "human energy field."[10] It was a simple but profoundly logical question that should have been raised twenty-five years ago when Krieger's article was first published. It also disarmingly pointed out the weakness of the vast majority of clinical studies, doctoral theses and assorted anecdotes that comprise the research literature on this technique. In order for Therapeutic Touch to work as advertised, *all* of the following propositions must be true:

1. An invisible human energy field must exist. (If invisible life energy and a human energy field do not exist, then Therapeutic Touch—and a number of other alternative therapies—do not warrant any serious attention in our society, except perhaps as a cautionary tale.)

2. The status of the human energy field must bear some relationship to a patient's health or illness. (If the human energy field does not reflect or affect one's state of health, then its existence would be an interesting finding but without any particular application to medicine or nursing.)

3. Whether or not the human energy field can be detected by instrumentation, it must be readily detectable by the human hand.

4. The combination of benign intention, meditative centering and hand movements over a patient's body, as taught by Therapeutic Touch practitioners, must be capable of changing the status of the human energy field. (If the human energy field does not actually interact with the human hand, then there is no point in making hand motions around a patient's body.)

5. Changes in the human energy field brought about by the above techniques must in turn bring about a demonstrable response in the patient with reasonable frequency, and that response must in some way be beneficial. (If nothing ever happens in response to Therapeutic Touch or if a benefit is detected after only one treatment out of a hundred, then this practice is a misdirection of time and resources. If patients routinely become worse after treatment, then Therapeutic Touch should be banned from hospitals and clinics.)

6. Whatever change is experienced or measured in the patient cannot be reasonably accounted for by a mechanism other than the one described by Therapeutic Touch practitioners.

Therapeutic Touch proponents would no doubt object to this reductionistic take on their practice. Yet these are reasonable deductions from a straightforward reading of their literature. It is instructive to think through these propositions and, for each of them, to ask two questions: "What if this isn't true?" and "How could we prove or disprove it?" The answer to the first question should be obvious: if any of these statements are not true, then the empress called Therapeutic Touch has no clothes, despite her heartfelt claims to the contrary, and the entire enterprise should be downgraded from a legitimate therapy to a large-scale misunderstanding. The second question is, for most of the propositions, somewhat more difficult to answer. For example, no scientific instrumentation or reputable study has documented the existence of life energy or a human energy field as proclaimed by Therapeutic Touch practitioners. One would think that this lack of objective evidence would serve to disprove the first proposition, yet it remains as an article of faith at the center of Therapeutic Touch and many other alternative therapies.

Indeed only three of the six propositions can be readily subjected to direct experimentation. Therapeutic Touch advocates proceed directly to proposition five and claim that their technique yields a wide spectrum of benefits. Critics stop at proposition five long enough to challenge whether a benefit has actually taken place and how often. Then they bear down on proposition six, contending that any changes observed can be readily explained by more prosaic mechanisms (for example, a patient's response to a nurse's attention or fascination with her movements). Emily Rosa, on the other hand, had the audacity to address proposition three, understanding that if Therapeutic Touch is valid, its practitioners must be able to demonstrate consistently the ability to detect a human energy field.

For Emily Rosa's experiment, twenty-one Therapeutic Touch practitioners (with experience ranging from one to twenty-seven years) agreed to participate, no doubt disarmed by the fact that the experimenter was a nine-year-old rather than a professional investigator from a conventional medical institution. The protocol, designed and explained by Emily herself, was straightforward. The practitioner would sit at a table behind a cardboard screen with cutouts at its base, through which she would insert her arms. She would be allowed to "center" or carry out any other mental preparation she felt appropriate. A cloth towel was draped over her arms to prevent any visual cues. Emily sat behind the screen, flipped a coin to determine which of the practitioner's hands would be chosen, and then placed her own hand palm down three to four inches above it. The practitioner was given an unlimited amount of time to decide which of her hands was under Emily's and would then give her answer. Each practitioner was given ten tries.

Fifteen practitioners were involved in an initial trial in 1996. All claimed to have used Therapeutic Touch successfully and described various perceptions in their hands that, they said, allowed them to evaluate and then manipulate a patient's energy field. Out of 150 tries, only 71 (47 percent) were correct, with individual therapists achieving from two to eight correct picks out of ten attempts. (The only practitioner who had correctly chosen eight times was retested and scored only six out of ten.) According to the most fundamental assumptions of Therapeutic Touch, all should have readily picked ten out of ten. A score of eight out of ten would have been statistically significant, however, because the odds of accomplishing this through random guessing would be more than twenty to one. But as a group, the practitioners would have generated a better score it they had merely flipped a coin on their side of the screen.

When informed of the disappointing results, each practitioner offered one or more explanations, including the following:

☐ Emily's hand left an energetic "memory" floating behind, and this made it increasingly difficult to distinguish the actual energy field from the memory. This would imply that everyone's first try should have been correct, but unfortunately eight out of fifteen practitioners were wrong on their first attempt.

☐ Emily should have "centered" herself and tried to transmit energy through her hand. However, Therapeutic Touch is explicitly understood to depend solely on the mindset of the practitioner and not that of the recipient. (This is particularly relevant to claims that this technique can benefit infants, animals, plants and even seeds.)

☐ Some participants claimed that their hands became "overheated" after a few trials and thus could not detect Emily's human energy field more accurately. But the sessions ranged in length from seven to nineteen minutes, while a typical Therapeutic Touch encounter lasts from twenty to thirty minutes.

☐ The participants should have had a chance to "warm up" by having a chance to feel Emily's energy field beforehand and choosing which of her hands would do the testing.[11]

This last objection was addressed the following year when thirteen practitioners, including seven from the first experiment, were tested before the cameras of the Public Broadcasting System. (A PBS producer had heard about Emily's experiment, which was subsequently featured on the program *Scientific American Frontiers*.) The practitioners "felt" Emily's energy field and chose the hand they preferred, but alas, the results were worse—only 53 of the 130 tries (a mere 41 percent) were correct. When informed of their second failure to pass Emily's simple test, several complained that the presence of the cameras and technical crew impaired their concentration. Whether the practitioners were distracted or not, the program aired and caught the attention of alternative medicine critic Stephen Barrett, M.D., who suggested that Emily's experiment should be submitted to the *Journal of the American Medical Association (JAMA)*. He joined Emily and her parents as a coauthor, and their article, "A Close Look at Therapeutic Touch," was accepted for publication.

The appearance of this study in the April 1, 1998, issue of *JAMA* was a major public relations setback for Therapeutic Touch. For the media, which has been generally friendly to alternative medicine, the story was irresistible: a fourth grader's ingenious science project had deflated the pretentious claims of a highly questionable practice. Emily began her day on April 1 with an appearance on NBC's *Today* show and was the talk of the nation by the end of the day. With the reputation of their practice on the line, Therapeutic Touch proponents quickly generated several objections for the press: Emily's experiment was not a true healing task, her energy field was off-kilter, medical journals care only about money and power, and so forth.

Dolores Krieger herself weighed in, declaring that the study was "poor in design and methodology" and that "innumerable" studies had demonstrated the value of Therapeutic Touch.[12] In fact, the introduction to the *JAMA* article included an exhaustive review of the research related to Therapeutic Touch and carefully outlined its unimpressive track record in controlled settings. Furthermore, Krieger had been personally invited by Emily Rosa to take a few minutes to participate in the experiment taped by PBS but sent a message that she "didn't have the time."[13] As might be expected, a torrent of hostile letters soon arrived at *JAMA*. These were dutifully printed and then capably answered by the authors of the April 1 study, who also noted that a million-dollar reward from the James Randi Educational Foundation was still awaiting the person who could conclusively demonstrate the presence of the human energy field.[14]

Despite the chorus of protest from practitioners and academics, Emily Rosa's simple experiment stands as a model of the kind of reality check that should be applied to a host of other alternative therapies. Unfortunately, even if a hundred Emilys of all ages came forward to challenge the basic assumptions of Therapeutic Touch, the faithful will fall back on the mantra of alternative medicine and postmodernism: "It works, and that's all that matters!" One of Emily's critics wrote to *JAMA* to declare that "the definitive test of a healing practice is whether healing takes place, not whether the practitioners have a flawless grasp on the natural forces at work."[15] In one sense this statement is correct: determining whether a healing has taken place is indeed of crucial importance (although not always as easy at it sounds). But if a patient feels better or in some other way improves following a session of Therapeutic Touch, determining or proclaiming what "natural forces" are at work is not at the sole discretion of the practitioner. Dolores Krieger and her followers would say that they have manipulated the patient's energy field. We could also propose any of the following explanations:

☐ The practitioner is channeling energy from the Ascended Masters.

☐ The practitioner is a conduit for healing rays from an advanced civilization in another galaxy.

☐ The practitioner is altering individual electrons within the patient's water molecules.

☐ The practitioner is driving malicious fairies and sprites away from the patient's body.

Getting Serious

These propositions could have been compiled from the thoughts of a schizophrenic. But from the standpoint both of plausibility and the likelihood of scientific validation, they are on absolutely equal footing with Krieger's conviction that health is advanced by adjusting a human energy field with well-intentioned hand passes. Postmodernism says that all of these explanations can have equal claims to validity, depending on how well crafted a story one can tell about them, how often they are repeated and how fervently their adherents believe them. Common sense says, "Get serious," and needs to say it more often.

Indeed there is one occasion in which Therapeutic Touch, homeopathy, *ayurveda* and the rest nearly always retreat—when things really *do* get serious. When a person is critically injured or acutely ill, even the most committed energy therapist or homeopath heads for that bastion of Western conventional medicine: the local emergency department.[16] When someone's life is really on the line, the promoters of *chi* and *prana,* meridians and *chakras*, extreme dilutions and hand passes all fold their cards and wait for a less risky occasion. If one has any doubt about this observation, consider what would ensue if a patient in the throes of a major heart attack or someone scraped broken and bleeding off the freeway after an auto wreck spent the first thirty minutes in the emergency room receiving a Therapeutic Touch treatment before anything else was done. The episode would make headlines, and malpractice attorneys would take note.

Speaking of attorneys, while as a group they are not always appreciated within the medical profession, their attention to such details as evidence, responsibility and standards of practice represent a de facto argument against the pretensions of postmodern medicine. Would anyone be sued for Therapeutic Touch malpractice? How would a jury decide if a nurse incorrectly assessed a patient's energy field? For that matter, is there any way to hold a homeopath accountable for making the wrong choice from the materia medica, or the traditional Chinese practitioner for misreading the twelve pulses at the wrist, or the ayurvedic doctor for drawing the wrong conclusion from a patient's tongue, or the iridologist for failing to predict kidney failure from the appearance of someone's iris? Accountability would imply not only that there is potentially a right or competent way to carry out any of these techniques but also that failing to do so might make a significant difference in a patient's health. If an alternative practice is immune from this type of accountability, why should it be taken seriously at all?

So far the primary malpractice issues relating to alternative medicine have been those of failing to recognize when someone needed "proper" (that is, conventional) care or of delaying the process of obtaining it. This would imply that in the world of truth and consequences, where responsibilities are taken seriously and results count, few people really expect much from alternative therapies. If conventional Western medicine has earned the public trust as the most viable approach to serious illness and trauma, it would seem inconsistent and irrational to toss it aside for less urgent problems. Conventional medicine certainly has a long way to go, but at least it is going *somewhere*—and has done so with demonstrable results.

One observation needs to be revisited before we leave the realm of postmodernism: when our physical safety is on the line, truth and objective reality suddenly become matters of prime importance. We previously noted that there is no "alternative" movement within aeronautical engineering. No one would volunteer to be the test pilot for a prototype aircraft designed around someone's subjective assessment of the energy flow emanating from the wings and fuselage. Postmodernism would say that such a design has as strong a claim on truth as one based on conventional aeronautics, but for the pilot the consequences of being wrong involve becoming one with the ground. Similarly, we would not want to ride an elevator, strap into a roller coaster, drive across a bridge or climb into a submarine if safety inspections consisted solely of a cadre of "sensitives" scanning these structures with their hands in order to find areas of congestion in undetectable energy fields. And we would look for a fast escape route if we found out that the only repair work was done by "structural healers" who enter a meditative state and wave their hands around the cables, beams, girders or hull with a strong intention to make them better.

We instinctively care an awful lot about truth and objective reality when our

lives are on the line, whether at an amusement park or in the emergency room.
This raises an important question. Jesus made it abundantly clear that there was no
profit in gaining the world (presumably including good health) and losing one's
soul (Matthew 16:26). That being the case, should we not also care deeply about
what is true—and what is not—in the spiritual realm? More specifically, given that
postmodernism's summary statement about reality, whether material or spiritual, is
"Whatever," do we dare allow this movement to impact our understanding of
God? As we will see in Dale Mabe's story in the next chapter, some forms of alternative medicine may be the agents by which this occurs.

The Postmodern

At last we know all truth is gray: no more
Faith's raucous rhetoric, this blinding trap
Of absolutes, this brightly colored map
Of good and bad: our ocean has no shore.
Dogmatic truth is chimera: deplore
All arrogance: the massive gray will sap
The sparkling hues of bigotry, and cap
The rainbow, mask the sun, make dullness soar.
    Yet tiny, fleeting hesitations lurk
    Behind the storied billows of the cloud
    Like sparkling, prism'd glory in the murk;
    The freedom of the gray becomes a shroud.
Where nothing can be false, truth must away—
Not least the truth that all my world is gray.
                D. A. Carson[17]

13

WHY I LEFT

A Former New Age Practitioner Tells His Story

T wenty years ago coauthor Dale Mabe, D.O., began a personal and professional journey during which he embraced New Age philosophy and practiced in a busy alternative medicine clinic. Ultimately he recommitted himself to a traditional biblical worldview and discontinued his involvement in many alternative practices. In this chapter he describes a number of his experiences and the evolution of his thinking about God and medicine.

Pulled in Two Directions

I was raised in a loving family in a small southern town by parents who provided all the love, support and understanding that one could hope for. I attended a Protestant church where I often heard the message of salvation. I accepted Christ when I was nine, but unfortunately this particular church really did not teach much about life after one's initial commitment to Christ. I was taught about Jesus' moral teachings but heard little about a daily walk with Christ or the nature of the Holy Spirit. Many of the virtues of simpler times were embodied within that church and community. There was a simple and genuine love for the Lord and care for those in need, providing a good and adequate framework for life within this community, but as I stepped out into the wider world, I was not prepared theologically for its many deceptions. I left the church when I was about thirteen, and as a result, my spiritual perspective entering young adulthood was rather shallow. Yet despite—or perhaps because of—my lack of a deeper relationship with God, I was yearning for something, for some sort of spiritual fulfillment. I became aware of a real lack of any spiritual power or evidence of the supernatural in my life.

Meanwhile, my enthusiasm for bodybuilding and staying fit led me to a local health food store. The abundance of health foods, remedies and supplements was surpassed only by the cornucopia of fascinating literature about all aspects of alternative spirituality. Also, the people with whom I became acquainted at the store were refreshing to me. They seemed much more spiritually alive than the people I had known up to that point. Their spirituality appeared to be an integral part of their lives, and it had become the core of who they were. Their lives seemed to be so much more filled with purpose and relevance. And they claimed to be Christians.

Ben was the first person with whom I established a relationship through the health food store. He had started his walk as a very sincere, committed Christian. He was loving, genuine, compassionate and patient—everything I imagined Jesus to be—and I found his demeanor to be deeply attractive. Ben was the person who first took me under his wing as a spiritual mentor. It was he who introduced me to the writings of Edgar Cayce and later to *A Course in Miracles*. My study of the Cayce materials seemed to be a perfect jumping-off point for me in more ways than one. I was taking a leap into an unknown but fascinating new realm of spirituality. Ben called himself a Christian and, like Cayce, had had a number of supernatural channeling experiences that he claimed he had not been seeking. In fact, Ben had been initially resistant to the idea that there was a spiritual dimension at all. He felt that God had brought about these channeling experiences, and in this way he justified his trafficking with the spirits. As I had received no grounding in spiritual discernment, I became a sponge for his teachings. Ben exposed me to a wealth of arcane spiritual knowledge that was light-years removed from what this country boy had experienced.

My search for nutritional information had initiated me into the world of New Age philosophy. If Ben taught me the possibilities and the lifestyle of New Age spirituality, Jan had a more profound impact on how I viewed life. I was seventeen and she was fifty-one—a courageous woman who had raised four children on her own after her husband had abandoned them. After her children were grown, she pursued her own education and earned a degree in existential psychology. This free, strong, independent woman seemed so worldly-wise, so spiritually self-contained, so loving. And she claimed to have a relationship with Jesus. But she was the first to teach me that whatever one believed was valid; indeed, she said that as human beings we are responsible to "create our own reality." (A solid grounding in

Scripture would have provided an echoing warning of the original lie: "You will be like God"). Any moral belief, any conduct was appropriate as long as it harmed no one else. Discomfort with the morally ambiguous was seen as puritanical squeamishness derived from an outmoded Western worldview. Other, more "enlightened" cultures around the world engaged in these behaviors without reservation, and so surely they were appropriate for all. As the sum of my knowledge of Scripture was encompassed by one idea—"You should accept Jesus as your Savior"— I was utterly unprepared to deal with the intellectual morass that was modern relativism. It was heady stuff for a heart-hungry seventeen year old—intoxicating and confusing.

The philosophies that I was absorbing from Ben and Jan produced intense internal conflict in me, a veritable babble of voices in my heart. With the eyes of an older man, I see in retrospect that the Holy Spirit himself was intervening, stirring up unrest, calling me back.

We serve a God whose wisdom and compassion toward his children is inexhaustible. And he uses whatever means he has at his disposal to influence us and rescue us from our foolishness. Even a pretty girl. Even another health food store, this one attached to a church. This independent fundamentalist church really knew Jesus in an intimate way. Their faith was integrated fully and genuinely into every aspect of their lives—a spiritual wholeness or completeness that I had been hungering for. I became enamored with Martha, one of the clerks. Before I knew it, we were dating, and I was attending her church. There I found individuals who really knew the Lord and had experienced his power in their lives—and not just on Sundays. Interestingly enough, as I grew in the knowledge of the truth, I had unconsciously ceased walking the strange spiritual paths I had been exploring. It was as if my heart, having found real spiritual food (John 6:48, 51), had ceased hungering and was finally content.

This church was becoming my home. And yet planted within the church were the seeds of its own destruction. I was increasingly confronted with issues that were disturbing but initially too vague to name. The deeper I grew into the church, the more disturbing the situation became. A spirit of control manifested itself among the church's members, at first subtle, then more and more emotionally coercive. Finally Martha and I were told that we should not be spending so much time with my family because "this church is your family." I knew then that I had to leave. Unfortunately, to my grief, Martha did not.

Still, that church was a great gift to me. Despite the sickness that had grown within it, God was mercifully carrying out his work in me. For the first time I understood that there really could be joy and power in the context of Christian experience. Unfortunately, the babble of confusion, the roar of competing voices in my soul, rose up again with a vengeance. Ben was first on the scene, picking his way through the emotional rubble that was my life. "The Christian church has such a narrow view of what Christianity is really about," he explained. "That's why they have hidden the existence of the Gnostic gospels all these years. Don't you see? If they had allowed the Gnostic gospels to enter the canon of Scripture, it would have eliminated the hierarchy of the organized church and undermined the reason for their very existence."[1] He made it seem as though the church's attempt to control me was part of a larger attempt to control the truth—a twisted conspiracy.

How could I ever trust again? If these loving, godly people were either accessories to a conspiracy against the truth or victims under its control, where did that leave me? What I had learned and experienced in the church had the ring of truth, and yet the church had become so sick. The things I was learning about soul awakening, Eastern meditation and energy meridians so conflicted with what I thought to be true in Christianity that the agony of emotional and spiritual confusion intensified and became unbearable. So I fled far beyond the confines of my North Carolina home.

A Final Plunge into Alternative Medicine—and a Final Escape

A few years after my initial exposure to Eastern ideas, I visited Boulder, Colorado. Boulder has a lot to commend itself in the heart of the naive and undiscerning. It sits, inlaid like a jewel, on the flanks of the Rockies, with a commanding view of the Great Plains below. It is an idyllic college community—green, eclectic, intellectually and spiritually diverse, a haven of political correctness. The community's gold standard is tolerance. Its common ground is spirituality. Everyone I met seemed to be intently pursuing some new and exotic spiritual path. For me, Boulder was a fascinating carnival of alternative spirituality. A week's visit made a lasting impression, and when I returned to Boulder a few years later to live, I immersed myself in its eclectic spirituality and worldviews. It was a relief to move to a place so different from home, a place where people were living out some form of spirituality in daily life, whether it was right or wrong.

Suddenly I had friends who were into alternative everything, including spirituality, social norms, politics, various healing practices—you name it. I was particularly drawn to Transcendental Meditation, transpersonal psychology and various "energy healing" modalities. I lived in a household consisting of a diverse collection of people: a Catholic monk, a Buddhist macrobiotic, a Sufi vegetarian, an atheist (and misanthropic) macrobiotic, a blue-green algae millionaire, a Quaker and Da Free John devotee, a yogi and an alcoholic Buddhist *kundalini* yoga master, to name a few. There was a selection of "paths" that claimed to develop power and potential and ultimately lead to "enlightenment." These paths also seemed more sophisticated than the one I had grown up with, and they provided ways for me to incorporate spirituality into my whole life, rather than just on Sunday morning.

The pervasive ideology that enveloped me in Boulder was the notion that truth is relative, and this premise reinforced the various philosophies, worldviews and even evolutionary theory to which I had been exposed in college. I concluded that my previous thinking that Jesus is the only way to God had been narrow-minded and judgmental, and I began to adopt the view of religious pluralism: "There are many paths to God and truth." It was all about process rather than con-clusion. Furthermore, once the idea of absolute, objective truth was replaced with the dictum that "you determine your own truth," anything could (at least theoret-ically) become possible—and nothing could be objectively knowable. In this worldview, scientific methodology loses its validating power, and feelings and experiences become the guide to knowledge. In many ways this made no sense to me, but I continued to lay aside my critical thinking in favor of what I was told was an "intuitive" path. I kept assuming that my lack of understanding was a pro-cess of growth, and so I continued to explore these ideas.

An important underlying attraction—one that helped settle my qualms about revising my basic understanding of truth and reality—was the feeling of love and total acceptance of everyone and everything that was expressed by those around me. Compassion, warmth and lack of pretense were clearly evident. The notion that we are all part of each other (not to mention the entire universe), and the emphasis on love that seemed to flow naturally from this assumption, had a real impact on me. In many ways it seemed an enticing alternative to Christianity's insistence on absolute moral standards and objective truth. (Jesus' bold claim "I am the way, the truth and the life" stood in stark contrast to "You will be like God.")

My experiences in Boulder both encouraged and deepened my involvement with alternative medicine. This was bolstered during my training in biochemistry and nutrition at the University of Colorado, where I found some allies in my efforts to integrate scientific and New Age worldviews. My adviser was interested in human energy fields, a concept that underlies many alternative therapy systems. Eventually I earned a D.O. (Doctor of Osteopathic Medicine) degree in Kansas City and then spent a year of postgraduate training at Denver Presbyterian Hospi-tal in family medicine. I began to see alternative therapies not merely as "alterna-tives" but as valid efforts by well-meaning people to correct many of the problems in conventional medicine—not the least of which was its apparent lack of interest in spirituality. To a significant degree, this void in modern medicine is now being filled with New Age spirituality.

Furthermore, I became aware that for many Western practitioners—and to some degree, for the health care system as a whole—compassion had been diluted by time pressures, technology and financial considerations. In contrast, proponents of the "new" medicine have consistently broadcast not only a genuine desire to heal (in the broadest sense, encompassing body, mind and spirit) but also boundless optimism. As a result, many of their ideologies and illogical assumptions are accepted at face value, and attempts to examine them on a more objective basis are often dismissed as narrow-minded. For many people, including Bible-believing Christians, the attraction boils down to a response to the way one is treated: "The acupuncturist/homeopath/energy therapist was so caring and interested in me as a person, while the clinic/ER/'gatekeeper' doctor just writes a prescription and rushes on to the next patient." In addition, many valid themes that are emphasized in holistic and alternative medicine—attention to nutrition, exercise, stress management and general self-care—are still not given the attention they deserve within mainstream medicine. Alternative practitioners are more likely to "lead by example," living healthier lives and generally conducting themselves in a more positive way than many of their conventional medical counterparts.

Because I saw legitimate problems with Western medicine, it became easy not only to promote unconventional practices as a viable alternative but also to deflect any criticism of them as attempts by the medical establishment to suppress a threat to its dominance—and income. (Many times I heard this argument used as a cover for what was in fact a lack of proof for alternative practices.) Eventually I joined a large clinic that actively promoted therapies such as chelation, intravenous vitamins, homeopathy, acupuncture point stimulation and a comprehensive alternative approach to health called "environmental medicine." Some of these approaches seemed to be promising, but they needed studies to substantiate their claims. My ideas about data collection seemed to fall on deaf ears. The notion that scientific validation was necessary did not seem important as long as patients felt better. There was also a climate of psychological coercion toward patients: "Others have felt better in response to these therapies, and you will too." I attended a number of conferences where the whole gamut of alternative medicine was on display: crystals, "high-powered water," aura-reading cameras—you name it. I heard and met a number of celebrities within the movement: Deepak Chopra, Andrew Weil and Larry Dossey among others.

Yet for all of its optimism and "good vibrations," after a while it became apparent that alternative medicine was not a realm of unbroken sweetness and light. For one thing, I began to notice that an active interest in the profit motive was not unique to the conventional medical establishment. A number of lectures and meetings in the alternative medicine circuit seemed to be more focused on boosting the practitioner's income than on enhancing the patient's health. There was also an uncomfortable emphasis in our own clinic on promoting vitamins and supplements, often to the tune of hundreds of dollars per month per patient, sold from the office not only with a healthy markup but also with a somber assurance that these were the only ones the patients should be taking.

My withdrawal from alternative medicine was ultimately driven by the same spiritual quest for truth that had led me into it. During this time I found myself calling on Christ for guidance, not only with my work but also with the more profound question of what was true and what was not. By this time I had been attending a theologically solid Christian Reformed church, attending a Bible study and listening to R. C. Sproul on the subject of truth.[2] I now was building the necessary intellectual foundation to discern truth from nontruth. Because of my earlier experience in Boulder, where I saw the fruits of relativistic spirituality, I noticed the same lack of grounding in truth being played out in alternative medicine. For the first time I began to understand why so many people who begin with a quest for alternative health approaches gradually become involved in a New Age worldview. The removal of the idea of discernible objective truth in the physical world (which also downgrades the importance of valid studies and collecting relevant data) allows for an easy entry into spiritual relativism and syncretism: "I have my truth, and you have your truth and all religions lead to God."

I saw that the pervasive notion of a universal energy, which could be channeled and manipulated for healing, was in essence an impersonal god—and not the God about whom Jesus spoke. The more grounded in Christianity I became, the more I realized what was amiss. I began to understand how spirituality built on the concept of absolute truth and a medical philosophy grounded on solid proof and combined with an attitude of compassion and service could interact and complement one another. As I attempted to share my insights with old friends, I received a tepid response: "I'm glad it works for you." This confirmed to me that within this movement there is a serious spiritual and practical blind spot—the inability to see that if something is true, something else that is blatantly contradictory to it cannot also be true.

Eventually the combination of my maturing Christian faith, disenchantment with New Age thinking and discomfort with the shaky foundations of alternative practices led me to leave the practice I had joined. Since that time I have been

involved in more conventional health care, but I continue to incorporate nutrition, diet, exercise and preventive medicine. Having worked on both sides of the
medical fence, I continue to be aware of strengths and weaknesses in both
approaches. As we have described elsewhere in this book, over the past few years
many barriers between conventional and alternative medicine have been breaking
down. It would appear, however, that the general direction of the resulting "cultural exchange" has been in one direction: alternative practices and thinking seem
to be impacting the conventional realm much more profoundly than the other
way around.

14

IS GOD A DEPENDENT VARIABLE?

Science, Spirituality & Sorcery

*T*he October 25, 1999, issue of the *Archives of Internal Medicine,* a mainstream scientific medical journal, contained a study that attempted to answer a provocative but seemingly very *un*scientific question: Is prayer for someone who is ill likely to make any difference in their recovery?[1] Over the course of a year, a team of researchers at the Mid America Heart Institute at Saint Luke's Hospital, Kansas City, randomly assigned 990 consecutive patients admitted to the Coronary Care Unit (CCU) to one of two groups. Both groups received the same quality and intensity of medical care normally delivered at this facility. For one group, however, the first name of each incoming patient—and no other information—was given to a team of five intercessors, who would then pray for the next twenty-eight days that the patient would have "a speedy recovery with no complications," along with anything else that seemed appropriate.

For this study fifteen teams of five intercessors had been recruited from the community by the researchers and represented a variety of Christian denominational and nondenominational backgrounds. (Other faiths, such as Judaism or Islam, were not represented in this study.) They were required to agree with the following mini-credo: "I believe in God. I believe that He is personal and is concerned with individual lives. I further believe that He is responsive to prayers for healing made in behalf of the sick." None of the patients were aware that they were being prayed for, and none of the physicians, nurses or other CCU staff were informed that the study was in progress. After the patients were discharged, a physician investigator reviewed and scored each chart using a point system devised for this study. Points were accumulated based upon the number and severity of events (including death) that took place during the hospital admission. The investigator assigning points did not know whether the patient had received prayer from an intercessor group.

When the scores were tallied and analyzed, the mean score for patients in the prayed-for group was 11 percent lower than that for the other group. There was no difference between the groups for number of days spent in the CCU or the hospital. The difference in scores was considered to be statistically significant, with the odds of it occurring by pure chance calculated to be twenty-five to one.

So this experiment showed that God answers prayer, right? Well, not exactly. Among their various conclusions, the authors made the following statement:

> Although we cannot know why we obtained the results we did, we can comment on what our data do not show. For example, we have not proven that God answers prayer, or that God even exists. It was intercessory prayer, not the existence of God, that was tested here. All we have observed is that when individuals outside of the hospital speak (or think) the first names of hospitalized patients with an attitude of prayer, the latter appeared to have a "better" CCU experience.[2]

Overall they concluded that this result "suggests that prayer may be an effective adjunct to standard medical care."[3]

Eight months later the June 26, 2000, issue of the *Archives* contained fifteen letters—an unusually large number for this type of journal—responding to the prayer study. The vast majority of the letters were highly critical of it. A number complained about the validity of the point system used to score the patients' course in the hospital, the statistics used to analyze it and the conclusions drawn from them. Some objected vigorously to the fact that the patients were not informed about the study, noting that it is likely that at least some would have declined to be involved, for any number of reasons. A few raised global, "What's the point?" types of questions. Only one actually thanked the authors for their efforts. The authors of the CCU prayer study responded to all of the objections, acknowledging a number of them as valid (especially some relating to experimental design). They concluded, however, by reiterating their contention that "since spiritual factors may play some role in healing, additional studies are needed to clarify the place of intercessory prayer in maintaining and restoring health."[4]

Also weighing in with his own critique of the critics was Larry Dossey, M.D., who was given a special commentary article in the same issue of the *Archives* that contained the bundle of hostile letters. Dossey scolded them with this caution:

"Although skepticism is an invaluable component of scientific progress, it can shade into a type of dogmatic materialism that excludes intercessory prayer in principle, as when Newton's critics condemned universal gravity as occult nonsense without weighing the evidence."[5]

The amount of space devoted to the subject of intercessory prayer in this issue of the *Archives* was extraordinary, offering yet another indication of the evolving impact of alternative therapies on conventional medicine and the culture at large. It also provided a brief introduction to a few of the combatants in an emerging controversy: the role of spirituality in health and medicine. Questions currently broiling in the medical literature, popular media and the Internet include the following:

☐ What role does spirituality play in a person's overall health?

☐ Do people with an active spiritual life have less illness (physical and emotional) and generally live longer than those who do not? Do those people have better outcomes when they do become ill or have surgery?

☐ What markers do we use to define and measure a person's spiritual life, especially for the sake of scientific inquiry? Church attendance? Prayer? Bible reading? Participation in small groups or other social functions related to a church or other religious group?

☐ Should physicians and other health care providers inquire about a patient's spirituality? Should church membership and prayer life be included in a medical history, along with occupation, marital status, tobacco and alcohol use?

☐ Should doctors recommend church attendance, prayer, meditation or other spiritually related activities to patients? If so, what churches—or for that matter, what religions—should be recommended?

☐ Does a person's individual prayer life affect his or her health?

☐ Can intercessory prayer for patients, whether at the bedside or across the country, be shown to be beneficial for them?

These are all extremely important questions, although at first glance it would seem that the answers—at least to some of them—would be self-evident. After all, with or without their doctors' advice, people have been praying for themselves and one another, attending religious services and making lifestyle changes (sometimes dramatic ones) based on their interactions with God all along. Do we really need the measured verbiage of a cadre of physicians and statisticians in a medical journal to convince us to pray for someone we care about or to attend a Wednesday night Bible study? A more important question to consider—one that we will revisit later in this chapter—is this: is it appropriate or reasonable to assign God the role of dependent variable in a scientific experiment? Can we design a test that will help us understand how God will behave under certain circumstances?

Everyone (including the authors of this book) has opinions and agendas relating to these topics, and in order to better understand the issues, it would be helpful to take a tour of the various viewpoints that are vying for our attention and allegiance. For the sake of easy identification, we will identify them by favorite catch phrases. The remainder of this chapter will also serve as a curtain call for a number of the individuals and practices we have discussed in previous chapters.

"Science and Religion Should Go Steady and Get Married"

This sentiment from grandmotherly psychic healer Olga Worrall during the heyday of the holistic health movement in the 1970s remains prominent throughout alternative medicine today, though expressed somewhat differently. It summarizes the heart and soul of Therapeutic Touch, the "quantum healing" teachings of Deepak Chopra, the life energy assessments of medical sensitives such as Carolyn Myss, the mysticism of *qi gong* and *feng shui,* and a host of other practices that claim to have found the link between science and religion through the manipulation of "invisible life energy." It motivates the proclamations that "Einstein proved we are all congealed energy" and that "quantum physics validates what the seers and yogis and spiritual masters of the East understood eons ago." It fires the imagination of those who believe that our consciousness, once unshackled from the notion that it has any limitations (such as being confined to our brain), can accomplish the miraculous. It is the language of the "materialist magician" described by C. S. Lewis in his classic satire *The Screwtape Letters,* the person who wants to cultivate supernatural abilities without any belief in, or accountability to, a higher authority.

In a number of ways this particular thrust of the alternative medicine movement is its most dishonest. We have noted that a number of therapies that portray themselves as "nonreligious" or "not promoting any particular religion" (for example, Therapeutic Touch) are in fact direct outgrowths of Vedism or Taoism or are a synthesis of Eastern mystical traditions. For more than a quarter century we have seen the efforts of Transcendental Meditation to package the repetition of the names of Hindu deities as a scientific approach to stress reduction. We have described Deepak Chopra's articulate nod to a variety of religious traditions while he systematically deconstructs them in his book *How to Know God.* We have heard Andrew Weil characterize himself as an "open-minded skeptic" and then inform us that optimum health involves a series of esoteric breathing exercises that are intended to improve the influx of *prana* into our bodies.

If these practitioners and their therapies would boldly and bravely proclaim that they are disseminating the teachings and performing the rituals of their chosen (Eastern) religious faith, we could at least have some honest dialogue about our various perspectives. Instead we continue to hear what almost sounds like a pitch from dozens of carnival barkers to tired and stressed Westerners: "Step right up and try the latest scientifically proven, all-natural way to relax, lose weight, improve energy and even spark up the old sex life." Once inside the midway tent, however, the "nonreligious" religious message invariably arrives: "You are energy, you are information, you are consciousness without boundaries, you are godlike, you are God."

Even yoga, that age-old staple of the health club and community center, has a lot more on its mind that a few stretching and breathing techniques. While a host of styles and practices beckon the budding practitioner, all yogic roads lead to Brahman. A manual clearly intended for use by beginners in the general populace, *The Sivananda Companion to Yoga,* states its purposes from the outset:

> The underlying purpose of all the different aspects of the practice of yoga is to reunite the individual self (jiva) with the Absolute or pure consciousness (Brahman)—in fact, the word yoga literally means "joining." Union with this unchanging reality liberates the spirit from all sense of separation, freeing it from the illusion of time, space and causation. It is only our own ignorance, our inability to discriminate between the real and unreal, that prevents us from realizing our true nature.[6]

Perhaps the introductory class at the YMCA did not mention anything about cosmic consciousness. But scratch just a little below the surface and you will find an elaborate system whose sole purpose is to convince you—no, to help you *experience*—that you and the Absolute are one and the same.

That perennial idea, the primal temptation from Genesis 3 ("You will not surely die. . . . You will be like God"), is the foundation for a multitude of alternative practices that continue to swell the science-marrying-religion camp. Behind their well-intentioned efforts to promote health for body, mind and spirit lies an age-old determination to obliterate any difference in nature, knowledge, power or glory between humanity and God. Since reason and normal waking consciousness consistently fail to support such an idea, elaborate wordplay and altered mental states must disarm, disable or detour around them. It is precisely this passion for depersonalizing and demoting God, deifying human beings and ultimately obliterating both in a supposedly inevitable cosmic "Oneness" that should cause those who believe in the veracity of the Old and New Testaments to avoid these practices and to resist their penetration into our culture.

Ironically, the healing systems whose proponents are so determined to unite science and (their) religion deconstruct not only God but science as well. Their spiritual underpinnings virtually guarantee this outcome in two ways. First, by insisting that there is no objective reality, that there is no real truth to be discovered, that the world around us and the bodies we inhabit are illusory (or maya), Eastern mysticism and postmodernism both effectively dismiss scientific inquiry as a monumental waste of effort. True "knowledge" apparently arrives only during altered states of consciousness (or through "stoned thinking," as Andrew Weil would call it). There is a certain cleverness and even a veneer of wisdom in this viewpoint. But left to its own devices, it would leave us dying of smallpox, diphtheria and a host of other plagues that are now preventable and treatable only because enough people decided that the world was in fact real and that its workings are knowable.

Second, the long-departed developers of both Taoism and Vedism, which undergird so many alternative therapies, made what appears from the twenty-first century to have been a short-sighted decision: they imagined a detailed and complex human physiology, involving invisible energies *(chi* and *prana)* flowing through equally invisible structures (meridians and *chakras).* Furthermore, they insisted that health and illness were the direct product of the quality of this flow and devised a complex system to manipulate it. Unfortunately, centuries of scientific and technological progress have come and gone without providing any objective evidence that *chi, prana,* meridians and *chakras* actually exist. (In more recent centuries homeopathy has found itself in precisely the same situation, pressing its case with religious fervor because scientific inquiry has failed to validate it.) Nevertheless, faithful followers continue to carry the torch for these therapies, proclaiming their usefulness for any and all conditions when much more straightforward explanations—most importantly, the body's normal recuperative abilities and the benefits of positive expectations—are readily available.

Standing in stark contrast to the antiscientific worldviews and the outmoded physiologies from the East is the Judeo-Christian Bible, which has long taken an undeserved rap for impeding scientific progress. In fact, just the opposite is true. While the Scriptures clearly declare that this world has a meter running, they never deny its reality. Instead they invite us to study God's creation, in which we will discover both his ingenuity and glory. David literally sang this idea at the beginning of Psalm 19:

> The heavens declare the glory of God;
>> the skies proclaim the work of his hands.
> Day after day they pour forth speech;
>> night after night they display knowledge.
> There is no speech or language

where their voice is not heard.
Their voice goes out into all the earth,
their words to the end of the world. (Psalm 19:1-4)

Many have blamed the Bible for impeding scientific progress by proclaiming such ideas as a flat earth and a geocentric (earth- rather than sun-centered) solar system. Sadly, in many cases over the centuries such errors were promulgated by the church, and those who dared disagree (such as Galileo) were even persecuted. But contrary to the clichés brought forward by its critics, the Bible does not specifically teach these ideas. For example, a passage such as Psalm 19:4-6, which describes the sun as rising at one end of the heavens and making its circuit to the other, is clearly set within an allegorical and poetic context. Galileo's argument was primarily with the long-entrenched cosmology of Aristotle and Ptolemy—not exactly prophets and apostles of Judaism and Christianity—to which the Catholic hierarchy had mistakenly pledged their allegiance. It is worth noting that many of the greatest scientists the world has ever known (such as Isaac Newton) were devout Christians who were eager to study and learn about the world around them.[7]

The Bible makes it abundantly clear that the world we live in and the bodies we inhabit will not last forever. It also clearly testifies that the physical universe is definitely not all there is and all there ever will be, as contemporary materialists would have us believe. But most important for our discussion, it describes a created order, a world whose workings are stable enough to be discoverable and knowable. Furthermore, those workings can be understood and verified by anyone with the capacity to do so, whether or not they believe in the one who created them. This premise both undergirds and encourages scientific inquiry, and (especially when fueled and guided by biblical admonitions to serve others and alleviate their suffering) it has led to the most significant advances in combating disease in human history.

Compared with the elaborate "invisible energy" systems of Taoism and Vedism, the Bible's almost complete silence on the subjects of human anatomy and physiology appears to be a stroke of genius. The Bible contains the dietary and public health admonitions that were important to the well-being of the nation of Israel as well as a host of teachings about prudent behavior that, if universally followed, would save the world untold disease and suffering. There are no tales of angels (or even the Holy Spirit) circulating in our bodies through some convoluted circuitry, nor are there detailed explanations linking symptoms to specific sins or guaranteeing cures when certain rituals are followed. The closest approximation to a biblical declaration about a particular body function is the repeated assertion in the Pentateuch that "the life of a creature is in the blood" (Leviticus 17:11, for example), a statement that is entirely correct from a physiologic perspective. Deprive any tissue of a steady flow of blood (and thus of life-sustaining oxygen), and it will die within minutes. Had the writer of these passages declared that "the life is in the bile" or "the life is in the urine," he would have caused untold harm to the reputation of the Scriptures thousands of years later.

There are, of course, many accounts of God and his enemies (specifically Satan and his demonic followers) affecting the health of human beings. But these stories invariably serve to illustrate broader themes, not define the ground rules for everyday health maintenance. There are no biblical recipes for potions, no biblical incantations that are supposed to bring heavenly energy into our bodies or keep devils at bay. The New Testament deals in a matter-of-fact way with demonic activity and at times describes Jesus calmly ending a siege of illness (including mental derangement) by driving malevolent "beings" out of a person (see Mark 5:1-20, for example). But these accounts serve primarily to point to three basic facts: (1) God's ultimate intention is for us to "have life, and have it to the full" (John 10:10); (2) Jesus had authority over physical and spiritual situations that were otherwise hopeless; and (3) demonic entities can indeed harass human beings. Yet even as these events unfold through the four Gospels and the book of Acts, and as the core teachings of Christianity are set forth in the Epistles that follow, there is no systematic teaching that we are to deal with illness by attempting to manipulate invisible forces or beings. We are to comfort those who are hurting and beseech God for their healing—period. No contemporary medical breakthrough or, for that matter, scientific discovery within the core of the atom or the far reaches of space contradicts those teachings.

"Prayer Is Good Medicine"

This phrase is actually the title of a popular book by Larry Dossey, M.D., whose name is now widely associated with promoting prayer as a viable and useful adjunct to conventional medicine—or perhaps an improvement on it. Whenever the combination of prayer and medicine is the topic of conversation, whether on a TV talk show (*Oprah* and *Good Morning, America,* among many others) or in a respectable medical journal (such as the discussion in the *Archives of Internal Medicine*), it is almost certain that Dossey's name will be mentioned or that he will be asked to offer his perspective. His prayer trilogy—the 1993 manifesto *Healing Words: The Power of Prayer and the Practice of Medicine,* the mini-devotional follow-up *Prayer Is Good Medicine* (1996) and the less well-known *Be Careful What You Pray For . . . You Might Just Get It* (1997)[8]—so enthusiastically promote the power and efficacy of prayer that Dossey has frequently garnered praise from conservative Christian writers.

Take, for example, the recent book *Healing Prayer* by Reginald Cherry, M.D., who hosts the program *The Doctor and the Word* on the Trinity Broadcasting Network. In building a case for the role of prayer in healing, Cherry references Dossey's *Healing Words* in a positive light. Dr. Cherry is but one of many evangelical writers who have endorsed Dossey's materials and offered them as evidence for what appears to be a positive trend in conventional medicine: *Finally doctors are understanding what the Bible teaches about prayer!*[9]

We have already noted that Dossey defended the researchers in the 1999 *Archives of Internal Medicine* study of intercessory prayer for coronary care unit patients. As it turns out, he was also profoundly impacted by another experiment in intercession that has been cited repeatedly in articles and books about prayer for more than a decade. This study was conducted by Randolph Byrd, M.D., in the coronary care unit of San Francisco General Hospital during the early 1980s.[10] This study was similar in many ways to the more recent Kansas City CCU study (which actually was an attempt to replicate it). Byrd, a cardiologist who has described himself as deeply committed both to Christ and to scientific inquiry, was reportedly troubled when a colleague made a disparaging comment about prayer for patients as "unscientific." After much prayer on his own, Byrd devised an experiment in which he would attempt to prove otherwise. Within a month his proposal was approved by the appropriate research committee at San Francisco General Hospital.[11]

Over a ten-month period beginning in August 1982, 393 patients admitted to the CCU were randomly assigned either to receive intercessory prayer (the "IP" group, which contained 192 patients) or to be in a control group (201 patients) who did not. One major difference between this and the Kansas City experiment was that Byrd's patients were informed about the study and were asked to give consent before participating. As it turned out, a small percentage of those entering the CCU over the course of the ten months did not want to be involved in the study. (The fact that the Kansas City study was carried out without the informed consent of the patients was a major target for criticism after it was published.)

Neither the patients, their physicians, the CCU staff nor Byrd himself knew to which group they would be assigned. The first name and diagnosis for each patient designated to receive prayer would be given to one of several prayer groups, each containing from five to seven people. All intercessors were self-identified as "'born again Christians (according to the Gospel of John 3:3) with an active Christian life as manifested by daily devotional prayer and active Christian fellowship with a local church."[12] They prayed daily for each member in the IP group, with specific requests for rapid recovery and prevention both of complications and death. (In this study it would appear that both the theological orientation and the prayer assignment of the intercessors were defined in greater depth than in the more recent Kansas City experiment.)

Overall, those who received prayer fared better than their counterparts in the control group in twenty out of twenty-nine predefined outcomes, which ranged in severity from needing antibiotics to having a cardiac arrest. However, the differences between the groups were considered statistically significant in only six out of the twenty outcomes. (Statistical significance is a calculation widely used in scientific literature to determine whether the results of an experiment are likely to be the result of pure chance. Usually this benchmark is achieved when analysis of the data suggests that the odds against the results being caused by chance are more than twenty to one.) For the other nine outcomes there was either no difference or nonsignificant differences favoring the control group.[13] Byrd's study also included a general assessment of the patients' hospital course and noted that 85 percent of the patients receiving prayer had a "good hospital course," compared to 73 percent of the controls. This difference also was statistically significant, but many critics subsequently challenged the validity of this assessment because it had been devised specifically for this experiment and was not used anywhere else.

Even among these measures for which the prayed-for group showed a statistically significant advantage, the magnitude of the benefit was not exactly overwhelming. For example, three patients in the prayer group received antibiotics versus sixteen in the control group. Based on these numbers, one could say that CCU patients who did not receive intercessory prayer were five times more likely to receive antibiotics than their counterparts in the control group. That sounds impressive until the numbers are expressed as a percentage of all of the patients involved: 1.6 percent needed antibiotics in the prayer group versus 8 percent in the control group—a difference of less than 7 percent.[14] In fact, all of the statistically significant improvements fell in the 5 to 7 percent range.

Thirteen of those who received prayer (6.7 percent) died, as opposed to seventeen of those who did not (8.4 percent), although this difference (1.7 percent) did not achieve statistical significance. There was also no difference between the groups in length of stay in the CCU or the hospital. Unfortunately, significant differences in recovery time and protection from death were two out of the three specific prayers offered by the intercessor groups, and it would appear that their efforts were not very successful—or were they? We will return to some important questions raised by the CCU prayer experiments in a moment.

Whatever else it might have accomplished, the Byrd experiment made a profound impact on Larry Dossey. According to the preface of his first book on prayer, *Healing Words,* learning of the study literally changed the direction of his practice. (It would also dramatically alter his writing career and public visibility.) In response to the Byrd study, Dossey searched through the scientific literature for other research that might validate the efficacy of prayer. What he discovered caught him by surprise:

> I found an enormous body of evidence: over one hundred experiments exhibiting the criteria or "good science," many conducted under stringent laboratory conditions, over half of which showed that prayer brings about significant changes in a variety of living things.
>
> I was astonished. I had begun my search believing it would turn up little. After all, if scientific proof for the healing effects of prayer existed, surely it would be common knowledge among scientifically trained physicians. I came to realize the truth of what many historians of science have described: A body of knowledge that does not fit with prevailing ideas can be ignored as if it does not exist, no matter how scientifically valid it may be. Scientists, including physicians, can have blind spots in their vision. The power of prayer, it seemed, was an example.[15]

It is these kinds of statements that have caused unsuspecting evangelical Christians to sit up and take notice. Unfortunately, they may not realize that much of the "scientific proof for the healing effects of prayer" that Dossey describes came from obscure sources (especially parapsychology journals) that are not highly regarded in the scientific community. More importantly, Christians who are encouraged by Dossey's endorsement of prayer are in for a big surprise when they discover how he defines God, how he defines prayer and what he thinks of Christian evangelism. The following passages speak for themselves.

☐ Regarding God and how he (or she or it) is to be addressed:

> Many terms are used throughout this book to refer to a Supreme Being. In most cases I have chosen as neutral a term as possible, such as *the Absolute.* . . . The Absolute is radically beyond any description whatsoever, including gender. With these limitations in mind, the reader may insert, in every instance that follows, his or her preferred name for the Absolute—whether *Goddess, God, Allah, Krishna, Brahman, the Tao, the Universal Mind, the Almighty, Alpha and Omega, the One.*[16]

☐ Regarding the nature of prayer and, more specifically, the most important reason for studying it "scientifically":

> *Prayer says something incalculably important about who we are and what our destiny may be.* As we shall see, prayer is a genuinely *nonlocal* event—that is, it is not confined to a specific place in space or to a specific moment in time. Prayer reaches outside the here-and-now; it operates at a distance and outside the present moment. Since

prayer is initiated by a mental action, this implies that there is some aspect of our psyche that also is genuinely nonlocal. If so, then something of ourselves is infinite in space and time—thus omnipresent, eternal and immortal. "Nonlocal," after all does not mean "really big" or "a very long time." It implies *infinitude* in space and time, because a limited nonlocality is a contradiction in terms. In the West, this infinite aspect of the psyche has been referred to as the soul. Empirical evidence for prayer's power, then, is indirect evidence for the soul. It is also evidence for shared qualities with the Divine—"the Divine within"—since infinitude, omnipresence, and eternality are qualities that we have attributed also to the Absolute.[17]

What this extended passage, and dozens of others like it in his other books, makes abundantly clear is that Dossey really belongs with the "marriage of science and religion" contingent, especially as he forthrightly echoes their "we are all God" message. But he is especially focused on what for decades has been called "psi" (that is, parapsychological) phenomena: telepathy, foreseeing the future and, most importantly, influencing others (or things) at a distance through our mental powers.

This picture of your mind as outside of your head may at first seem foreign. But as we shall see, "nonlocal" or "infinite" describes a natural part of who we are. Its expressions include sharing of thoughts and feelings at a distance, gaining information and wisdom through dreams and visions, knowing the future, radical breakthroughs in creativity and discovery, and many more. And this part of your mind can be used today in healing illness and disease.[18]

Dossey has in many ways become a standard bearer for the age-old pursuit of psychic abilities, but he has also managed to ingratiate himself with the general public by substituting the more acceptable (and safe) word *prayer* for "absent healing" or "psychic healing." When he refers to prayer, he is not talking about what goes on at the Wednesday night service at First Baptist or at the Wailing Wall in Jerusalem. His vision of prayer is not the humble communication between a human being and his or her Creator but rather the extension of our "nonlocal" (that is, infinite) consciousness instantly across time and space, a sort of psychic e-mail. And if a prayer seems to be answered, it isn't because God Almighty, Creator of heaven and earth, intervened on our behalf. "Answers to prayer" are just demonstrations of the incredible capabilities of our nonlocal consciousness.

Imagine that, as you read these words, a part of your mind is not present in your body or brain or even in this moment. Imagine that this aspect of your consciousness spreads everywhere, extending billions of miles into space, from the beginning of time into the limitless future, linking us with the minds of one another and with everyone who has ever lived or will live. This is the infinite piece of your consciousness.[19]

Dossey's acquisition of the term "nonlocal" from physics, by the way, is analogous to Deepak Chopra's borrowing the term "quantum healing" to prop up *ayurveda,* and it serves the same purpose: adding the respectability of contemporary science to the discussion. This cultivation of scientific credibility becomes even more important as he delves into some unsettling implications of his contention that our nonlocal consciousness can affect things and people at any distance (or apparently in any time frame, including past and future). Obviously not all of us harbor lovely thoughts about one another. What havoc might our stray "prayers" wreak if they intend someone else's undoing? To address the "negative" aspects of prayer (including such unsavory things as curses and hexes), Dossey in 1997 published *Be Careful What You Pray For . . . You Just Might Get It.* This is a field guide of sorts to the dark side of our nature, including suggestions for limiting the harm that it might unleash and protecting ourselves from incoming invisible malevolence.

And what about those who object to Dossey's ascribing to the word *prayer* meanings and implications that are clearly at odds with the common and traditional understanding of this word? What specifically does Dossey have to say to those who might propose that all prayers are not created equal?

> It is not the Absolute who is threatened by the scientific evidence favoring prayer, only our own arrogance and pride and the special status that some religions have claimed for themselves. Prayer experiments level the praying [*sic*] field. They show that prayer is a universal phenomenon belonging to every faith and creed, and these studies, therefore, affirm tolerance.[20]

That Dossey is specifically referring to conservative Christianity as the wellspring of "arrogance and pride" is clear from his caustic remarks about "fundamentalists" who condemned the contents of *Healing Words* as "New Age" and "occultic." He holds even greater scorn for physicians who might have the audacity to discuss their faith with their patients. "I have come to believe that patients do not wish, by and large, to bring their religion into their relationship with their physician. Something about mixing religions and the practice of medicine seems as odious and dangerous as letting church and state mingle."[21]

After describing two uncomfortable encounters with doctors who "used Christian principles in their medical practice," Dossey issued this verdict:

> I believe the physicians should not use their medical authority as a platform for espousing their private religious beliefs. Patients, especially when severely ill, are often terribly vulnerable to anything a physician suggests, which makes it all too easy for physicians to prey on them in the name of their personal religious credo. Quite simply, it is a shameful abuse of power.[22]

It is indeed ironic that the physician-author (not to mention executive editor of the journal *Alternative Therapies*) who is so anxious to see prayer become a staple of routine medical care can suddenly sound like the most vociferous materialist whenever conservative Christianity comes anywhere near the conversation. Why the hostility? The preface to *Healing Words* provides some insight, as Dossey describes his experiences as a child and teenager caught up in central Texas revivalism. He was planning to become a minister, but his twin brother talked him into doing his undergraduate work at the University of Texas in Austin. When his adolescent faith collided with scientific materialism, the contest wasn't even close. "Under its withering influence," he recalls, "and aided by my discovery of Bertrand Russell, Aldous Huxley, and other intellectual giants, my religious fervor wilted like a central Texas cotton field in September. I became an agnostic."[23]

But during medical school he discovered Buddhism and Taoism and later took up meditation:

> I read widely and insatiably the works of Eastern mystics and Western commentators. I was delightfully surprised to discover that their core teachings were not just Eastern but universal, appearing also in the esoteric traditions of the major Western spiritual traditions. . . . I gradually adopted an eclectic philosophy that was more spiritually satisfying than anything I had grown up with.[24]

To drive home even more forcefully his contempt for the spiritual traditions from which he fled as a college and medical student, take one last look at the imagery he uses to represent the prayer focus of conservative Christianity. Having become intrigued as a practicing internist with the evidence for the efficacy of healing prayer (that is, psychic healing), he felt that he should begin to pray for his patients.

> But how? I felt I could not pray the way I'd learned as a child. The old images of prayer I had grown up with—pleading with an elderly, robed, bearded, white male figure who preferred English—were hopelessly unsatisfying. As a child I'd made endless lists of everyone I could think of who was needy, which I obsessively and joylessly recited to the Almighty almost daily.[25]

This poignant story of a child's faith strangled by legalism and then buried by collegiate materialist rhetoric, only to be reborn in Eastern mysticism, certainly helps explain Dossey's current viewpoints on prayer. But it also serves as a reminder that his ideas about healing prayer can in no way serve as a resource for Christians who have a genuine interest in this subject.

"Prayer, or Any Promotion of Religion, Has No Place in Medical Care"

This camp's members are the skeptics, throwers of wet blankets on promoters of alternative therapies or, for that matter, on anyone who harbors a thought that something (or Someone) might exist beyond the measurable realm of the material universe. Yet some of the members of the skeptics' camp might challenge the idea that they exist primarily to rain on other people's parades. A position statement in *Skeptic,* the official (and quite well-crafted) periodical of an organization called, appropriately enough, The Skeptics Society, offers this perspective:

> Some people believe that skepticism is rejection of new ideas, or worse, they confuse "skeptic" with "cynic" and think that skeptics are a bunch of grumpy curmudgeons unwilling to accept any claim that challenges the status quo. This is wrong. Skepticism is a provisional approach to claims. It is the application of reason to any and all ideas—no sacred cows allowed. In other words, *skepticism is a method, not a position.* Ideally, skeptics do not go into an investigation closed to the possibility that a phenomenon might be real or that a claim might be true. When we say we are "skeptical," we mean that we must see compelling evidence before we believe. Skeptics are from Missouri—the "show me" state. When we hear a fantastic claim we say, "that's nice, prove it." . . . The key to skepticism is to continuously and vigorously apply the methods of science to navigate the treacherous straits between "know nothing" skepticism and "anything goes" credulity.[26]

When evaluating alternative practices, from magnetic therapies to *ayurveda,* the skeptics provide a stimulating and useful perspective that is conspicuously absent from conventional medical journals and even scarce within the Christian community. (Organizations such as the Spiritual Counterfeits Project and the Christian Research Institute, which chronicle the ebb and flow of worldviews within our culture, are notable exceptions.) Magazines and journals such as *The Skeptical Inquirer* (published by the Committee for the Scientific Investigation of Claims of the Paranormal, or CSICOP), the *Scientific Review of Alternative Medicine* and the above-noted *Skeptic* provide research and analysis that truly belong in *JAMA* and the *New England Journal of Medicine.* They shun the credulous, this-appears-to-work-so-we-must-accept-it attitude of many mainstream medical journals and dare to question the foundational assumptions of some of the most popular therapies in the public square. All of these groups have full-service websites and cross-fertilize on the Internet with medical watchdog groups, such as Quackwatch and The National Council for Reliable Health Information (formerly the National Council Against Health Fraud), which provide useful assessments of alternative practices.

But the skeptics also tend to be enmeshed with materialistic naturalism ("The universe is all there is and all there ever will be") and are often vocal proponents of a religion-is-bad-for-everyone mentality. Thus the skeptics' websites typically link to other sites belonging to groups such as Atheists United, Freedom from Religion Foundation, The Council for Secular Humanism and the American Humanist Association. A website run by the "Internet Infidels" serves as a jumping-off point for these and other organizations that seem intent primarily on running religion out of Dodge. The "About Us" page on the Internet Infidels site (<www.infidels.org>) contains this decidedly unfriendly sentiment:

> Our mission is to defend and promote metaphysical naturalism, the view that our natural world is all that there is, a closed system in no need of an explanation and sufficient unto itself. To that end we publish the very best secular books, essays, papers, articles and reviews. We also stand as a bulwark against the forces of superstition, especially the radical religious right, whose proponents would have us fear knowledge rather than embrace it.[27]

Not surprisingly, the skeptical-materialist camp takes a dim view of the integration of spirituality into medical practice, especially if it might involve discussions between physicians and their patients about spiritual or religious topics. What has raised the eyebrows of some observers is a rising tide of research in the professional literature, as well as articles in the popular press, suggesting that religious involvement, expressed as both as personal commitment and participation in religious services, has a positive impact on overall health, recovery from illness or surgery, and longevity. What has raised their hackles as well is the prospect that doctors might encourage religious activity among their patients.

The most prominent organization disseminating information that supports the benefits of religion is the National Institute for Healthcare Research (NIHR), whose vision statement describes it as "an educational and research organization committed to exploring and communicating the dynamic relationship of spirituality with health."[28] NIHR's president, David Larson, M.D., is a Christian with strong academic credentials. A psychiatrist, geriatrician and epidemiologist, he has also worked as a senior researcher at the National Institutes of Health, the Department of Health and Human Services and the National Institute of Mental Health. He and his coresearchers have compiled detailed summaries of research literature suggesting that religious commitments offer benefits in dealing with problems ranging from cancer and heart disease to drug abuse, alcoholism and depression.[29] For example, a recent meta-analysis of forty-two studies encompassing more than 125,000 people, compiled by NIHR research director Dr. Michael McCullough, has indicated that religious involvement increases the likelihood of living longer by nearly 30 percent. Larson, who also served as coauthor for this study, noted, "A lack of religious belief or practices stood out as a health risk for earlier death to the same degree as heavy alcohol consumption, exposure to organic solvents in the workplace, and hostility."[30]

NIHR materials encourage physicians to at least make an appraisal of their patients' spiritual commitments, much as they would inquire about their occupational and family background.

> The goals of a spiritual history are to realize the patient's definition of spirituality and to make the appropriate referral if needed. Medical professionals who are uncomfortable with taking a spiritual assessment should be reminded it is far less intimate than the sexual history and other parts of the patient assessment. It is extremely helpful to know the patient's coping methods before revealing bad news. . . . A spiritual assessment can be taken as part of the social history section of the standard history and it need not take more than two minutes.[31]

Gathering such information makes perfect sense within the context of a thorough medical evaluation, especially when serious problems are under consideration. But it also squares with recent survey data:

> Statistics from a 1990 Gallup Poll reveal that religion, one expression of spirituality, plays a central role in the lives of many Americans. According to the poll, 95 percent of Americans believe in God, 57 percent pray daily, and 42 percent attended a place of worship in the last week. Other surveys indicate that 75 percent of Americans say religion is central to their lives and a majority feel that spiritual faith can help them recover from illness. . . . Another recent survey found that 75 percent of patients believed that their physicians should address spiritual issues as part of their medical care.[32]

All of these factors considered, one could readily argue that it is time to begin reversing the materialistic, mechanistic tide that has gradually turned conventional medicine into a purely secular enterprise. Shouldn't physicians take a more active role in encouraging the faith factor?

A contingent of critics (who harbor what would appear to be a degree of antagonism toward religion) has forcefully argued otherwise. In a strongly worded article in the *New England Journal of Medicine* entitled "Should Physicians Prescribe Religious Activities?"[33] Columbia University psychologist Richard P. Sloan, Ph.D., and a group of coauthors—including, ironically, a number of chaplains—have essentially proposed a "wall of separation" between religion and medical practice, much like the one between church and state that some feel is vital to our national welfare. Sloan and the others raise four objections, all of which, at face value, have some merit:

The studies linking religion and health are not what they are cracked up to be. A potential weakness of the studies cited by NIHR and others is the validity of the measures used to gauge a person's religious commitment. For example, some have used church attendance as a marker, but all of us have known regular churchgoers whose behavior and health habits outside the sanctuary suggest little commitment to what is taught inside. (Most evangelical Christians are familiar with the old adage that sitting in church every Sunday doesn't make you a Christian any more than working in the garage every Saturday makes you a car.) Also, using church attendance as a measure for religious commitment might exclude those who are too incapacitated to attend services and thus artificially enhance the appearance of health among those who come regularly.

Identifying a valid measure for religious commitment is certainly more difficult than finding one for diabetes or obesity. But Dr. Larson and colleagues at NIHR are not naive about the qualities of good versus sloppy research, and they continue to address this issue in their publications. For example, in the meta-analysis of studies linking religious activity to longevity, McCullough and coauthors "excluded those that looked only at religious affiliation—like Christian, Jewish or Moslem—and instead focused on studies that included some measure of religious involvement. For instance, the measures included how often one attends religious services, how personally important one ranks one's religious faith, or the degree to which one finds strength or comfort from one's relationship to God."[34]

Indeed, while the verdicts of common sense are not always borne out by scientific research, accepting the likelihood that religious commitment would benefit health, at least for some, does not require a major leap of faith. Virtually all religious traditions, for example, strongly discourage drunkenness, sexual promiscuity, random violence and other forms of riotous living. Presumably at least some who hear these messages take them to heart and act accordingly, thereby reducing the risk of several important health problems. This does not take into account the potential impact of faith on attitudes and emotions. In his letter to the Galatians the apostle Paul describes the fruit of the Spirit as "love, joy, peace, patience, kindness, goodness, faithfulness, gentleness and self-control" (Galatians 5:22-23). This is a concise picture of emotional well-being, which a growing body of evidence suggests would contribute to physical health as well.

There is always danger in pressing the connection between health and spirituality too vigorously. Does this connection imply that the person beset with chronic or terminal illness is "unspiritual"? (This issue also arises for those who insist that the Bible teaches that physical healing is universally available to believers in Christ who have enough faith, and that illness is the product of—or at least is perpetuated by—sin and unbelief.) Nevertheless, the kinds of studies cited by NIHR and others, and the conclusions they draw from them, are not judgmental. They merely serve to raise our awareness of the potential contribution of religious commitment to human health.

Doctors are not competent to engage in a discussion of religion with their patients. Sloan and his coauthors argue that cultural and religious diversity in the United States is increasing so rapidly that broaching the subject of spirituality is a major challenge, one that physicians are apparently not capable of handling appropriately.

> Assessing the spirituality of patients and providing spiritual care require skill and at least an implied covenant between the provider and the recipient of such care. Although one might argue that physicians may also participate in this covenant with patients, the results of a study of physicians, nurses, patients and family members suggest otherwise. The authors point out that the "religious backgrounds, beliefs, activities and coping behaviors of patients and families were notably different from those of health care providers, particularly physicians." Addressing patients' spiritual concerns across these gulfs is a complicated and sensitive matter. For all these reasons, it is not clear that physicians should engage in religious discussions with patients as a way of providing comfort.[35]

This argument is a convoluted—and ultimately pretentious—exhortation to exclude even a discussion of faith from the bedside or the exam room. Another section of this article says in essence that such conversations should be "left to the professionals," that is, chaplains and community clergy "who have received systematic postseminary training and clinical supervision in such areas as pastoral psychology, ethics, and multicultural pastoral care and who are endorsed by their denominations."[36] In other words, "Butt out, Doctor—you're just the mechanic here."

To put this into perspective, consider the fact that primary care practitioners are commonly expected to recognize and deal with a variety of complicated and sensitive subjects, including depression, domestic violence and child abuse, as a part of everyday practice. The management of these problems, of course, will vary considerably with the skill and experience of the physician. Depression, for example, is often recognized and treated in the primary care office. In fact, a physician would be considered remiss if he or she did not consider this as a possible diagnosis in a patient presenting a list of symptoms such as fatigue, insomnia and irritability. If we applied Dr. Sloan's line of reasoning to conversations about depression, physicians would not only refer all such patients immediately to psychiatrists and full-time counselors, but they would actually avoid bringing up the topic in the first place.

Obviously physicians are not going to be competent or comfortable handling all (or even some) of these issues, and an important element of their art involves knowing when and how to refer them elsewhere with finesse and sensitivity. In reality, the biggest obstacle that faces physicians when broaching spirituality, or any other element of what is called the personal/social component of a patient's status, is not necessarily competence but time. As we discussed in chapter four, conventional physicians are notorious for being rushed during their appointments, and so having a conversation about a patient's religious faith would be a luxury in most offices. What Dr. Larson and NIHR (among others) are pointing out is that these topics have relevance to a person's overall health and to specific medical conditions, and to ignore them sells the patient short.

Doctors have no business recommending any religious activities to their patients. Even if they were convinced that the scientific literature shows that religious commitments enhance health, Dr. Sloan and coauthors would have grave reservations about doctors recommending that their patients somehow increase or enhance their religious activities. They worry that such admonitions, no matter how tactfully offered, could represent a coercive intrusion into a person's private convictions.

> Marital status is associated with health, but physicians do not dispense advice regarding marriage. There is evidence that early rather than late childbearing may reduce the risk of various cancers, but we would recoil at a physician's recommendation that a young woman, either married or single, have a child to reduce her risk of cancer. These matters are personal and private, even if they are related to health. Many patients regard their religious faith as even more personal and private than their health.[37]

They also note that for some people religion may represent a source of personal turmoil. What if the patient is embroiled in conflict over an interfaith marriage or a family disagreement that arises from religious doctrine or teaching about behavioral choices? If those issues were raised during a medical visit, might the result be detrimental rather than beneficial?

Concerns over coercion and overstepping of boundaries are certainly valid. No one wants to hear a sermon during a pap smear or to harbor an uneasy feeling that the doctor has a religious agenda that overrides providing quality care. But that argument cuts both ways: no patient should ever have his or her faith and spiritual commitments undercut by a skeptical physician. One of us (Paul Reisser) has heard complaints from more than one young woman who was ridiculed by a gynecologist or ER physician for making a decision to remain sexually abstinent until marriage. Such comments are not only unconscionable but also highly unprofessional.

It should be noted that this entire argument raised by Dr. Sloan and others assumes—quite correctly—the spiritual neutrality of conventional medicine. And it is a little ironic that while the skeptics gleefully debunk mystical and pseudoscientific ideas in many alternative therapies, they never raise the issue of religious coercion or subterfuge by their practitioners. We have already gone to some lengths to demonstrate that many alternative therapies come with spiritual baggage attached. Even if the provider denies any specific intention to "convert" the patient, the simple act of describing how adjusting the flow of *chi* or *prana* will improve health is a de facto pitch for a Taoist or Vedic worldview. Wouldn't it be more ethical for a doctor to be forthright about discussing a patient's religious commitments during the course of an evaluation?

The vigorous pursuit of the personal and private line of reasoning also raises suspicion. This is the language of those who are generally antagonistic to religious expression, who would just as soon keep everyone's spiritual commitments in the closet and so private and personal that they never have any effect on daily decisions or discourse. One has to ponder the significance of the fact that Dr. Sloan included the major points of his *New England Journal of Medicine* article in a November 1999 address given at the annual convention of the Freedom from Religion Foundation.[38]

Whether skeptics and opponents of religion like it or not, some doctors and some of their patients are going to enter into conversations about spiritual matters, at least some of the time. This is not so much the byproduct of a rising tide of public and professional interest in the connection between spirituality and health (although such interest will no doubt increase the number of these conversations). Rather, it is a normal response to illness, especially serious illness, to look beyond human resources for help and to think about the big picture: *So I'm not immortal after all? Does my life have a meter running? What really matters, anyway?* We should not find it surprising that in primitive societies the roles of healer and priest reside in the same individual (that is, the shaman), even if we would have concerns about the medical and spiritual orientation of such an individual.

While physicians may not have the interest, let alone the time, to probe such questions in detail on a routine basis, the basic spiritual assessment suggested by NIHR makes perfect sense, especially in a primary care setting where (hopefully) long-standing relationships develop. In some situations such information will be critical to providing appropriate care. For example, as already mentioned, primary care physicians are now frequently involved in the assessment and management of depression. For many people this problem has an endogenous (biochemical) component, which is usually responsive to one of several medications. While these drugs are safe and never addicting, some patients are unwilling to try them because they are convinced that to do so would be unspiritual. *I shouldn't need a drug to feel normal,* they may think. *I should be able to snap out of this with more prayer and Bible study.* A physician who is not aware of the patient's spiritual concerns may never know why the prescription was not taken. But a sympathetic and respectful discussion could help the patient use *all* of the appropriate avenues to resolve the depression—medication, professional counseling and spiritual resources, including prayer, group support and pastoral input.[39]

"God Is Responsive to Prayers, but We Should Not Put Him to a Test"

As we have seen, the Kansas City study on the effects of prayer on patients in the coronary care unit and the 1988 San Francisco study that inspired it have provoked a wide range of energetic responses: "Amen!" from Christians who are happy to see prayer validated scientifically. "Ditto!" from writers such as Larry Dossey who view prayer as psychic e-mail. "Bunk!" from skeptics who challenge the validity of the experimental design. And "Keep your prayers to yourself!" from materialists who find religion distasteful. We would like to propose one more viewpoint: "Do not put the Lord your God to the test."

While we have no reason to doubt the sincerity of those who conducted the studies or those who are encouraged by them, this type of research raises a number of important issues.

How do we measure the efficacy of prayer, and what conclusions might we draw from our measurement? What if every patient who received intercessory prayer experienced immediate healing, while those who did not receive prayer had a stormy course in the CCU? Would that prove that God exists? It might—but what kind of deity would this be? Probably not the sovereign Creator, the maker of heaven and earth described in the Scriptures. The Bible describes many ways in which we have the privilege of interacting with God, but none of them involve our being in command of him. He is not a cosmic butler responding to a human aristocrat, nor a harried parent working to satisfy a demanding toddler. And he is definitely not the "dependent variable" whose behavior will conform to an experimental protocol designed by those he created in the first place. In an incisive essay entitled "The Efficacy of Prayer," C. S. Lewis made this observation:

> Now even if all the things that people prayed for happened, which they do not, this would not prove what Christians mean by the efficacy of prayer. For prayer is request. The essence of request, as distinct from compulsion, is that it may or may not be granted. And if an infinitely wise Being listens to the requests of finite and foolish creatures, of course He will sometimes grant and sometimes refuse them. Invariable "success" in prayer would not prove the Christian doctrine at all. It would prove something much more like magic—a power in certain human beings to control, or compel, the course of nature.[40]

Such complete success in prayer would almost certainly arouse a universal human impulse to be in charge, to exert power, to command not only the world we can see but the unseen world as well. You can almost hear the buzz on the talk shows and in the Internet chat rooms: "What did the intercessors say? What's their secret? What's their formula? Can I have it?" Attempting to manipulate supernatural forces using any kind of formula (even in the form of a prayer) is called sorcery and is roundly condemned in both Old and New Testaments (see, for example, Deuteronomy 18:10-14 and Galatians 5:19-20).

What if the experiments described in this chapter showed no advantage whatsoever for those who received prayer? What if they fared more poorly than the controls? Would these outcomes prove that God does not exist or that he is malevolent? We could come up with a number of explanations and hypotheses, none of which could be tested using controlled studies. For example, perhaps God felt sorry for the people who were not receiving prayer and decided to help them instead. For that matter, neither of the CCU studies could control for the likelihood that the control patients were also the objects of prayer, either their own or those offered by friends and loved ones who deeply cared about their welfare. One could easily argue that such prayers might have been more earnest—and thus more effective—than those offered by the intercessor groups who knew virtually nothing about the patients for whom they were praying. This question was addressed—almost prophetically—by C. S. Lewis in the above-noted essay on prayer, published more than forty years ago:

> I have heard it suggested that a team of people—the more the better—should agree to pray as hard as they knew how, over a period of six weeks, for all the patients in Hospital A and none of those in Hospital B. Then you would tot up the results and see if A had more cures and fewer deaths. And I suppose you would repeat the experiment at various times and places so as to eliminate the influence of irrelevant factors.
>
> The trouble is that I do not see how any real prayer could go on under such conditions. . . . You cannot pray for the recovery of the sick unless the end you have in view is their recovery. But you can have no motive for desiring the recovery of all the patients in one hospital and none of those in another. You are not doing it in order that suffering should be relieved; you are doing it to find out what happens. The real purpose and the nominal purpose of your prayers are at variance. In other words, whatever your tongue and teeth and knees may do, you are not praying. The experiment demands an impossibility.[41]

We have not mentioned another disturbing possibility: what if someone devises an experimental prayer protocol in which the intercessors are beseeching Krishna or Baal or even Molech for intervention? Should we set up prayer competitions, pitting Christians against Hindus or Muslims against Buddhists to see whose deity is the most powerful or attentive? We might be tempted to view Elijah's confrontation with the prophets of Baal as a precedent for such an event, but he was clearly on assignment from God, and Elijah knew that the outcome was a foregone conclusion (1 Kings 18). Were we to set up such a contest, would we not be violating the spirit, if not the letter, of Deuteronomy 6:16? Jesus quoted this command—"Do not put the Lord your God to the test"—during his temptation in the wilderness, when Satan suggested that he throw himself from the highest point of the temple to see whether God might save him (Matthew 4:7). Even granting that those conducting experiments on intercessory prayer have noble aspirations, it is difficult not to hear the murmurings of a test below the surface: "C'mon, God, let's prove that prayer really works."

While this chapter is certainly not an all-encompassing treatise about prayer and its many benefits, suffice it to say that we see prayer as having a depth and breadth that far surpasses the narrow parameters of any experimental protocol. Quoting once again from C. S. Lewis:

> The very question "Does prayer work" puts us in the wrong frame of mind from the outset. "Work": as if it were magic, or a machine—something that functions automatically. Prayer is either a sheer illusion or a personal contact between embryonic, incomplete persons (ourselves) and the utterly concrete Person. Prayer in the sense of petition, asking for things, is a small part of it; confession and penitence are its threshold, adoration its sanctuary, the presence and vision and enjoyment of God its bread and wine. In it God shows Himself to us. That He answers prayers is a corollary—not necessarily the most important one—from the revelation. What He does is learned from what He is.[42]

EPILOGUE

Conventional medicine's greatest asset has been its reliance on scientific methodology to pursue the nature and causes of disease, discover and test therapies and develop powerful technologies. Its greatest weakness now lies in the deployment of its products and services, and it is in this arena that it has the most to learn from many alternative practices. Conventional medicine has pushed itself into the fast lane, where it is too rushed, too expensive and too driven by technology and invasive procedures. It could stand to pay attention to alternative medicine's interests in prevention, teaching the basics and building therapeutic relationships between practitioners and patients. Moving in this direction would indeed be desirable, but it would also represent a major course correction, requiring fundamental changes in attitude among the recipients of health care as well as those delivering it. What conventional medicine must *not* do is abandon the thinking processes that have led to such unprecedented progress over the past century. Reforming the delivery process is a far cry from abandoning reason and rigorous standards.

Believers in Scripture and its good news about Jesus' life, death and resurrection on our behalf have no enemy in the scientific method. They should be on the forefront of scientific inquiry and should be the most cautious (and skeptical) analysts of alternative practices. Unfortunately, all too often the reverse has been the case. Christians have been prone to harbor suspicions of science (perhaps identifying it with critics of their faith, especially evolutionists) and have been all too eager to embrace ideas relating to health that are not only irrational but also at times hostile to the Scriptures. In particular, some have become involved with therapies purporting to manipulate invisible "life energies," apparently not noticing their deep roots in Vedism, Taoism and monism, or perhaps naively believing that this baggage can be extracted from a more fundamental and spiritually neutral truth.

Western medicine, having accomplished so much with its intellect and technology, is at constant risk of losing its heart and soul. Alternative medicine is connecting with hearts and souls but all too frequently seems intent on abandoning reason and common sense. And in its pursuit of health for the whole person—body, mind and spirit, as its literature never tires of reminding us—many of its most prominent therapies drive their patients and the public toward Eastern mysticism. This leaves the Christian who would like to explore health options beyond the boundaries of conventional medicine in a bit of a quandary: how might this be done without leaving reason behind or, worse, compromising a commitment to the basic teachings of Scripture? Here are few parting thoughts to consider:[1]

1. *Learn about how your body works.* Borrow some books from the library or take a course in basic physiology at a local college. (An important advisory—if the material involves meridians or *chakras,* you need to look elsewhere.)

2. *Learn some basics about the fundamental differences between the teachings of the Scriptures and the precepts of competing worldviews,* especially those from the East and the New Age movement. Why spend time on other "isms" when there is so much to learn from the Scriptures? Because a little knowledge of their vocabulary and assumptions may prevent a spiritual misadventure. We would recommend, as a starting point, reading James Sire's excellent summary *The Universe Next Door* (InterVarsity Press, 1997) or logging on to the Spiritual Counterfeits Project website and subscribing to its excellent newsletters and journal.

3. *Taking herbs and supplements will not compromise your faith* (although they may take a bite out of the budget). But remember—talk is cheap. It's much easier to make extravagant claims than to prove them. If a product sounds too good to be true, it most likely is.

4. *We've said it before and will say it again: stay away from techniques that claim to manipulate invisible "life energy."* Their "science" is nonexistent and their spiritual roots uniformly lead to a conclusion that we are all God (by some other name).

5. *Learn to meditate.* Contemporary evangelical Christianity has essentially lost track of this practice, abandoning it to Eastern traditions. This is a tragic miscalculation. In our Western churches and in our Western Christian media we are buried in a twenty-four-hour torrent of words, interrupted occasionally by music. We are

intimidated by silence, whether in our services or our living rooms.

Eastern meditation is driven by the goal of emptying the mind and experiencing an altered state of consciousness. Biblical meditation is all about getting quiet long enough to focus intently on our God, his creation, his laws, his love and a thousand other topics—and perhaps hearing from him as well. Bible study, which is both important and highly regarded in evangelical circles, may or may not involve meditation. Throughout Scripture we are not only admonished to meditate but also repeatedly informed of its manifold benefits. (Read Psalm 1, for example.) But most of us are so overscheduled, overstressed, overbooked and overtired that the closest we ever come to a meditative state is when we settle into a hot bath at the end of a long day. (This could actually be an appropriate time to meditate if we would take the opportunity to do so.)

For those who desire to pursue this practice, we would recommend Richard Foster's classic *Celebration of Discipline* (which also includes an excellent chapter on prayer) as well as the forty-day devotional *Meditation: A Practical Guide to a Spiritual Discipline* by Thomas McCormick and Sharon Fish.[2]

6. At the risk of sounding narrow-minded, we recommend staying away from yoga, even when it would seem to be nothing more than simple stretching and breathing exercise. The word *yoga* is derived from the Sanskrit term for "yoke" or "union," and yogic exercises are ultimately intended to produce an experience of union with Brahman, the impersonal god of Hinduism. The widespread availability of yoga classes in health clubs and physical education programs has unfortunately given these practices an air of innocence and spiritual neutrality they scarcely deserve.

While we believe that the practice of martial arts, for instance, can be taught and mastered in a form that is separated from its spiritual underpinnings, the same cannot be said for yoga. In martial arts various physical actions, whether offensive or defensive in nature, can be taught in isolation from Eastern philosophy, but yoga seems inextricably tied to the philosophy and religion behind it. Christian researchers John Weldon and Clifford Wilson summarized this problem as follows:

> The goal of yoga is the same as Hinduism—Hindu God-realization, i.e., for the yoga devotee to realize that he is one with Brahman, the highest impersonal Hindu God. The physical exercises of yoga are designed to prepare the body for the psychospiritual change vital to inculcating this idea into the consciousness and being of the person. Hence talk of separating yoga practice from theory is meaningless. From a Christian perspective, whether the two can safely be divided is doubtful. "I do yoga, but Hinduism isn't involved," is an incorrect statement.[3]

The term "Christian yoga," then, seems to be an oxymoron. If the purpose of yoga, by definition, is to join with Brahman through the practice of mastering breathing techniques aimed at harnessing *prana*, then there can be no doubt that this conflicts directly with the teachings of Christianity as well as a great many other religions. In our assessment a viable alternative to yoga would be stretching exercise that is not tied to any religious philosophy.

7. *Don't forget the benefits of aerobic exercise.* As simple an activity as walking for a half-hour daily has been shown to offer protection against a variety of significant health problems.

8. *Coming full circle, be a wise consumer of conventional medicine.* Hopefully you can establish a relationship with a practitioner who will listen to you, answer your questions and discuss options—including alternatives—evenhandedly.

Notes

Chapter 1: A Nation Takes Notice

[1] All of these quotes are take from transcripts of the lectures given at the Physician of the Future Conference in 1976 and published as the *Journal of Holistic Health* (San Diego: Association for Holistic Health, 1977).

[2] A similar boom in alternative therapies has been unfolding, sometimes at greater speed, in other developed countries with well-entrenched Western medical systems, including Canada, Western Europe and Australia.

[3] *The Medical Advisor: The Complete Book of Alternative and Conventional Treatment* (Alexandria, Va.: Time-Life, 1996).

[4] This number undoubtedly reflects the number of times the phrase was mentioned on any particular website *and* on the multiple pages that make up such a site. Nevertheless, the number of alternative medicine sites on the Internet has grown exponentially over the course of just a few years.

[5] National Institutes of Health, "Exploratory Centers for Alternative Medicine Research," RFA: OD-94-004, *NIH Guide* 23, no. 15 (1994).

[6] The ten centers and their areas of research are (1) Bastyr University, Seattle, Washington (specialty: HIV/AIDS); (2) Beth Israel Hospital, Harvard Medical School, Boston, Massachusetts (specialty: general medical conditions); (3) Columbia University College of Physicians and Surgeons, New York, New York (specialty: women's health issues; cofunded by the Office of Research on Women's Health, NIH); (4) Kessler Institute for Rehabilitation, West Orange, New Jersey; the University of Medicine & Dentistry, Newark, New Jersey (specialty: stroke and neurological conditions; cofunded by the National Institute of Child Health and Human Development, NIH); (5) Hennepin County Medical Center, University of Minnesota Medical School, Minneapolis, Minnesota (specialty: addictions); (6) Stanford University, Palo Alto, California (specialty: aging); (7) University of California at Davis (specialty: asthma, allergy and immunology); (8) University of Maryland School of Medicine Baltimore, Maryland (specialty: pain; cofunded by the National Institute of Arthritis and Musculoskeletal and Skin Diseases, NIH); (9) University of Texas Health Science Center, Houston, Texas (specialty: cancer; cofunded by the National Cancer Institute, NIH); and (10) University of Virginia School of Nursing, Charlottesville, Virginia (specialty: pain).

[7] John E. Porter, "OAM Funding: A Shared Responsibility," *Alternative Therapies in Health and Medicine* 1, no. 3 (1995): 80. The emphasis has been added.

[8] Wayne B. Jonas and Jennifer Jacobs, *Healing with Homeopathy: The Natural Way to Promote Recovery and Restore Health* (New York: Warner, 1996).

[9] James M. Gordon, "Alternative Medicine and the Family Physician," *American Family Physician* 54 (1996): 2205-12. Gordon was previously mentioned as a passionate advocate of alternative medicine who served as chairman of the Program Advisory Council for the Office of Alternative Medicine. *American Family Physician* received a number of letters critical of the November 1996 alternative medicine article. Subsequently it has published more balanced and informative articles on this subject, focusing primarily on herbal therapies.

[10] David Eisenberg et al., "Trends in Alternative Medicine Use in the United States, 1990-1997: Results of a Follow-up National Survey," *Journal of the American Medical Association* 280 (1998): 1569-75;

David Eisenberg et al., "Unconventional Medicine in the United States: Prevalence, Costs, and Patterns of Use," *New England Journal of Medicine* 328 (1993): 246-52.

[11]Eisenberg and his coauthors identified these as sixteen specific interventions that were "neither taught
. widely in U.S. medical schools nor generally available in U.S. hospitals." The therapies were, in order of most to least frequently used, as follows: relaxation therapies, chiropractic, massage, imagery, spiritual healing, commercial weight loss programs, lifestyle diets (e.g., macrobiotics), herbal therapies, megavitamin therapy, self-help groups, energy healing, biofeedback, hypnosis, homeopathy, acupuncture, folk remedies.

[12]Harvard Medical School has presented a series of seminars entitled "Spirituality and Healing in Medicine," as well as a fourteen-cassette video course (with a 370-page syllabus) called "Alternative Medicine: Implications for Clinical Practice," directed by David Eisenberg, M.D.

[13]M. S. Wetzel, D. M. Eisenberg and T. J. Kaptchuk, "Courses Involving Complementary and Alternative Medicine at U.S. Medical Schools," *Journal of the American Medical Association* 280 (1998): 784-87.

[14]Examples of prominent medical schools and centers with on-site alternative medicine programs or clinics include the following: (1) Beth Israel Deaconess Medical Center, Center for Alternative Medicine Research, Boston, Massachusetts; (2) Cedars/Sinai Medical Center, Integrative Medicine Program, Los Angeles, California; (3) Columbia University College of Physicians and Surgeons, the Rosenthal Center for Complementary and Alternative Medicine, New York, New York; (4) Duke University, Office of Integrative Medicine Education, Duke Center for Integrative Medicine; (5) University of Maryland School of Medicine, Complementary Medicine Program; (6) Stanford University, Complementary Medical Clinic, Stanford, California; (7) Thomas Jefferson University Hospital, Center for Integrative Medicine; (8) University of California at Los Angeles, Center for East-West Medicine.

[15]"Scientists and Physicians Gather in Philadelphia for 'Science Meets Alternative Medicine,' " Committee for the Scientific Investigation of Claims of the Paranormal <www.csicop.org/articles/19990226-altmed/>.

[16]Daniel P. Eskinazi, "Factors That Shape Alternative Medicine," *Journal of the American Medical Association* 280 (1998): 1621-23.

[17]"National HMO Study Promises Future for Alternative Health Care" (March 10, 1999), Landmark Healthcare <www.landmarkhealthcare.com/releases/pr031099.htm>.

[18]Shari Roan and David Olmos, "Alternative, Conventional Care Forge Uneasy Alliance," *Los Angeles Times,* September 2, 1998, p. 1.

[19]"Recognizing the Value," Oxford Health Plans <www.oxhp.com/altmed/1_overview.html>.

[20]"Did You Know?" Oxford Health Plans <www.oxhp.com/altmed/skptc.html>.

[21]The passage of the Dietary Supplement Health and Education Act of 1994 clearly reflected congressional responsiveness to public interest in supplements as well as the personal convictions of many representatives. Congress has also considered the Access to Medical Treatment Act, which would allow patients to be treated by any practitioner with any form of therapy (whether or not approved, certified or licensed) as long as the practitioner actually examines the individual.

[22]"National HMO Study."

Chapter 2: What Are Alternative Therapies?

[1]David Eisenberg et al., "Trends in Alternative Medicine Use in the United States, 1990-1997: Results of a Follow-up National Survey," *Journal of the American Medical Association* 280 (1998): 1569-75; David Eisenberg et al., "Unconventional Medicine in the United States: Prevalence, Costs, and Patterns of Use," *New England Journal of Medicine* 328 (1993): 246-52.

[2]"Complementary and alternative medicine covers a broad range of healing philosophies, approaches, and therapies. It generally is defined as those treatments and health care practices not taught widely in medical schools, not generally used in hospitals, and not usually reimbursed by medical insurance companies." NIH National Center for Complementary and Alternative Medicine Clearinghouse, "Frequently Asked Questions," October 1998, p. 1.

[3]Daniel P. Eskinasi, "Factors That Shape Alternative Medicine," *Journal of the American Medical Association* 280 (1998): 1621-23.

[4]James E. Dalen, " 'Conventional' and 'Unconventional' Medicine: Can They Be Integrated?" *Archives of Internal Medicine* 158 (1998): 2179-81.

[5]NIH National Center for Complementary and Alternative Medicine Clearinghouse, "Considering Complementary and Alternative Therapies?" October, 1998. Other general information publications (which also can be downloaded from NCCAM's website) are "Frequently Asked Questions" and "Classification of Complementary and Alternative Health Care Practices."

[6]Marcia Angell and Jerome P. Kassirer, "Alternative Medicine—The Risks of Untested and Unregulated Therapies," *New England Journal of Medicine* 339 (1998): 839-41. When this editorial was published, Dr. Kassirer was editor-in-chief and Dr. Angell was executive editor of the *New England Journal of Medicine.*

Chapter 3: A "Reality Check" Tour of Alternative Medicine

[1]D. L. Sackett, W. M. C. Rosenberg, J. A. M. Gray, R. B. Hayes, W. Scott, "Evidence-Based Medicine: What It Is and What It Isn't," *British Medical Journal,* January 13, 1996, pp. 71-72.

[2]*Complementary/Alternative Medicine: An Evidence-Based Approach* (ed. J. Spencer and J. Jacobs [St. Louis: Mossby, 1999]) is a compendium funded by the NIH's National Center for Complementary and Alternative Medicine. A newer book written from a Christian perspective, *Alternative Medicine: A Christian Handbook* by Walter Larimore and Donal P. O'Mathuna (Grand Rapids, Mich.: Zondervan, 2001) also utilizes an evidence-based approach to evaluating a number of alternative therapies.

[3]C. Maxwell Cade and Nona Coxhead, *The Awakened Mind: Biofeedback and the Development of Higher States of Consciousness* (New York: Delacorte, 1979).

[4]James Dillard and Terra Ziporyn, *Alternative Medicine for Dummies* (Foster City, Calif.: IDG, 1998), p. 162.

[5]The origin in the technique is generally credited to a nineteenth-century Swedish athlete, Peter Heinrik Ling. "Massage Therapy: Key Questions and Answers," American Massage Therapy Association <www.amtamassage.org/about/faq.htm>.

[6]Herbert Benson, *The Relaxation Response* (New York: William Morrow, 1975).

[7]The question of TM's religious nature became a public policy issue during the 1970s, when efforts were made to introduce this practice into public schools.

[8]These include *The Mind/Body Effect* (New York: Simon & Schuster, 1979); *Beyond the Relaxation Response* (New York: Times, 1984); *The Wellness Book: The Comprehensive Guide to Maintaining Health and Treating Stress-Related Illness* (New York: Fireside, 1993), written with Eileen M. Stuart; and *Timeless Healing: The Power and Biology of Belief* (New York: Scribner, 1996).

[9]David Eisenberg et al., "Trends in Alternative Medicine Use in the United States, 1990-1997: Results of a Follow-up National Survey," *Journal of the American Medical Association* 280 (1998): 1569-75; T. J. Kaptchuk and D. Eisenberg, "Chiropractic: Origins, Controversies and Contributions," *Archives of Internal Medicine* 158 (1998): 2215-24.

[10]Kaptchuk and Eisenberg, "Chiropractic," pp. 2215-24.

[11]S. Bigos, O. Bowyer, B. Baren et al., *Clinical Practice Guideline No. 14: Acute Low Back Problems in Adults,* AHCPR publication 95-0642 (Rockville, Md.: U.S. Department of Health and Human Services, 1994).

[12]NIH Consensus Development Panel on Acupuncture, "Acupuncture," *Journal of the American Medical Association* 280 (1998): 1518-1524.

[13]Dillard and Ziporyn, *Alternative Medicine for Dummies,* pp. 249-50; Benson and Stuart, *Wellness Book,* pp. 341-42.

[14]See B. Wilson, M.D., "The Rise and Fall of Laetrile" <www.quackwatch.com/01QuackeryRelated Topics/Cancer/laetrile.html>.

[15]Needless to say, it is important to remember that the likelihood of cure or containment will depend enormously on the type and extent of the tumor, not to mention the individual characteristics of the person who has it.

[16]I. J. Lerner and B. J. Kennedy, "The Prevalence of Questionable Methods of Cancer Treatment in the United States," *CA* 42 (1992): 181-91.

[17]Stephen Barrett and Victor Herbert, "Questionable Cancer Therapies" (July 26, 1999), Quackwatch

<www.quackwatch.com/01QuackeryRelatedTopics/cancer.html>.

[18]Ibid.

[19]G. A. Gellert, R. M. Maxwell and B. S. Siegel, "Survival of Breast Cancer Patients Receiving Adjunctive Psychosocial Support Therapy: A Ten-Year Follow-up Study," *Journal of Clinical Oncology* 11 (1993): 66-69. Although Dr. Siegel was listed as a coauthor of this study, which failed to validate the notion that E-CaP patients would live longer than their nonparticipating counterparts, he subsequently indicated that the study was carried out by a student and was not properly designed (see Barrett and Herbert, "Questionable Cancer Therapies," p. 11.)

[20]Stephen Barrett, "Iridology" (September 1999), Quackwatch <www.quackwatch.com/01QuackeryRelatedTopics/iridology.html>.

[21]A. Simon et al., "An Evaluation of Iridology," *Journal of the American Medical Association* 242 (1979): 1385-87.

[22]The Federal Trade Commission (FTC), along with consumer protection and public health agencies in twenty-five countries, has conducted two "Health Claim Surf Days," one in 1997 and one in 1998, in which thousands of websites and Usenet newsgroups were visited for information about six diseases: heart disease, cancer, AIDS, diabetes, arthritis and multiple sclerosis. These identified approximately eight hundred websites and numerous newsgroups that were promoting unsubstantiated products and services. In June 1999 the FTC announced formal charges and settlement agreements involving four Web-advertised companies, two of which were promoting magnetic therapy devices.

[23]See, for example, D. W. Ramey, "Analysis: Magnetic and Electromagnetic Therapy," *The Scientific Review of Alternative Medicine* 2, no.1 (1998). Dr. Ramey, a veterinarian, carefully addresses claims made regarding magnetic therapy for both humans and animals, especially racehorses, on whose behalf a thriving magnet business has developed.

[24]C. Vallbona, D. F. Hazlewood and J. Gabor, "Response of Pain to Static Magnetic Fields in Postpolio Patients: A Double-Blind Pilot Study," *Archives of Physical and Rehabilitation Medicine* 78 (1997): 1200-3; J. D. Livingston, "Magnetic Therapy: Plausible Attraction?" *Skeptical Inquirer*, July-August 1998; E. A. Collacott et al., "Bipolar Permanent Magnets for the Treatment of Chronic Low Back Pain: A Pilot Study," *Journal of the American Medical Association* 283 (2000): 1322-25.

[25]A. T. Barker et al., "Pulsed Magnetic Field Therapy for Tibial Non-Union," *The Lancet* (1984): 994-96.

[26]Some readers may recall the popularity of Carlos Castaneda, author of several books (such as *The Teachings of Don Juan*) purportedly documenting his experiences with the Native American shaman known only as "Don Juan." For his alleged experiences and research, Castaneda was awarded a Ph.D. in anthropology from UCLA in 1973. One article exposing the flaws in Castaneda's works reported that "careful research and investigation uncovered gaping holes, inconsistencies, and outright fabrications in the convoluted stories Castaneda told" (Bob Passantino, "Fantasies, Legends, and Heroes: What You Know May Not Be So and How to Tell the Difference" [1990], Answers in Action <www.answers.org/apologetics/Fantasy.html>).

Chapter 4: What Draws People to Alternative Therapies?

[1]J. Astin, "Why Patients Use Alternative Medicine," *Journal of the American Medical Association* 279 (1998): 1548-53.

[2]Andrew Weil, *Spontaneous Healing* (New York: Fawcett Columbine, 1995), p. 221. The emphasis is in the original text.

[3]We are well aware that physcian's assistants and nurse practitioners play an ever-expanding role in providing medical services, especially in primary care settings. As such they face many, if not most, of the same difficulties that challenge mainstream physicians. For the sake of simplicity, throughout this discussion (and in others relating to patient care in this book) we will use the terms *physician* and *doctor* when referring to the broader sweep of conventional health care providers.

[4]G. Leonard, "The Holistic Health Revolution" in *The Journal of Holistic Health* (San Diego: Association for Holistic Health, 1977), p. 81.

[5]Arnold Relman and Andrew Weil, "Is Integrative Medicine the Medicine of the Future? A Scholarly Debate" (Tucson, Arizona: Program in Integrative Medicine, April 9, 1999).

[6]Herbert Benson, *Timeless Healing* (New York: Scribner, 1996).

[7]In using the term "remembered wellness" to indicate the effect of belief and expectation, Benson was primarily attempting to depart from the pejorative implications of the phrase "placebo effect," which assumes either manipulative hokum or an inert research tool. What "remembered wellness" means, however, is not exactly intuitive. Benson proposes that we all have beneficial physiological responses programmed into our central nervous system as a memory of life events in which healing or improvement took place. A more straightforward term for this phenomenon, which also encompasses the importance of negative beliefs, might be "the belief and expectation response."

[8]Benson, *Timeless Healing,* pp. 107, 109.

[9]Ibid., p. 35.

Chapter 5: Going with the Flow

[1]George Lucas, *Star Wars* screenplay, 1977.

[2]Leigh Brackett and Lawrence Kasdan, *The Empire Strikes Back,* screenplay, 1980.

[3]Mary Henderson, *Star Wars: The Magic of Myth* (New York: Bantam, 1997), pp. 197-98.

[4]Bill Moyers, "Of Myth and Men," *Time,* April 26, 1999, <www.time.com/time/magazine/article/0,9171,23298-2,00.html>.

[5]John Ankerberg and John Weldon, *Can You Trust Your Doctor? The Complete Guide to New Age Medicine and Its Threat to Your Family* (Brentwood, Tenn.: Wolgemuth & Hyatt, 1991), p. 46.

[6]Irving Oyle, *Time, Space and the Mind* (Millbrae, Calif.: Celestial Arts, 1976), p. viii.

[7]Donna Eden, *Energy Medicine* (New York: Jeremy P. Tarcher/Putnam, 1998), pp. 15-16. Dr. Oyle made the same "log into flame" error in his book (see previous footnote), and Ms. Eden has unwittingly perpetuated it.

[8]Stephen Barrett, "Electrodiagnostic Devices," Quackwatch <www.quackwatch.com/04ConsumerEducation/electro.html>.

[9]Eden, *Energy Medicine,* pp. 295-316.

[10]Jane Thurnell-Read, *Geopathic Stress: How Earth Energies Affect Our Lives* (Rockport, Mass.: Element, 1995).

[11]Sylvia Bennett and Jonathan Bennett, "Space Clearing," Feng Shui Living <www.fengshui-living.com/space_clearing.htm>.

[12]Eden, *Energy Medicine,* p. 9. The emphasis is in the original text.

[13]William A. Tiller, "Creating a New Functional Model of Body Healing Energies" in *Journal of Holistic Health* (San Diego: Word Shop, 1978), p. 46.

[14]Quoted in A. Nietzke, "Portrait of an Aura Reader," *Human Behavior,* February 1979, p. 31.

[15]Evarts G. Loomis, "The Healing Center of the Future" in *The Journal of Holistic Health* (San Diego: Association for Holistic Health, 1977), p. 73. Capitalization is in the original text.

[16]Jack Gibb, "Psycho-sociological Aspects of Holistic Health" in *Journal of Holistic Health* (San Diego: Association for Holistic Health, 1977), p. 44; Shirley MacLaine, *Out on a Limb* (New York: Bantam, 1983).

[17]Hank Hanegraaff of the Christian Research Institute has written detailed reviews of the issues raised by a number of faith healing and positive confession ministries. See his *Christianity in Crisis* (Eugene, Oreg.: Harvest House, 1993) and *Counterfeit Revival* (Dallas: Word, 1999).

[18]M. J. Nightingale, "Air and Light" in *A Visual Encyclopedia of Unconventional Medicine,* ed. Ann Hill (New York: Crown, 1979), p. 92.

[19]Quoted in L. A. Clark, *Help Yourself to Health* (New York: Pyramid, 1972), p. 106.

[20]Eden, *Energy Medicine,* p. 133.

[21]Carolyn Myss, *Why People Don't Heal, and How They Can* (New York: Harmony, 1997).

[22]K. Dychtwald, "Sexuality and the Whole Person" in *The Holistic Health Handbook* (Berkeley, Calif.: And/Or Press, 1978), p. 304.

[23]Quoted in Nikhilananda, *Vivekananda: The Yogas and Other Works* (New York: Rama Krishna-Vivekananda Center, 1953), pp. 592-93, 598.

[24]NIH Consensus Development Panel on Acupuncture, "Acupuncture," *Journal of the American Medical Association* 280 (1998): 1518-24.

[25]Ilza Veith, introduction to Huang Ti, *Huang Ti Nei Ching Su Wen (The Yellow Emperor's Classic of Internal Medicine), trans.* Ilza Veith (Berkeley: University of California Press, 1966), p. 4.

[26]G. Stux and B. Pomeranz, *Acupuncture: Textbook and Atlas* (Berlin: Springer-Verlag, 1987), p. 37.

[27]Ibid.

[28]David Eisenberg, *Encounters with Qi: Exploring Chinese Medicine* (New York: W. W. Norton, 1995), p. 52. As we discuss later in this chapter, David Eisenberg was also the primary author of the two important surveys of alternative medicine described in chapter one.

[29]G. Ulett, *Beyond Yin and Yang: How Acupuncture Really Works* (St. Louis: Warren H. Green, 1992), p. 10; Bill Moyers, *Healing and the Mind* (New York: Doubleday, 1993), p. 260.

[30]Ibid., p. 12.

[31]Eisenberg, *Encounters with Qi*, p. 125.

[32]T. M. Murphy and J. J. Bonica, "Acupuncture Analgesia and Anesthesia," *Archives of Surgery* 112 (1977): 898.

[33]M. Austin, *Acupuncture Therapy* (New York: ASI, 1972), p. 119.

Chapter 6: Variations on a *Chi* Theme

[1]D. S. Walther, *Applied Kinesiology: Synopsis* (Pueblo, Colo.: Systems DC, 1988), p. 135.

[2]An exhaustive treatment of this concept was set forth in John Diamond, *Behavioral Kinesiology* (New York: Harper & Row, 1979). This book was subsequently rereleased with a more reader-friendly title: *Your Body Doesn't Lie.*

[3]John Maguire, "TFH Scores Big at Anthony Robbins' Mastery University," Touch for Health <www.63.238.164.100/health/masruniv.htm>.

[4]"Reiki FAQ: What Is Reiki?" excerpted from William Lee Rand, *Reiki: The Healing Touch* (Southfield, Mich.: Vision, 1991), posted at <www.reiki.org/FAQ/WhatIsReiki.html>.

[5]Ibid.

[6]William Lee Rand, "Becoming a Reiki Master," The International Center for Reiki Training, posted at <www.reiki.org/reikinews/reikin3.html>.

[7]A. Woodham and D. Peters, *Encyclopedia of Healing Therapies* (London: Dorling Kindersley, 1997), p. 99.

[8]Yugui Guo, "Introduction to Qi Gong," at<www.acupuncture.com/QiGong.htm>.

[9]Wallace Sampson and Berry Beyerstein, "Traditional Medicine and Pseudoscience in China: A Report of the Second CSICOP Delegation," parts 1 and 2, *Skeptical Inquirer* (July-August 1996; September 1996).

[10]"The Mystery of Ch'i," part 1 of *Healing and the Mind*, Public Affairs Television, 1993. Second paragraph from Bill Moyers, *Healing and the Mind* (New York: Doubleday, 1993), p. 297.

[11]Sampson and Beyerstein, "Traditional Medicine and Pseudoscience." Since the only people who were shown "challenging" Master Shi were his own dedicated students, one must wonder what might have happened if the producers of *Healing and the Mind* had offered a hefty reward to any appropriately trained person who could upend the old gentleman.

[12]"Mystery of Ch'i."

[13]A. Gordon, J. H. Merenstein, F. D'Amico and M. A. Hudgens, "The Effects of Therapeutic Touch on Patients with Osteoarthritis of the Knee," *The Journal of Family Practice* 47 (1998): 271-77; J. G. Fauuhgan and E. A. Lagace, "Science and the Alternative," *The Journal of Family Practice* 47 (1998): 262-63.

[14]F. A. Pattie, *Mesmer and Animal Magnetism: A Chapter in the History of Medicine* (Hamilton, N.Y.: Edmonston, 1994), p. 39. Quoted in Thomas S. Ball and Dean D. Alexander, "Catching Up with Eighteenth Century Science in the Evaluation of Therapeutic Touch," *Skeptical Inquirer* 22, no. 4 (1998).

[15]Pattie, *Mesmer and Animal Magnetism*, p. 41.

[16]Fauuhgan and Lagace, "Science and the Alternative," p. 263.

[17]John J. Bonica, "Therapeutic Acupuncture in the People's Republic of China," *Journal of the American Medical Association* 228 (1974): 1545-50. Other more recent estimates have suggested higher numbers, ranging from 30 to 40 percent. See George A. Ulett, *Beyond Yin and Yang* (St. Louis, Mo.: Warren H. Green, 1992), p. 21; James Dillard and Terra Ziporyn, *Alternative Medicine for Dummies* (Foster City,

Calif.: IDG, 1998), p. 155.

[18]NIH Consensus Development Panel on Acupuncture, "Acupuncture," *Journal of the American Medical Association* 280 (1998): 1518-24. Altogether, 2,302 references from January 1970 through October 1997 were reviewed.

[19]Bonica, "Therapeutic Acupuncture in the People's Republic of China," p. 1549. The emphasis is in the original text.

[20]NIH Consensus Development Panel, "Acupuncture," p. 1520.

[21]Ulett, *Beyond Yin and Yang*, pp. 43-44.

[22]Quoted in S. T. Botek, "One Doctor's Acupuncture Odyssey," *Medical Tribune*, May 2, 1984.

[23]Ulett, *Beyond Yin and Yang*, p. 54.

[24]The use of acupuncture for specific problems, especially chronic pain, by a qualified individual who is trained in conventional anatomy and physiology, and who is consciously working within that realm would be an exception.

[25]Brooks Alexander, "Holistic Health from the Inside," *Journal of the Spiritual Counterfeits Project*, August 1978, p. 16.

Chapter 7: Going Natural

[1]Donna Abu-Nasr, "New Chips Laced with Herbs to Promote Well-being" (September 24, 1998) <www.athleticscanada.com/HEALTHNews/980924_mentalhealth.html>.

[2]David Eisenberg et al., "Trends in Alternative Medicine Use in the United States, 1990-1997: Results of a Follow-up National Survey, " *Journal of the American Medical Association* 280 (1998): 1569-75.

[3]Pamela Donegan, "A Skeptic's Guide to Supplements," *Hippocrates* 13 (July-August 1999): 39-45.

[4]For example, L. G. Miller, "Herbal Medicinals: Selected Clinical Considerations Focusing on Known or Potential Drug-Herb Interactions," *Archives of Internal Medicine* 158 (1998): 2200-2211; T. Zink and J. Chaffin, "Herbal 'Health' Products: What Family Physicians Need to Know," *American Family Physician* 58 (1998): 1133-40; M. Johns, "Herbal Remedies: Adverse Effects and Drug Interactions," *American Family Physician* 59 (1999): 1239-44. The Johns article is accompanied by a patient information sheet that lists side effects and possible drug reactions for a number of common herbs.

[5]Ephedrine's cousin pseudoephedrine is widely used as a decongestant in many nonprescription (Sudafed) and prescription cold remedies. It is generally better tolerated than ephedrine but may have similar side effects if taken in excessive doses.

[6]Eisenberg et al., "Trends in Alternative Medicine Use," pp. 1569-75.

[7]J. Lazarou, B. H. Pomeranz and P. N. Corey, "Incidence of Adverse Drug Reactions in Hospitalized Patients: A Meta-analysis of Prospective Studies," *Journal of the American Medical Association* 279 (1998): 1200-1205.

[8]Bruce Pomeranz, "Alternative Medicine and the Raison d'Etre for Alternative Medicine," *Alternative Therapies in Health and Medicine* 2 (1996): 85-91.

[9]Shari Roan, "Alternative Medicine: The 18 Billion Dollar Experiment," *Los Angeles Times*, September 1, 1998.

[10]*Consumer Reports*, November 1995, pp. 698-705.

[11]Donegan, "Skeptic's Guide to Supplements," pp. 39-45.

[12]Mark Blumenthal et al., eds., *The Complete German Commission E Monographs* (Boston: Integrative Medicine, 1998).

[13]Donegan, "Skeptic's Guide to Supplements," pp. 39-45.

[14]Mayo Clinic, "Herbal Remedies, There's No Magic," (March 27, 1997) <www.physiciansdirectory.com/articles/9703/htm/herbs.htm>.

[15]"What Does the Public Need to Know About Dietary Supplements?" (June 1997) The Food and Nutrition Science Alliance <www.ift.org/resource/news/news_rel/FANSA/sc_h06.shtml>. FANSA's member organizations are the American Dietetic Association, the American Society for Clinical Nutrition, the American Society for Nutritional Sciences, and the Institute of Food Technologists.

[16]Andrea Peirce, *The American Pharmaceutical Association Practical Guide to Natural Medicines* (New York: William Morrow, 1999); Varro E. Tyler, *Herbs of Choice: The Therapeutic Use of Phytomedicinals* (Bir-

mingham, N.Y.: Haworth/Pharmaceutical Products, 1994); Varro E. Tyler, *The Honest Herbal* (Birmingham, N.Y.: Haworth/Pharmaceutical Products, 1993); D. O'Mathuna and W. Larimore, *Alternative Medicine: The Christian Handbook* (Grand Rapids, Mich.: Zondervan, 2001).

[17]Many parents are appropriately concerned about the potential risks of drugs, especially repeated rounds of antibiotics, for their children, and some see herbal preparations as a gentler alternative for common conditions such as colds and stomachaches. Nevertheless, herbal expert Varro Tyler, Ph.D., has cautioned against widespread use of these remedies in young children, at least until more data is available: "As a conservative in the area, I'd say that herbal remedies should not be administered to babies and children. There are simply no data on the safety and efficacy in children, and there's no reliable information about dosage." Quoted in B. Holcomb, "Herbal Remedies: Are They Safe for Your Child?" *Parents,* December 1999, p. 144.

[18]"USP Publishes Nine New Botanical Monographs," U.S. Pharmacopeia (November 2, 1998) <www.usp.org/aboutusp/releases/pr_9827.html.

Chapter 8: Andrew Weil

[1]Dr. Weil.com <www.drweil.com>.

[2]Quoted in Arnold S. Relman, "A Trip to Stonesville," *The New Republic,* December 14, 1998.

[3]Andrew Weil, *A New Approach to Medicine,* audiocassette series (Ukiah, Calif.: New Dimensions Foundation, 1997).

[4]Andrew Weil, *Spontaneous Healing* (New York: Fawcett Columbine, 1995), pp. 13-14.

[5]Andrew Weil, *The Natural Mind: An Investigation of Drugs and the Higher Consciousness,* rev. ed. (Boston: Houghton Mifflin, 1986), p. x.

[6]Ibid., p. 120.

[7]Ibid., p. 121.

[8]Ibid., pp. 131-32.

[9]Ibid., p. 149.

[10]Ibid., pp. 153-54.

[11]Ibid., p. vii.

[12]Andrew Weil, "Any Basis for the Blood-Type Diet?" May 17, 1999, <www.drweil.com/archiveqal0,2283,1532,00.html>.

[13]Weil, *Spontaneous Healing,* p. 185.

[14]Ibid., p. 242.

[15]Weil, *New Approach to Medicine.*

[16]Weil, *Natural Mind,* p. 140.

[17]Many voices in the alternative movement, including Dr. Weil's, tend to criticize the use of drugs to lower blood pressure, on the grounds that they do not address the underlying cause(s) of the problem. But in the real world of people with hypertension who cannot solve this problem on their own (with or without weight loss, exercise or relaxation techniques), there is ample evidence that successful lowering of high blood pressure with medication reduces the risk of three serious complications: heart attack, stroke and kidney failure.

[18]Weil, *Natural Mind,* pp. 142-43.

[19]Ibid., p. 146. Koch's Postulates, named for nineteenth-century German bacteriologist Robert Koch, played a significant role in the understanding of the relationship between specific microorganisms and disease. They are the following: (1) The organism must consistently be isolated from those with the illness. (2) The organism must be grown in vitro, that is, in a test tube or culture plate (outside of the body). (3) When the organism is inoculated into a susceptible test animal, the typical illness develops. (4) The organism is again isolated from that test animal.

[20]Ibid., p. 144.

[21]Ibid., p. 166.

[22]Andrew Weil, *Eating Well for Optimum Health* (New York: Alfred A. Knopf, 2000).

[23]Ibid., p. 175.

[24]Ibid., p. 176.

[25]Ibid., p. 278.

[26]Ibid., p. 280.

[27]Arnold Relman and Andrew Weil, "Is Integrative Medicine the Medicine of the Future? A Scholarly Debate" (Tucson, Arizona: Program in Integrative Medicine, April 9, 1999).

[28]Weil, *New Approach to Medicine.*

[29]Weil, *Spontaneous Healing,* p. 247.

[30]Weil, *New Approach to Medicine.*

[31]Dr. Weil's endorsement reads: "If medicine is to come back into alignment with the great healing traditions and satisfy the needs and desires of those who are sick, it must rediscover the truths that Bob Fulford expresses." Andrew Weil, dust jacket endorsement to Robert C. Fulford, *Dr. Fulford's Touch of Life* (New York: Simon & Schuster, 1996).

[32]Fulford, *Dr. Fulford's Touch of Life.*

[33]Weil, *Spontaneous Healing,* pp. 205-6.

[34]Ibid., pp. 207-8.

[35]Weil, *New Approach to Medicine.*

[36]Huxley's book *The Doors of Perception* provides vivid accounts of his experimentation with mescaline. The title was excerpted from the poem "The Marriage of Heaven and Hell" by William Blake (1757-1827): "If the doors of perception were cleansed every thing would appear to man as it is: infinite." (Incidentally, the popular 1960s rock band The Doors took its name from this quote as well.)

[37]Weil, *Natural Mind,* p. 180.

[38]Relman and Weil, "Is Integrative Medicine the Medicine of the Future?"

[39]For example, during a medical roundtable broadcast on a major Christian TV network in May 2000, the physicians present vigorously condemned the use medications such as Prozac and Zoloft to treat depression, while speaking favorably about St. John's wort for the same purpose. Yet all of these products, whether pharmaceutical or herbal, serve the same basic function, that of affecting neurotransmitter levels in the brain.

[40]"What Does the Public Need to Know About Dietary Supplements?" (June 1997) The Food and Nutrition Science Alliance <www.ift.org/resource/news/news_rel/FANSA/sc_h06.shtml>.

[41]G. Gugliotta, "Health Concerns Grow Over Herbal Aids," *The Washington Post,* March 19, 2000.

Chapter 9: Deepak Chopra

[1]M. Willson, *The Music Man* (Frank Music Corporation and Rinimer Corporation, 1950).

[2]David Eisenberg et al., "Trends in Alternative Medicine Use in the United States, 1990-1997: Results of a Follow-up National Survey," *Journal of the American Medical Association* 280 (1998): 1569-75; David Eisenberg et al., "Unconventional Medicine in the United States: Prevalence, Costs, and Patterns of Use," *New England Journal of Medicine* 328 (1993): 246-52. It is likely that the absence of *ayurveda* in the 1998 study resulted from its not being reported in the 1993 study. Data for the earlier survey had been collected in 1990, when *ayurveda* was still relatively obscure. In 1998 Dr. Eisenberg and his coauthors were clearly seeking to chart the change in popularity of various therapies over time.

[3]W. W. Mills, "Ayurvedic Medicine" (1997), Sonoma County Medical Association <www.scma.org/magazine/scp_newformat/scp970304/mills.html>.

[4]Hari Sharma, "Maharishi Ayur-Veda: An Ancient Health Paradigm in a Modern World," *Alternative and Complementary Therapies* 1 (1995): 364-72.

[5]Deepak Chopra, *Ageless Body, Timeless Mind: The Quantum Alternative to Growing Old* (New York: Harmony, 1993), p. 269.

[6]James Dillard and Terra Ziporyn, *Alternative Medicine for Dummies* (Foster City, Calif.: IDG, 1998), p. 112.

[7]V. Lad, "An Introduction to Ayurveda," *Alternative Therapies* 1 (1995): 57-63.

[8]Ibid.

[9]Andrew Weil, *Spontaneous Healing* (New York: Fawcett Columbine, 1995), p. 239.

[10]Roy Porter, *The Greatest Benefit to Mankind* (New York: W. W. Norton, 1997), p. 139.

[11]Deepak Chopra, *Perfect Health: The Complete Mind/Body Guide* (New York: Harmony/Random House, 1991).

[12]The National Institutes of Health, "Ayurvedic Medicine," in *Alternative Medicine: Expanding Medical*

Horizons: A Report to the National Institutes of Health on Alternative Medical Systems and Practices in the United States (Chantilly, Va.: NIH Publications, 1992).

[13]Mills, "Ayurvedic Medicine."

[14]Tal Brooke, "Deepak Chopra: The Wizard of Boundless Healing," *SCP Journal* 21 (1997): 4-13.

[15]Chopra.com <www.chopra.com/aboutdeepak.htm>.

[16]The Watchman website <www.watchman.org/profile/choprapro.htm> and the New Religious Movements website <cti.itc.virginia.edu/~jkh8x/soc257/nrms/Chopra.html> are two that contain this information.

[17]Deepak Chopra, *Return of the Rishi: A Doctor's Story of Spiritual Transformation and Ayurvedic Healing* (Boston: Houghton Mifflin, 1988), pp. 105, 108-9, 125.

[18]Sharma, "Maharishi Ayur-Veda."

[19]Deepak Chopra, *Quantum Healing: Exploring the Frontiers of Mind/Body Medicine* (New York: Bantam, 1989), pp. 3-4.

[20]Ibid., p. 6.

[21]The favorable quote from the *New England Journal of Medicine* on the cover of *Quantum Healing* would, at first glance, suggest an endorsement by that eminent journal. But the quote actually came from an unsolicited review of the book written by John W. Zamarra, M.D., who, unbeknownst to the *Journal's* editors, had long-standing ties to TM.

[22]Hari Sharma, Brihaspati D. Triguna and Deepak Chopra, "Letter from New Delhi. Maharishi Ayur-Veda: Modern Insights into Ancient Medicine," *Journal of the American Medical Association* 265 (1991): 2633-37; A. Skolnick, "Maharishi Ayur-Veda: Guru's Marketing Scheme Promises the World Eternal 'Perfect Health,' " *Journal of the American Medical Association* 266 (1991): 1741-46. The same issue of *JAMA* that contained the Skolnick article also contained a lengthy "Letters to the Editor" section in which conventional physicians, ex-TM initiates and prominent alternative medicine critics (such as Wallace Sampson, M.D.) ridiculed the article and the fact that it was published in a respectable journal. A favorable mention of pulse diagnosis within the article was a particularly irresistible target. "Where is their double-blind study," asked Tim Gorski, M.D., "wherein it is shown that Ayurvedic practitioners can accurately 'diagnose diseases . . . such as diabetes, neoplastic disease, musculoskeletal diseases and asthma' by palpation of the radial pulse? Just think of all the laboratory analyses, surgery, x-rays and spirometry that could be dispensed with if they could prove such claims." A counterpunch to these attacks was delivered in a number of favorable letters written, as might be expected, by practitioners of *ayurveda* and TM, including some with direct connections to the Maharishi's organization.

[23]J. Knapp, "Deepak Chopra Interview" (February 6, 1997), Trancenet <www.trancenet.org/chopra/interview/>. It is worth noting that the Trancenet website is routinely critical of TM and Chopra. (The area of the site focusing on Chopra is called "Shameless Mind," a play on his bestselling *Ageless Body, Timeless Mind*.) This interview, however, was characterized by Knapp as a "halting beginning" and a "most unusual step," in which Chopra had "chosen to meet a critic and begin a direct conversation."

[24]Weil, *Spontaneous Healing*, pp. 239-40.

[25]J. Leland, C. Power and L. Reibstein, "Deepak's Instant Karma," *Newsweek*, October 20, 1997, p. 54.

[26]Chopra.com <www.chopra.com>. The quote was prominently displayed at the top of the website's home page.

[27]Quoted in Tony Perry, "So Rich, So Restless," *Los Angeles Times Magazine*, September 7, 1997, p. 28.

[28]Tony Perry, "So Rich, So Restless," *Los Angeles Times Magazine*, September 7, 1997, pp. 27-28.

[29]Leland, Power and Reibstein, "Deepak's Instant Karma," p. 52.

[30]Deepak Chopra, *The Seven Spiritual Laws of Success: A Practical Guide to the Fulfillment of Your Dreams* (San Rafael, Calif.: New World Library, 1994), pp. 69, 4, 5.

[31]Deepak Chopra, *The Wisdom Within: Your Personal Program for Total Well-Being* (New York: Crown, 1997).

[32]Ibid.

[33]Deepak Chopra, *Journey into Healing: Awakening the Wisdom Within You* (New York: Harmony/Random House, 1994), p. 153-54.

[34]Chopra, *Ageless Body, Timeless Mind*, p. 3.

[35]Chopra, *Seven Spiritual Laws of Success,* pp. 55-56, 85, 2-3.

[36]Ibid., pp. 28-29.

[37]For example, Chopra's website <www.chopra.com> noted that the weeklong Seduction of Spirit seminar earns forty-four contact hours of continuing education credit for counselors from the National Board of Certified Counselors.

[38]As of May 6, 2000, all of these seminars and many more were listed at <www.chopra.com>.

[39]Deepak Chopra, *Creating Health: How to Wake Up the Body's Intelligence* (Boston: Houghton Mifflin, 1987), pp. 223-24.

[40]Deepak Chopra, *The Seven Spiritual Laws for Parents: Guiding Your Children to Success and Fulfillment* (New York: Harmony/Random House, 1997), p. 14.

[41]Chopra, *Ageless Body, Timeless Mind,* pp. 3-4.

[42]Ibid., p. 4.

[43]Chopra, *Seven Spiritual Laws of Success,* pp. 67, 69.

[44]Deepak Chopra, *Creating Affluence: Wealth Consciousness in the Field of All Possibilities* (San Rafael, Calif.: New World Library, 1993), p 19.

[45]Chopra, *Journey into Healing,* p. 34.

[46]Chopra, *Ageless Body, Timeless Mind,* pp. 6-7.

[47]Ibid., p. 7.

[48]Victor Stenger, "Quantum Quackery," *Skeptical Inquirer,* January-February 1997, <www.csicop.org/si/9701/quantum-quackery.html>.

[49]Phil Molé, "Deepak's Dangerous Dogmas," *Skeptic* 6, no. 2 (1998): 38-45.

[50]Lucy Lidell, *The Sivananda Companion to Yoga* (New York: Fireside/Simon & Schuster, 1983), p. 98.

[51]See chapter three, pp. 36-37, for further discussion of Dr. Benson and the relaxation response.

[52]Deepak Chopra, *How to Know God: The Soul's Journey into the Mystery of Mysteries* (New York: Harmony/Random House, 2000), p. 95.

[53]Ibid., p. 164.

[54]Jagad Guru Shankracharya, endorsements to Chopra, *How to Know God.*

[55]Deepak Chopra, "A Welcome from Deepak," How to Know God <www.howtoknowgod.com/about>.

[56]Chopra, *How to Know God,* pp. 53-54.

[57]Ibid., pp. 55-56.

[58]Ibid., p. 57.

[59]Ibid.

[60]Ibid.

[61]Ibid., pp. 138-39.

[62]Ibid., p. 112.

[63]Ibid., p. 114.

[64]Ibid., p. 145

[65]Ibid., p. 170.

[66]Chopra, *Seven Spiritual Laws for Parents,* pp. 20-21, 31, 57, 68.

[67]Chopra, *Creating Affluence,* p. 38.

[68]Chopra, *Seven Spiritual Laws of Success,* pp. 17-18.

[69]Chopra, *How to Know God,* p. 151.

[70]Ibid.

[71]On a special website devoted to this book, <www.howtoknowgod.com>, Chopra has a question-and-answer section that includes an elaborate and highly inventive interpretation of John 14:6. Needless to say, he concludes that Jesus really didn't say, or at least didn't mean it when he said, "No one comes to the Father except through me."

[72]An excellent treatment of the question of judgment from a Christian perspective may be found in Robert M. Bowman Jr., *Orthodoxy and Heresy: A Biblical Guide to Doctrinal Discernment* (Grand Rapids, Mich.: Baker, 1992), chapter three.

[73]"Ask Dr. Chopra" (May 23, 1998), Chopra.com <www.chopra.com/askdeepak.htm>. The emphasis has been added.

[74]Chopra, *Journey into Healing,* p. 159.

Chapter 10: Postmodernism & Medicine
[1]D. A. Carson, "Why Are Fire Engines Red?" in *Exegetical Fallacies* (Grand Rapids, Mich.: Baker, 1984), p. 91.

[2]Blaise Pascal, *Pensées,* trans. A. J. Krailsheimer (New York: Penguin, 1966), p. 256.

[3]A detailed analysis of postmodernism is beyond the scope of this book, but this formidable task has been ably tackled by others, notably James Sire in his excellent worldview catalog entitled *The Universe Next Door* (Downers Grove, Ill.: InterVarsity Press, 1997) and by Douglas Groothuis in his book *Truth Decay: Defending Christianity Against the Challenges of Postmodernism* (Downers Grove, Ill.: InterVarsity Press, 2000). Other worthwhile books dealing with postmodernism include the following: J. R. Middleton and B. J. Walsh, *Truth Is Stranger Than It Used to Be: Biblical Faith in a Postmodern Age* (Downers Grove, Ill.: InterVarsity Press, 1995); Dennis McCallum, ed., *The Death of Truth: What's Wrong with Multiculturalism, the Rejection of Reason and the New Postmodern Diversity* (Minneapolis: Bethany, 1996); and Timothy R. Phillips and Dennis L. Okholm, *Christian Apologetics in the Postmodern World* (Downers Grove, Ill.: InterVarsity Press, 1995).

[4]Alan G. Padgett, "Christianity and Postmodernity," *Christian Scholar's Review* 26, no. 2 (1996), <www.hope.edu/resources/csr/XXVI2/padgett/>.

[5]Sire, *Universe Next Door,* pp. 175-84.

[6]Lael Arrington, *Worldproofing Your Kids* (Wheaton, Ill: Crossways Books, 1997).

[7]Dennis McCallum, *Focal Point* (spring 1997): 5.

[8]Francis J Beckwith and Gregory Koukl, *Relativism: Feet Firmly Planted in Mid-Air* (Grand Rapids, Mich.: Baker, 1998), p. 28.

[9]Ibid., p. 27.

[10]Sire, *Universe Next Door,* p. 185.

[11]Harold O. J. Brown, *The Sensate Culture* (Dallas: Word, 1996), p. 202.

[12]Donal P. O'Mathuna, "Postmodern Impact: Health Care" in Dennis McCallum, ed., *The Death of Truth* (Minneapolis: Bethany House, 1996), pp. 62-63. The italics are in the original text.

Chapter 11: Homeopathy
[1]Dana Ullman, *Discovering Homeopathy: Medicine for the Twenty-First Century* (Berkeley, Calif.: North Atlantic, 1991), p. 40.

[2]Ibid., p. 6.

[3]For example, Dana Ullman is willing to give immunizations at least some credit for the reduction of previously common childhood diseases. But Connecticut homeopath Vinton McCabe blames vaccinations for a host of violent, addictive and even sexually assaultive behaviors. Vinton McCabe, *Let Like Cure Like* (New York: St. Martin's, 1997), pp. 251-57.

[4]Ullman, *Discovering Homeopathy,* pp. 6-7.

[5]McCabe, *Let Like Cure Like,* p. 28.

[6]Ullman, *Discovering Homeopathy,* p. 11.

[7]Robert Ullman, N.D., and Judyth Reichtenberg-Ullman, N.D., *Homeopathic Self-Care: The Quick and Easy Guide for the Whole Family* (Rocklin, Calif.: Prima, 1997), pp. 306-10.

[8]Ibid., p. 12.

[9]Douglas Stalker and Clark Glymour, eds., *Examining Holistic Medicine* (New York: Prometheus, 1985).

[10]Stephen Barrett, "Homeopathy: The Ultimate Fake" (February 24, 2000), Quackwatch <www.quackwatch.com/01QuackeryRelatedTopics/homeo.html>.

[11]Ibid.

[12]D. Ramey, W. Wagner, R. H. Imrie and V. Stenger, "Homeopathy and Science: A Closer Look," University of Hawaii <www.phys.hawaii.edu/vjs/www/med/homeop.html>.

[13]Steven Novella, "Homeopathy," *The Connecticut Skeptic* 1, no. 3 (summer 1996), available online at Healthcare Reality Check <www.hcrc.org/contrib/novella/homeop.html>. The description of the tadpole experiment and the odd conclusions of its designers are attributed to Wim Betz, a European physician and former homeopath who is now an outspoken critic of this practice. It is also glowingly

recounted, including a conclusion that homeopathic remedies can apparently transmit their effects through glass, by Dana Ullman in his audiotape series *Homeopathic Healing* (Boulder, Colo.: Sounds True Audio, 1995), tape three.

[14] Ullman, *Discovering Homeopathy,* p. 15.

[15] McCabe, *Let Like Cure Like,* p. 16.

[16] Barrett, "Homeopathy."

[17] Ullman, *Discovering Homeopathy,* p. 17.

[18] Ibid., pp. 23-24. In reviewing these various unconventional techniques, Ullman takes a rather relaxed posture regarding not only their departure from traditional homeopathic principles but also the use of methodologies such as the pendulum or arm pulling.

[19] For example, homeopathic literature frequently cites a 1994 study published in the mainstream journal *Pediatrics* that apparently showed that homeopathic treatment of infectious diarrhea in Nicaraguan children was more effective than standard rehydration therapy (J. Jacob et al., "Treatment of Childhood Diarrhea with Homeopathic Medicine: A Randomized Clinical Trial in Nicaragua," *Pediatrics* 93 [1994]: 719-25). One rarely hears, however, about a follow-up article that described numerous methodological flaws in the diarrhea study (W. Sampson and W. London, "Analysis of Homeopathic Treatment of Childhood Diarrhea," *Pediatrics* 96 (1995): 961-64).

[20] E. Ernst and M. Pittler, "Alternative Therapy Bias," *Nature* 365 (1997): 480.

[21] J. Aulas, "Homeopathy Update," *Prescrire International* 15 (1996): 674-84, quoted in Ramey et al., "Homeopathy and Science."

[22] K. Linde et al., "Are the Clinical Effects of Homeopathy Placebo Effects? A Meta-analysis of Placebo-controlled Trials," *The Lancet* 350 (1997): 834-43.

[23] Ramey et al., "Homeopathy and Science."

[24] Ibid.

Chapter 12: Therapeutic Touch

[1] L. Rosa, E. Rosa, L. Sarner and S. Barrett, "A Close Look at Therapeutic Touch," *Journal of the American Medical Association* 279 (1998): 1005-10.

[2] Dolores Krieger, *The Therapeutic Touch: How to Use Your Hands to Help or Heal* (Englewood Cliffs, N.J.: Prentice-Hall, 1979), p. 4.

[3] Ibid., p. 13.

[4] Ibid.

[5] Ibid., pp. 49-50.

[6] Rosa et al., "A Close Look at Therapeutic Touch." Other benefits referenced in a table in this article include the following: "breaks fever," "decreases inflammation," "helps skin grafts to seed," "helps children make sense out of the world," "treats measles and many different forms of cancer," "promotes bonding between parents and infants" and "helps to evaluate situations where diagnosis is elusive."

[7] Krieger, *Therapeutic Touch,* pp. 70-71, 77, 80.

[8] Rosa et al., "Close Look." All of the facts in this quotation are accompanied by citations in the article. It should be noted that the National League for Nursing is no longer the primary accrediting body for nursing programs.

[9] J. F. Quinn, "Therapeutic Touch as Energy Exchange: Replication and Extension," *Nursing Science Quarterly* 2 (1989): 79-87, cited in Sharon Fish, *Christian Research Journal,* summer 1995, pp. 28-38. Fish's outstanding article for the Christian Research Institute is highly recommended for anyone interested in Therapeutic Touch and its implications.

[10] Al Hinman and Andrea Richards, "Fourth-grade science project casts doubt on 'Therapeutic Touch' " (April 1, 1998), CNN <www.cnn.com/HEALTH/9804/01/therapeutic.touch/>.

[11] Rosa et al., "Close Look."

[12] Ibid.

[13] "Healing Touch—Emily Rosa," *Scientific American Frontiers,* "Ask the Scientists," <www.pbs.org/safarchive/3_ask/archive/qna/3282_erosa.html>.

[14] Letters to the Editor, *Journal of the American Medical Association* 280 (1998): 1905. James Randi is a professional illusionist ("The Amazing Randi") and long-time hero in skeptic circles for his work in

exposing bogus paranormal phenomena and other "miracles."

[15]J. Lee, Letter to the Editor, *Journal of the American Medical Association* 280 (1998): 1905.

[16]One exception to this rule is the true believer in Christian Science, who may put his or her life on the line by refusing conventional care and attempting to straighten out the erroneous thinking of "mortal mind."

[17]D. A. Carson, "The Postmodern," *First Things* 93 (May 1999). Used by permission. Available online at <www.firstthings.com/ftissues/ft9905/poetry.html#the>.

Chapter 13: Why I Left

[1]For a thoughtful overview of the Gnostic gospels, see "Gnosticism and the Gnostic Jesus" by Douglas Groothuis, originally published in the *Christian Research Journal* and available online at <www.iclnet.org/pub/resources/text/cri/cri-jrnl/web/crj0040a.html>.

[2]R.C. Sproul's website may be found at <www.gospelcom.net/ligonier/>.

Chapter 14: Is God a Dependent Variable?

[1]W. S. Harris et al., "A Randomized, Controlled Trial of the Effects of Remote, Intercessory Prayer on Outcomes in Patients Admitted to the Coronary Care Unit," *Archives of Internal Medicine* 159 (1999): 2273-78.

[2]Ibid.

[3]Ibid.

[4]Editor's correspondence, *Archives of Internal Medicine* 160 (2000): 1870-78.

[5]Larry Dossey, "Prayer and Medical Science: A Commentary on the Prayer Study by Harris et al., and a Response to Critics," *Archives of Internal Medicine* 160 (2000): 1735-38.

[6]Lucy Lidell, *The Sivananda Companion to Yoga* (New York: Fireside/Simon & Schuster, 1983), p. 15.

[7]For further reading on this subject, see Henry Morris's book *Men of Science, Men of God: Great Scientists Who Believed the Bible* (San Diego: Creation-Life Publishers, 1982).

[8]Larry Dossey, *Healing Words: The Power of Prayer and the Practice of Medicine* (New York: HarperSanFrancisco, 1993); Larry Dossey, *Prayer Is Good Medicine* (New York: HarperSanFrancisco, 1996); Larry Dossey, *Be Careful What You Pray For . . . You Might Just Get It* (New York: HarperSanFrancisco, 1997).

[9]Reginald Cherry, *Healing Prayer* (Nashville: Thomas Nelson, 1999). Dr. Cherry is not the first Christian to misunderstand Dossey's materials, and he probably will not be the last. His positive reference to Dossey's book *Healing Words* was no doubt an oversight, because Dr. Cherry otherwise completely shuns New Age approaches to healing throughout his book.

[10]Randolph C. Byrd, "Positive Therapeutic Effects of Intercessory Prayer in a Coronary Care Unit Population," *Southern Medical Journal* 81 (1988): 826-29.

[11]H. Wolinksy, "Prayers Do Aid Sick, Study Finds," *Chicago Sun-Times,* January 26, 1986, p. 30; J. Sherrill, "The Therapeutic Effects of Intercessory Prayer," *Journal of Christian Nursing* (1995): 21-23; Larry Dossey, *Reinventing Medicine* (New York: HarperSanFrancisco, 1999), pp. 55-56.

[12]Byrd, "Positive Therapeutic Effects of Intercessory Prayer," quoted in Gary P. Posner, "God in the CCU? A Critique of San Francisco Hospital Study on Intercessory Prayer and Healing," *Free Inquiry* (spring 1990), available online at Internet Infidels <www.infidels.org/library/modern/gary_posner/godccu.html>.

[13]The six outcomes for which the patients receiving prayer did significantly better (statistically speaking) involved reduced need for antibiotics and for diuretics (medications that remove excess water from the body) as well as fewer episodes of pneumonia, congestive heart failure, cardiac arrest and intubation (the insertion of a tube in the airway to allow for assisted breathing).

[14]One could also make the argument that those receiving prayer were not actually protected from bacterial infections but rather from doctors who were prone to order antibiotics too readily.

[15]Dossey, *Healing Words,* p. xv.

[16]Dossey, *Prayer Is Good Medicine,* pp. xiii–xiv.

[17]Dossey, *Healing Words,* p. 6. The emphasis is in the original text.

[18]Dossey, *Reinventing Medicine,* pp. 24-25.

[19]Ibid., p. 24.

[20]Dossey, *Prayer Is Good Medicine,* p. 19.

[21]Dossey, *Healing Words,* p. xx.

[22]Ibid., p. xxi.

[23]Ibid., pp. xvi–xvii.

[24]Ibid., p. xvii.

[25]Ibid., p. xviii.

[26]"What Is a Skeptic?" *Skeptic* 6, no. 2 (1998): 5. The emphasis is in the original text.

[27]"About Us," Internet Infidels <www.infidels.org/infidels/>.

[28]"Mission and Vision," National Institute for Healthcare Research, <www.nihr.org/about/index.html>.

[29]David B. Larson and Susan S. Larson, *The Forgotten Factor in Physical and Mental Health* (Rockville, Md.: National Institute for Healthcare Research, 1994); David B. Larson, James B. Swykers and Michael E. McCullough, eds., *Scientific Research on Spirituality and Health* (Rockville, Md.: National Institute for Healthcare Research, 1998).

[30]McCullough et al., "Religious Involvement and Mortality: A Meta-analytic Review," *Health Psychology* 19 (2000); David B. Larson, "Summing 42 Studies—Chances of Living Longer Rise by 29% for Religiously Active," National Institute for Healthcare Research <www.nihr.org/researchreports/livinglonger.html>.

[31]Christina M. Puchalski, "Research Review: The Importance of the Spiritual Assessment," National Institute for Healthcare Research <www.nihr.org/media2/smc_spiritualassess.html>.

[32]Ibid.

[33]Richard P. Sloan et al., "Should Physicians Prescribe Religious Activities?" *New England Journal of Medicine* 342 (2000): 1913-16.

[34]Larson, "Summing 42 Studies."

[35]Sloan et al., "Should Physicians Prescribe Religious Activities?" Interestingly, the study referenced in this quote came from NIHR, whose leadership would no doubt take exception to the conclusions that Sloan and the others drew from it. The study in question is H. G. Koenig et al., "Religious Perspectives of Doctors, Nurses, Patients and Families," *Journal of Pastoral Care* 45 (1991): 254-67.

[36]Ibid.

[37]Ibid.

[38]Richard P. Sloan, "Religion, Spirituality and Medicine" (speech delivered at the twenty-second annual convention of the Freedom From Religion Foundation, November 6, 1999), available online at Freedom From Religion Foundation <www.ffrf.org/fttoday/jan_feb00/sloan.html>.

[39]Many Christians who would shun antidepressant medications because "they don't rely on God to solve the problem" should ponder whether they would take antibiotics for a serious infection or insulin for diabetes. For that matter, is a farmer not relying on God because she uses fertilizer, or a fisherman not relying on God because he uses hooks and bait? Every line of endeavor has its tools, and we should thank God routinely that we have the intelligence and resources to create them. We also need to rely on him for wisdom to use them properly, not to mention for the ultimate outcome. No tool works every time.

[40]C. S. Lewis, "The Efficacy of Prayer," in *The World's Last Night and Other Essays* (New York: Harcourt Brace Jovanovich, 1960), pp. 4-5.

[41]Ibid., pp. 5-6.

[42]Ibid., p. 8.

Epilogue

[1]We also recommend Walter Larimore and Donal P. O'Mathuna, *Alternative Medicine: A Christian Handbook* (Grand Rapids, Mich.: Zondervan, 2001) as a useful resource for addressing this question.

[2]Richard Foster, *Celebration of Discipline* (New York: Harper & Row, 1978); Thomas McCormick and Sharon Fish, *Meditation: A Practical Guide to a Spiritual Discipline* (Downers Grove, Ill.: InterVarsity Press, 1983).

[3]John Weldon and Clifford Wilson, *Occult Shock and Psychic Forces* (San Diego, Calif.: Master Books, 1980), p. 71.

Index

Accupath 1000, 84
acupressure, 35, 101
acupuncture, 39-40, 97-99
  conditions treated by, 40
  ear (auriculotherapy) 100
  hand, 100
  NIH Consensus Panel Statement, 40
  pain relief, 112-16
  possible mechanisms of action, 114-16
Ageless Body, Timeless Mind, 164, 174, 177-78, 180-81, 184
Agency for Health Care Policy and Research statement on acupuncture, 39
aging, 64
agni (in *ayurveda*), 165
allopathy, 207
Alternative and Complementary Therapies, 15
alternative medicine
  and "baby boomers," 65-68
  books regarding, 10
  categories, 26-31, 32-59
  definitions, 24-31
  descriptive terminology, 18-19
  entry into cultural mainstream, 9-23
  evidence for, 21-22, 28-29
  herbal remedies, 126-39
  insurance coverage, 19-21
  and malpractice, 231-33
  "Marriage of Science and Religion," 245-49
  medical conferences, 18
  medical school curricula, 18-19
  media coverage, 10-11
  and the National Institutes of Health, 11-13
  "natural medicine," 123-39
  postmodernism, 196-202
  reasons for widespread interest, 60-77
  skeptics, 255-57
  spiritual implications, 116-22, 245-49
  spiritual underpinnings,

22-23, 237-41
  spirituality and health, 257-63
  wise use of, 266-69
Alternative Therapies in Health and Medicine, 15, 130
Alpert, Richard, 141
American Academy of Family Physicians, 14-15
American Association for Ayurvedic Medicine, 172
American Cancer Society, 48, 50
American Dietetic Association, 135
American Family Physician, 14-15
American Humanist Association, 257
American Medical Association, 16
Anatomy of the Spirit, 88
Angell, Marcia, 28-29, 202
animal magnetism, 38
  investigation by French royal commission, 109-10
Ankerberg, John, 80
antineoplastins, 50
applied kinesiology, 43, 101-2
Archive journals, 16
Archives of Internal Medicine
  study on prayer in CCU, 242-45
Association for Holistic Health, 87
Atheists United, 257
"at-one-ment," 9, 120
auriculotherapy, 100
ayurveda, 11, 26, 162-95
  and consciousness change, 167-68
  dietary treatments, 166-67
  efficacy in India, 168
  herbal remedies, 166-67
  origins, 163-65
  pulse diagnosis, 165
  similarities to traditional Chinese medicine, 164-68
  tongue diagnosis, 165-66
Barrett, Stephen, 212, 214-15
Bastyr University, 12
Be Careful What You Pray For . . . You Might Just Get It, 249, 254
Beckwith, Francis J., 199-

200
Benson, Herbert
  and placebo effect, 72-74
  and "relaxation response," 36-37
  and Transcendental Meditation, 36-37, 170
  critique by Deepak Chopra, 187
Beth Israel Deaconess Medical Center, 37
Beyond Yin and Yang: How Acupuncture Really Works, 115
biblical worldview, 8-9, 22-23, 57-58, 88-89
  and scientific research, 245-49
  contrasted with Eastern/New Age worldview, 117-21
  regarding nature, 157-58
  regarding prayer, 263-65
biofeedback, 34
Bloomfield, Harold, 8
Blue Cross, 20, 34-35
Bonica, John J.
  investigation of acupuncture pain relief, 113-14
Brooke, Tal, 168
Brown, Harold O. J., 201
Bruyere, Rosalyn, 87
Burton, Lawrence, 50
Burzynski, Stanislaw, 50
Byrd, Randolph, 250-52
Caisse, Rene, 49
calcium supplementation, 135
Campbell, Joseph, 79-80
CanCell, 50
cancer treatments, 48-51
  clinics in Mexico, 48
  dietary changes, 44, 48-49
  "headliner" therapies, 48
  herbs and supplements, 49
  "metabolic" treatments, 50
Candida albicans, 46, 47, 146
Carson, D. A., 233
Cayce, Edgar, 57, 235
Celebration of Discipline, 268
cell-specific cancer therapy, 50
chakras, 83, 85, 90-91, 165
chelation therapy, 55

Cherry, Reginald, 250
cinchona bark, 204, 205
ch'i, 39-40, 81-89, 94-99
  existence of, 40
  flow of, 94-95
  in massage, 35
  in traditional Chinese medicine, 91-99
  spiritual implications, 116-22
  therapies based upon, 100-107
Chinese medicine. *See* traditional Chinese medicine
chiropractic, 37-39
  "straights" versus "mixers," 38-39, 55
  "Christ consciousness," 9, 88
chondroitin, for arthritis, 45
Chopra, Deepak, 11, 26, 162-95
  and affluence, 178
  Ageless Body, Timeless Mind, 164, 174, 177-78, 180-81, 184
  books, 168-69, 178-79
  critique of worldview, 180-95
  How to Know God, 172, 175, 187-92, 193
  and media coverage, 174-75
  medical training, 169
  and meditation, 177, 186-87
  misinterpretations of Bible, 189-92
  and objective reality, 180-82
  Quantum Healing, 171, 172, 176
  and quantum theory, 182-87
  seminars, 179
  spiritual worldview, 175-95
  and Transcendental Meditation, 169-74
  The Wisdom Within (CD-ROM), 174, 176-77
Chopra Center for Well Being, 168, 174, 179
Clark, Larry, 49
colon cleansing, 46
Committee for the Scientific Investigation of Claims of the Paranormal (CSICOP), 256-57
  investigation of *qi gong,* 105
Commission E, 133, 138